FIRST AID ON BOARD

The ultimate visual guide to medical emergencies at sea

Nina Olofsson, Pär Olofsson and Olle Landsell

ADLARD COLES

LONDON • OXFORD • NEW YORK • NEW DELHI • SYDNEY

ADLARD COLES
Bloomsbury Publishing Plc
50 Bedford Square, London, WC1B 3DP, UK
Bloomsbury Publishing Ireland Limited,
29 Earlsfort Terrace, Dublin 2, D02 AY28, Ireland

BLOOMSBURY, ADLARD COLES and the Adlard Coles logo are trademarks of
Bloomsbury Publishing Plc

First published in Great Britain 2026

A catalogue record for this book is available from the British Library

Library of Congress Cataloguing-in-Publication data has been applied for

ISBN: PB: 978-1-3994-2584-1; ePub: 978-1-3994-2585-8; ePDF: 978-1-3994-2582-7

2 4 6 8 10 9 7 5 3 1

MIX
Paper | Supporting responsible forestry
FSC® C010615

Designed and typeset in Myriad Pro by Tom Storr
Printed and bound in India by Thomson Press India Private Limited

To find out more about our authors and books visit www.bloomsbury.com and sign up for our newsletters

For product safety related questions contact productsafety@bloomsbury.com

CONTENTS

INTRODUCTION

Modern developments in boating life pose new challenges from a medical perspective. The number of recreational boats venturing far beyond their home waters and even around the globe is steadily increasing, as is the number of people extending their boating season and sailing year round.

Healthcare on board is worthy of our care and attention.

The weakest link – the people on board, the crew – is exposed to new stresses and risks as we venture beyond the horizon. The purpose of this book is to update our knowledge on how to prevent and manage various acute medical illnesses and injuries on board. Naturally, the needs vary greatly depending on whether you are sailing close to a port, in very remote and desolate areas, or out on an ocean. In the latter cases, a high level of self-sufficiency is needed. Knowing how to act during a severe medical condition can be life-saving, even in situations near urban areas.

Our advice is based on extensive experience as physicians in acute specialties – surgery/vascular surgery, anaesthesiology, intensive care and pain management – as well as our experience as long-distance sailors and rescue crew. The principles described reflect how we ourselves would likely act in various situations. As is often the case in medicine, there are multiple ways to solve a problem, and other physicians may recommend different solutions.

We place great importance on 'thinking ahead' to ensure enjoyable cruising experiences. Preventing accidents or illnesses as much as possible is, of course, the best approach in every scenario. The weekend boat trip, boating holiday or long-distance voyage can be the wonderful experience you hoped for if medical issues are avoided. It must be emphasised that many, or even the majority, of accidents and illnesses can be prevented.

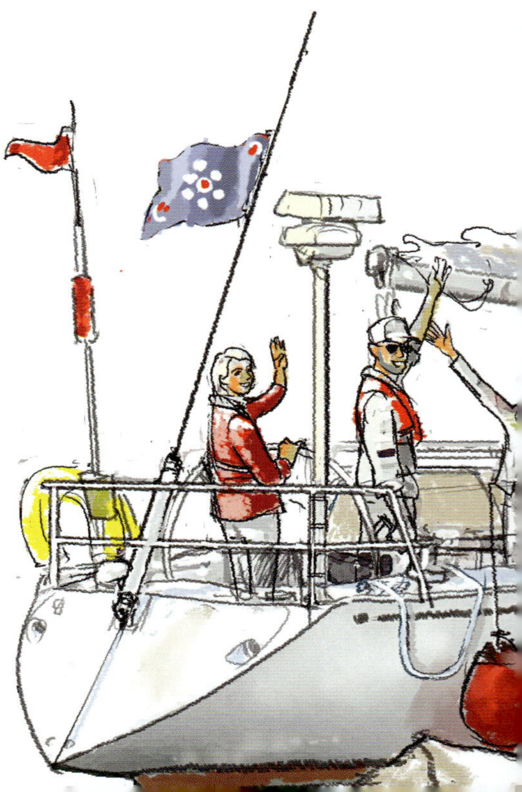

This book focuses on acute and unexpected medical incidents.

We have endeavoured to tailor the content to be useful for all categories of sailors and boaters, regardless of how fast, how far, or where they sail (or take their motorboat). We have also included simple diagnostic examinations that may be valuable on board. Our advice is primarily directed towards people who are medically laymen with no access to professional equipment like oxygen, injections or surgical instruments.

Considering these circumstances, it is important to emphasise the need for education and training as well as access to advice and support from medical expertise. Consequently, access to modern communication equipment is an important prerequisite when planning adventurous voyages by boat. If the on-board equipment includes a ship's dispensary with strong antibiotics, narcotic analgesics or other medications for treatment of acute illnesses, it is advised to consult a physician about diagnosis, indication and dosage prior to administration. If such advice is not available, you have to rely on your own knowledge and experience and make potentially very difficult decisions about issues affecting others. It is also important to thoroughly brief the crew on the particular risks involved when travelling on a leisure craft at sea.

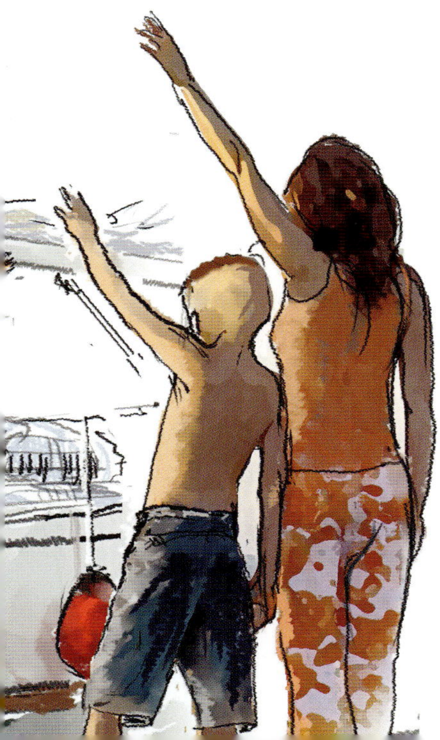

The content is divided into 27 sections. Each chapter generally follows the same structure:

A brief introduction: with relevant and important background to the topic, including basic anatomy.

Signs and symptoms

A description of common symptoms and findings during examination of importance for establishing a preliminary diagnosis.

Immediate action

What to do once a reasonable diagnosis is available.

Treatment

Options for self-care on board, and when to evacuate and seek hospital care urgently.

Far from help

Many conditions can successfully be managed on board; others present very difficult medical and ethical challenges.

Prevention

A most important part, as many medical emergencies can be prevented.

Specific advice is also included for situations where medical assistance is far away, whether in a remote archipelago with unreliable communication and challenging weather, or during an ocean crossing with perhaps two weeks remaining until landfall.

In a true acute situation, it is a great advantage if crucial manoeuvres are well practised. It is too late to read a manual in the acute situation! It has to be emphasised that exercises and training in first aid is an extremely important part of preparations.

It is the captain's responsibility to educate the crew about the emergency equipment available, where to find it and how to use it.

1. SEASICKNESS

Individual risk of becoming seasick varies significantly.

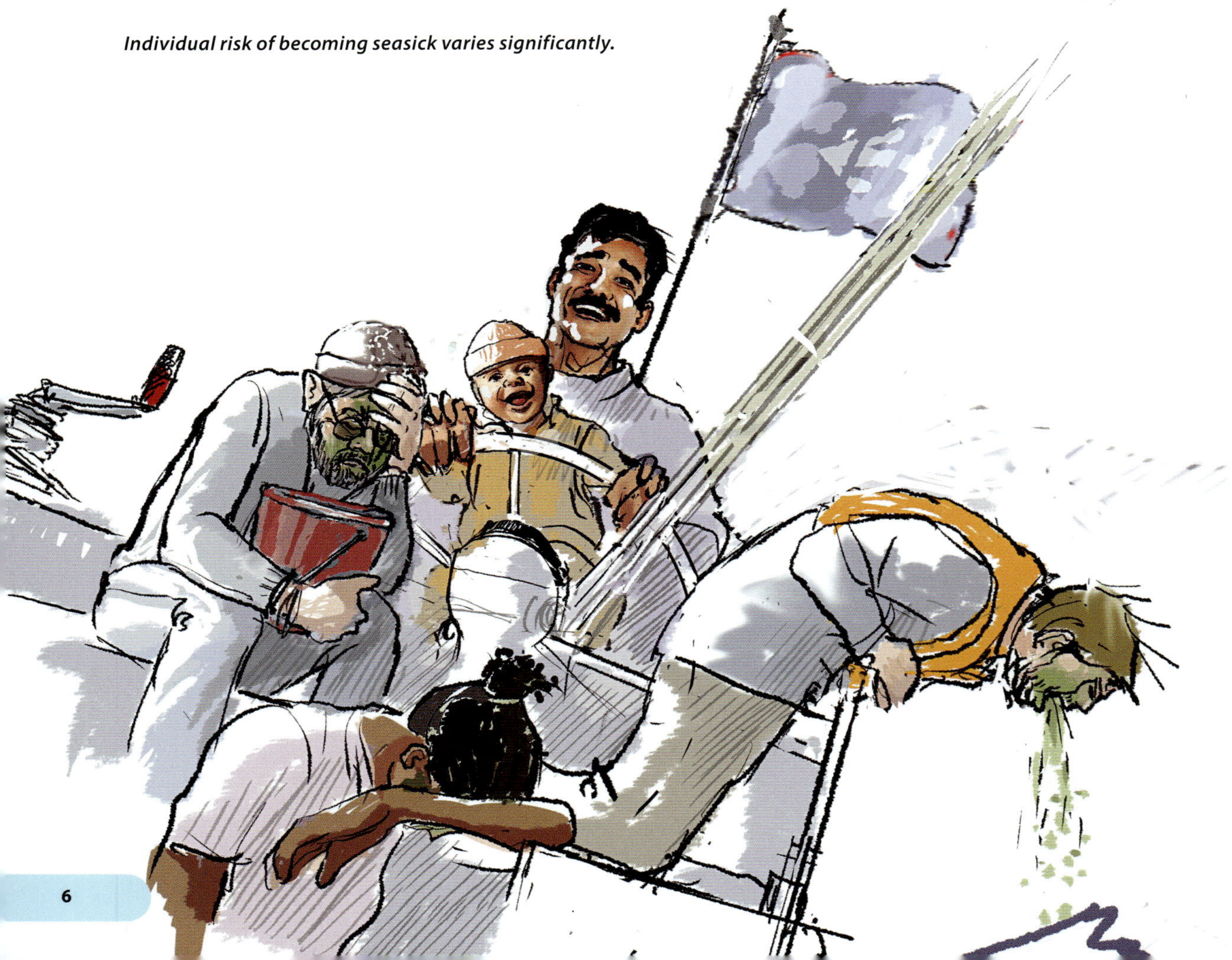

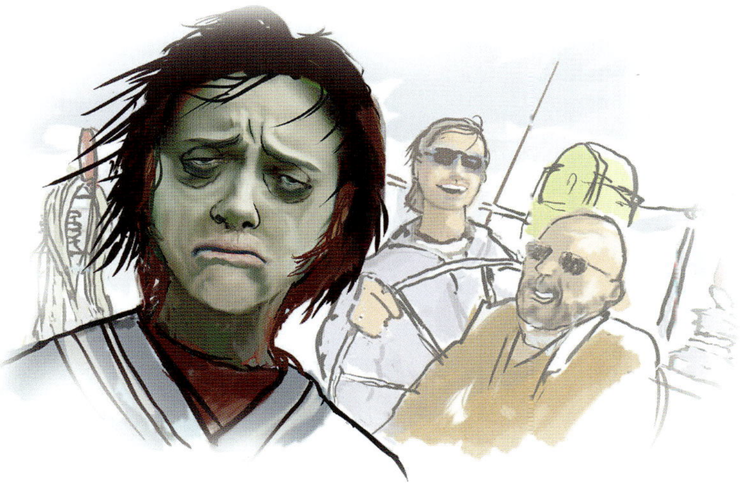

Be cautious of developing seasickness. Be proactive, and give help to crew showing signs of not being well.

Most people, even seasoned crews, may experience discomfort or nausea during the first hours/days after leaving port. For the majority, the nausea subsides after one to three days, but about 3 per cent may develop severe seasickness that persists, and these individuals are advised to avoid longer ocean voyages. Approximately 1 per cent are naturally resistant and never experience seasickness.

Seasickness is the most common medical issue at sea, often becoming serious if left untreated. It occurs when signals from the balance organs and visual impressions no longer match; the uncoordinated movement of the boat relative to the horizon confuses the brain, leading to rapid exhaustion. Factors like anxiety, fear and cold may also worsen symptoms.

Each individual experiences seasickness differently, so it is essential to find personal strategies to counteract it. Experiencing seasickness is normal, and there is no reason to feel embarrassed. Effective strategies include medications, home remedies and learned behaviours.

Signs and symptoms

- Fatigue and yawning, dizziness. The person may become quiet, cold and pale.
- Discomfort, nausea, stomach churning, retching and vomiting.
- Severe vomiting can lead to dehydration (see page 94).
- Extreme symptoms may include complete apathy, hallucinations, and an inability to function as a crew member.

Immediate action

Prompt attention and care are essential when treating seasickness. Offer the affected person a stable seat with a clear view of the open horizon, wrap them in a warm blanket or jacket and give them something to eat and drink.

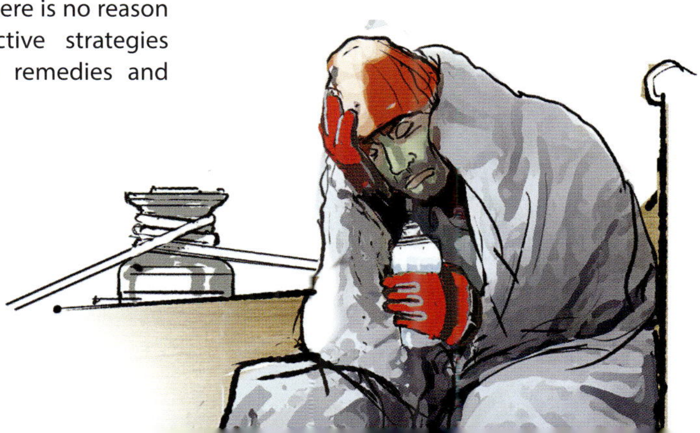

Prevent seasickness from getting worse.

Severe seasickness requires close support and help from the crew. Keep hydrated to avoid risk of dehydration.

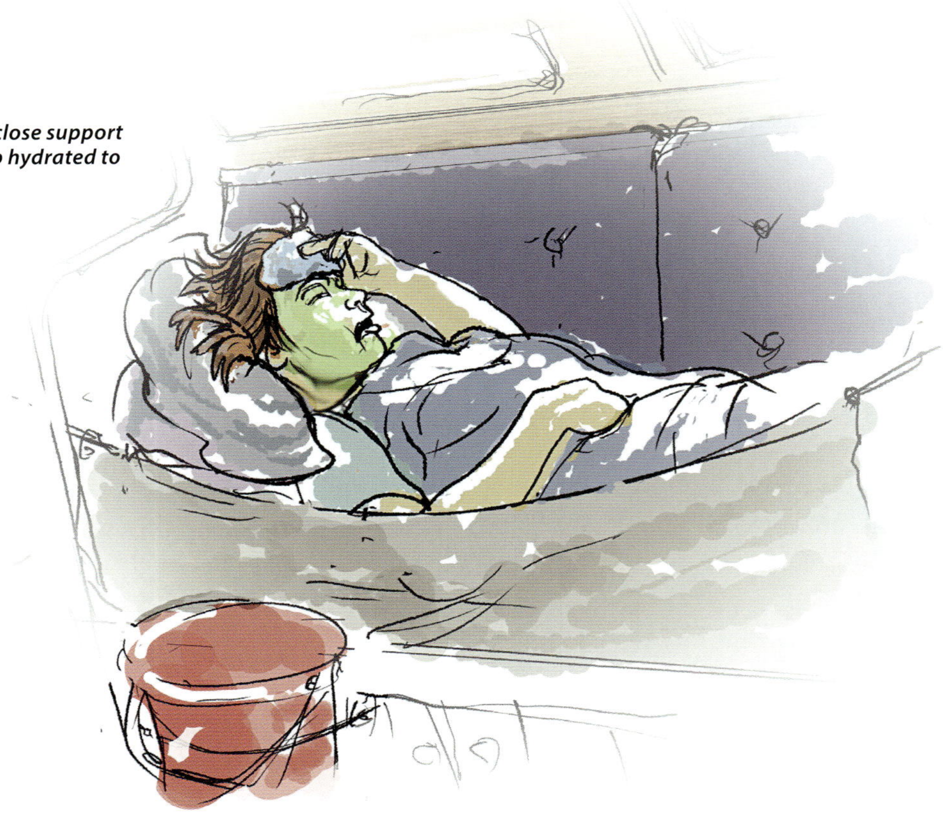

Treatment

Treatment and prevention methods of seasickness often overlap. Once symptoms have started, the medication and other remedies (described below under 'Prevention') may still help but are most effective when taken a few hours before embarking.

If medication is considered, tablets may be thrown up when vomiting. A better choice is, for example, a chewing gum with dimenhydrinate, an antihistamine and antiemetic, or a chewable tablet with hyoscine (such as Kwells). The advantage is that treatment can start even if sailing has already begun and after nausea has started.

Far from help

If the person becomes severely ill, they may need to lie down in a stable area of the boat, typically amidships where there is the least movement. Place pillows or sail bags around them for stability, and encourage sleep, reassuring them of the crew's support. A few hours of rest combined with treatment may improve their condition. Be aware of vomiting and the need for rehydration. If near shore, consider returning to port; if at sea, some sedative, for example diazepam or promethazine, may be required to break the cycle of nausea and vomiting.

Prevention

Medication treatment/prevention of seasickness.

Active substance	Route of administration	Dose	Type
Hyoscine hydrobromide	Patch	1 every 72 hours Start 24 hours prior	Anticholinergic
Dimenhydrinate 20 mg	Chewing gum	Max 4 gums/day	Antihistamine
Mechlozine dihydrochloride (Mechlozine) 25 mg	Oral tablet	1 every 8 hours	Antihistamine Antiemetic
Cyclizine 50 mg	Oral tablet	1 every 8 hours	Antihistamine
Promethazine 25 mg	Oral tablet	1 every 8 hours	Antihistamine
Cinnarazine 25 mg	Oral tablet	1 every 8 hours	Antihistamine
Diphenhydramine	Oral tablet	1 every 8 hours	Antihistamine, Stimulant

Most medications against seasickness are preventive and should be taken before symptoms occur. All may cause side effects such as fatigue, dry mouth, visual disturbances and urinary issues (in older men). The severity of side effects varies by individual and medications. We recommend a discussion with your GP and everyone on board to try out which medication has the least side effects, before heading out to sea. Many of them are available over the counter; others need a prescription. Some medications are contraindicated in, for example, glaucoma, urinary problems and asthma.

Home remedies considered effective against seasickness (try the one that suits you best):

- fresh or pickled ginger
- ginger biscuits or ginger tablets from health food shops
- whole cloves (spice) before setting out
- acupressure with wristbands or fingertip pressure

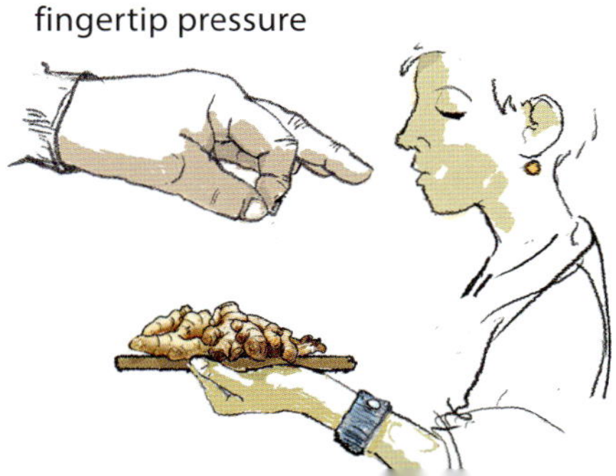

Other strategies to counteract seasickness and prevent its occurrence:

- Be well rested and dress warmly.
- Focus on the horizon to provide a reference point to help the sense of balance.
- Stay as active as possible, such as steering the boat.
- Eat and drink frequently, in small amounts.
- Avoid going below deck during the first few hours.
- Prepare meals beforehand to minimise time spent in the galley.
- Start longer passages in daylight to allow easier adaptation.
- Plan your trip; avoid starting in strong winds and high seas.

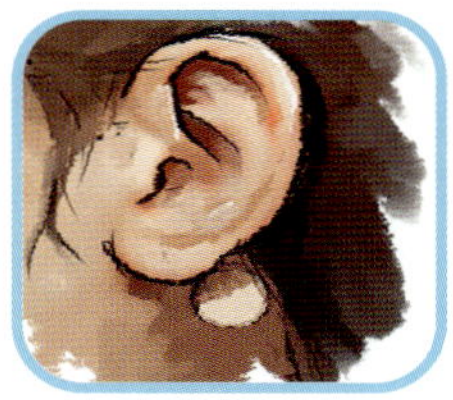

Proper placement of a patch against seasickness.

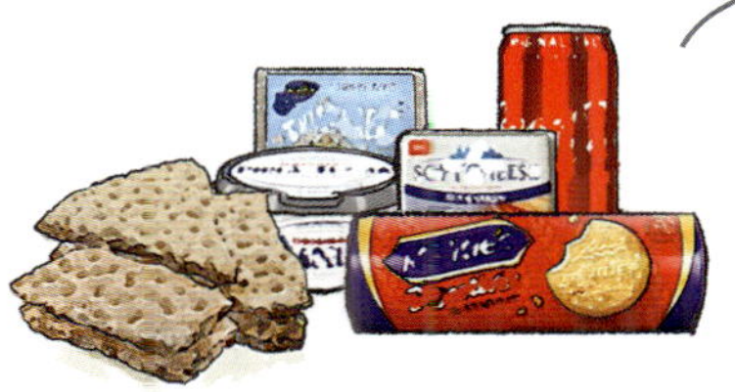

Easy access to snacks and drinks is important to prevent seasickness.

Acupressure wristbands, fingertip pressure (distraction methods) and all forms of ginger are reported to prevent seasickness.

2. FIRST AID

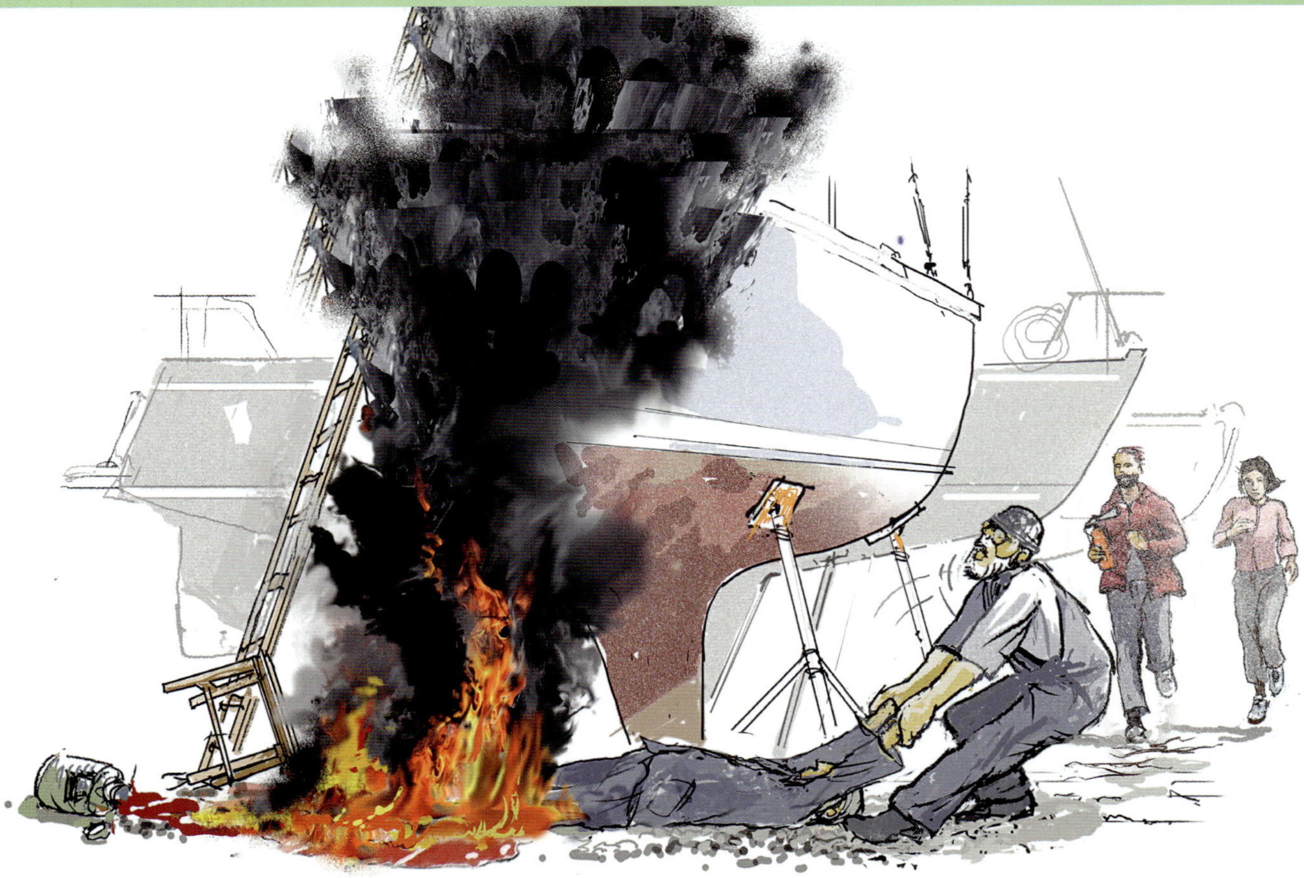

Immediate danger, act swiftly and then follow DRABC procedure!

FIRST AID GOALS

The goals of first aid are to:

- Save lives
- Prevent an injury or acute illness from worsening
- Provide pain relief
- Transport the patient to hospital

When it comes to healthcare and responding to acute medical issues on board a leisure boat, conditions can vary greatly. These range from being moored in a marina, anchored at a favourite island, sailing in waters with a maximum of 12–24 hours to reach a doctor, to being at sea on a longer ocean crossing where professional medical help may be two or more weeks away. Despite the vastly different circumstances, they inevitably share common healthcare aspects; some situations can be resolved entirely on board, while others require temporary measures to continue to port for professional medical assistance. Certain acute conditions, however, will require immediate life-saving interventions and urgent transport to hospital. In the case of obvious or suspected severe injury/illness, consider seeking early support from healthcare professionals on how to proceed.

HOW TO FIND HELP

- Mobile phone: Call 112 in an emergency in the UK and all EU countries, 911 in the US and parts of Asia
- Sat phone: Call local MRCC (Maritime Rescue Co-ordination Centre)
  VHF: Channel 16
- Radio: 2182 kHz (MF)/ 8291 kHz (HF)
- EPIRB: If there is an EPIRB on board, remember to activate it in a serious situation
- SAR contacts: If you have access to internet, you will get a relevant SAR contact list of RCC (Rescue Co-ordination Centres) worldwide, including contact information. https://sarcontacts.info

DRABC

The DRABC concept has been chosen as a base for our recommendations on how to act in a medical situation when life is at stake. DRABC is compliant with recommendations of European and other international organisations working on the continuous improvement of life-saving techniques. Different rescue organisations have different versions (L-ABCDE, ABCDE, DRSABCDE) but basically with the same message. In advanced trauma care and military first aid, CABC is used, where the first C stands for 'catastrophic bleeding'.

Immediate action

If a serious accident occurs on board, prioritise your own safety! If you become injured, you will not be able to help others. Follow the DRABC, a concept used internationally by emergency services for making an initial assessment in emergencies. It also forms a good basis for emergency calls.

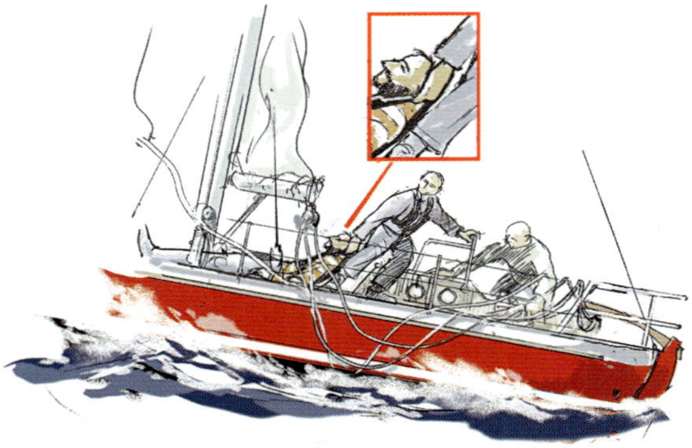

D – DANGER: Move the casualty to a safer place if the location poses a danger to you and/or the injured person, such as under a swinging boom or in proximity to fire with a risk of explosion.

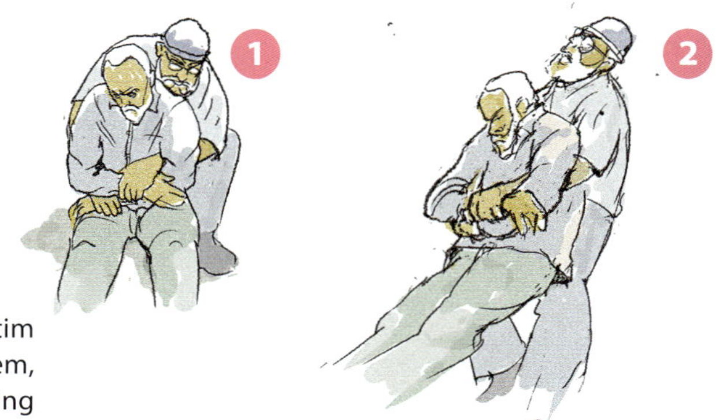

Pull on the clothes or use a fireman's lift. It is a difficult and heavy job! Practise!

R – RESPONSE: Is the victim conscious? Try talking to them, shouting for response, or using pain stimuli if there is no answer. If still unresponsive, the person is unconscious.

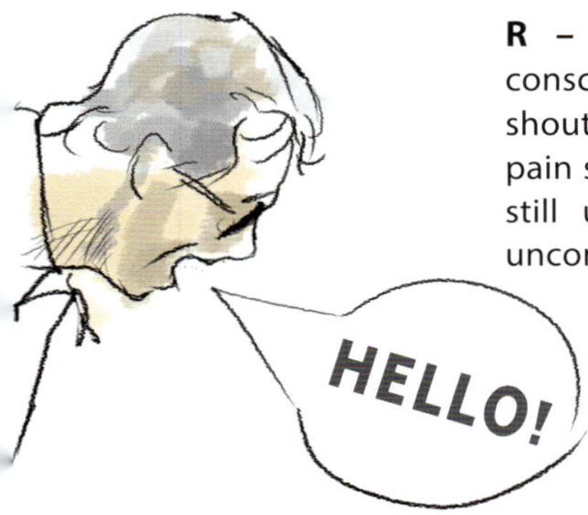

Shout, call the person's name! Use the AVPU classification (see page 135).

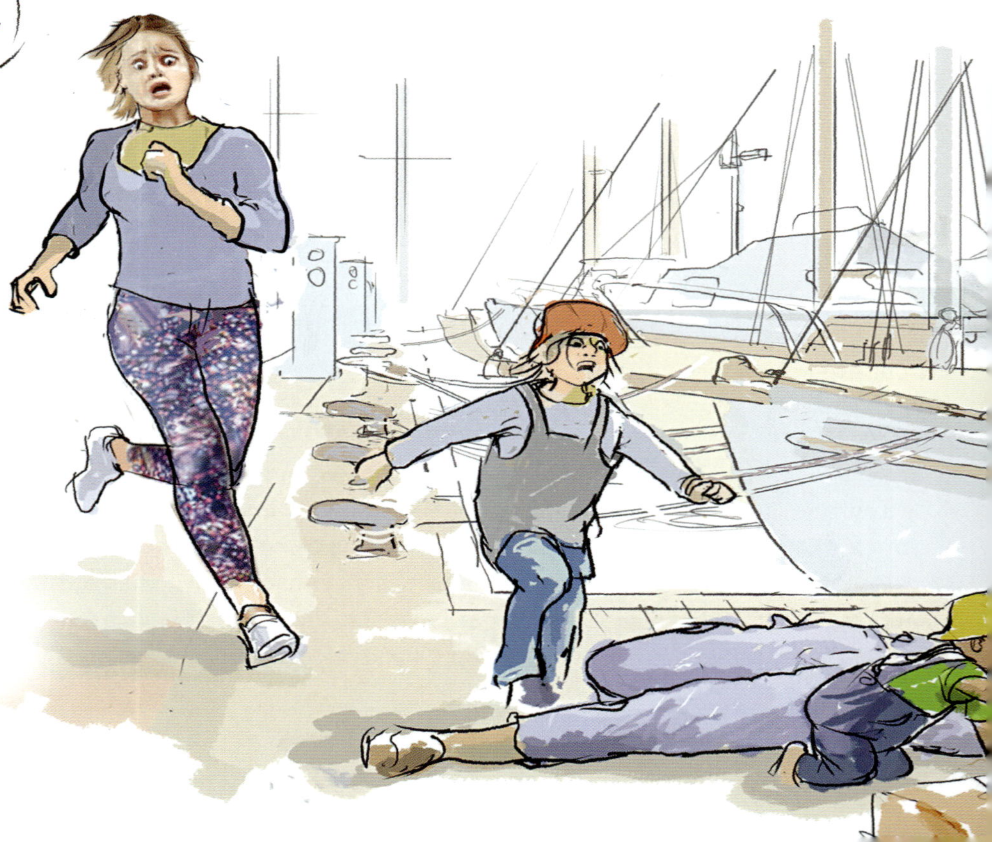

An emergency can happen at any time.

PAIN STIMULI

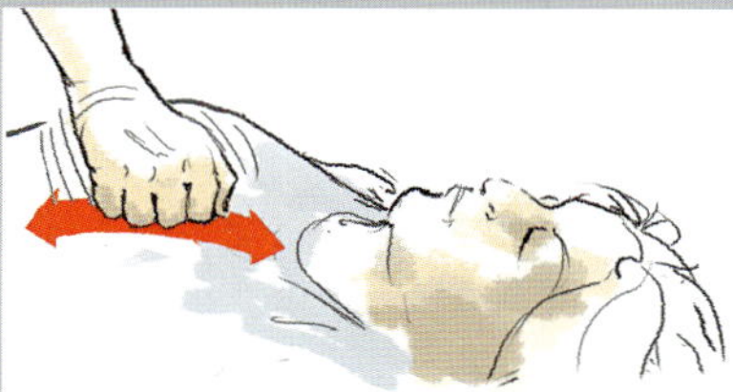

Pain stimulus. Scrub hard on the breastbone!

Other methods for pain stimulation

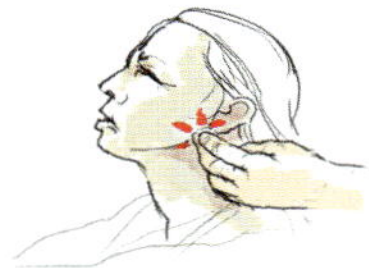

Press hard on the mandibular angle.

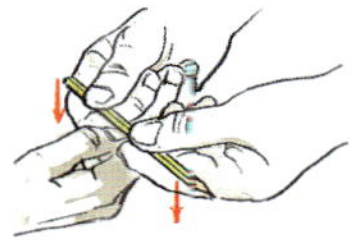

Squeeze a thumb or fingernail with a pen.

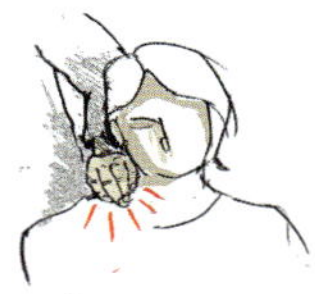

Squeeze the clavicle and the muscles above.

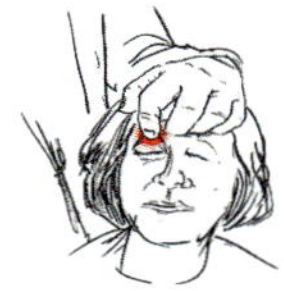

Press hard on the upper margin of the orbit.

A – AIRWAY: Check if the person can breathe, and if the airways are clear. Maintaining an open airway is always the highest priority. Secure an open airway by lifting the jaw upwards/backwards ('jaw lift') and clearing the mouth of foreign material. A person can only survive about three minutes without oxygen.

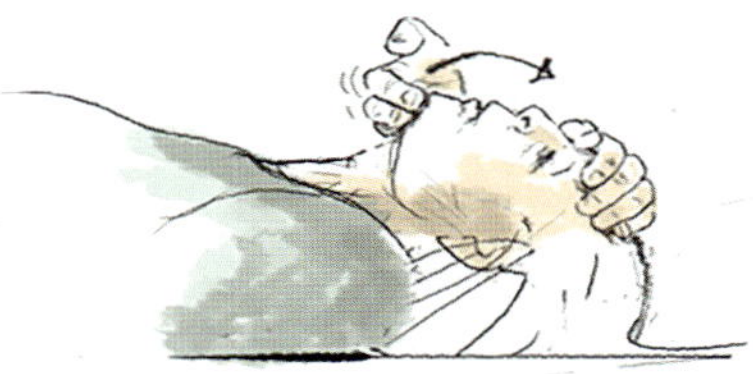

Jaw lift. Two fingers under the chin and a hand on the forehead tilting the head backwards.

B – BREATHING: Observe the rate and nature of breathing. Normal breathing in an adult is 10–20 breaths per minute and without abnormal sounds – for example, gurgling, whistling/wheezing or snoring. Listen for breath sounds, feel for airflow and observe chest movements.

Ear close to the mouth. Do you feel or hear any breaths from the mouth?

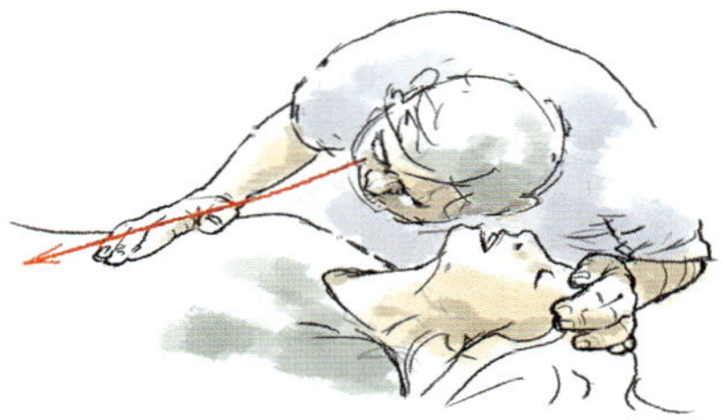

Put a hand on the chest. Can you see or feel any movement?

Look, listen, feel! Can you see or feel movements of the chest? Do you hear a weak sound of breathing, or do you feel the flow of air against your cheek? Are there any unusual sounds?

C – CIRCULATION: Check for internal bleeding. For trauma to the abdomen, chest, thighs or pelvis, assess for signs of internal bleeding (pallor, cold sweat, pain). Check the pulse to see if it is weak, slow or rapid.

Stop external bleeding, see page 21.

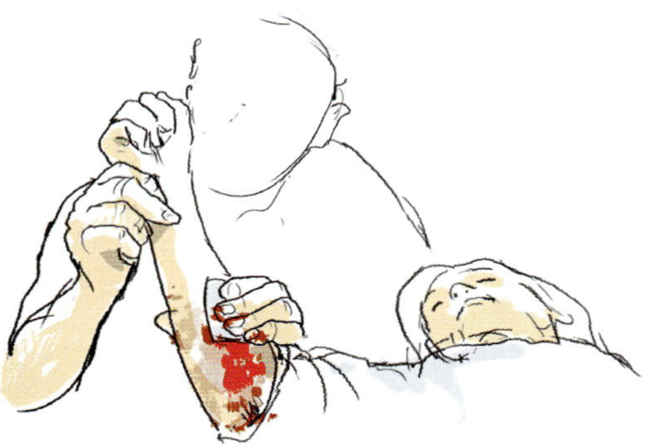

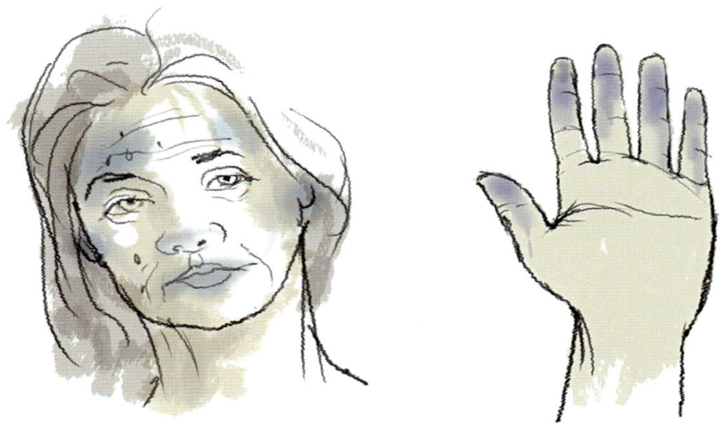

Signs of shock: cyanosis and cold sweat. Abnormally rapid or slow pulse.

CARDIOPULMONARY RESUSCITATION (CPR)

When to suspect cardiac arrest? If someone collapses on the jetty near you, and the cause is unknown, you have 10 seconds to decide if the person is conscious or unconscious and is breathing or not.

1. CONSCIOUSNESS: Try waking the person by loudly calling their name, shaking them, or by applying pain stimuli (see page 13). Rub your knuckles against the breastbone or pinch the nose or ear.

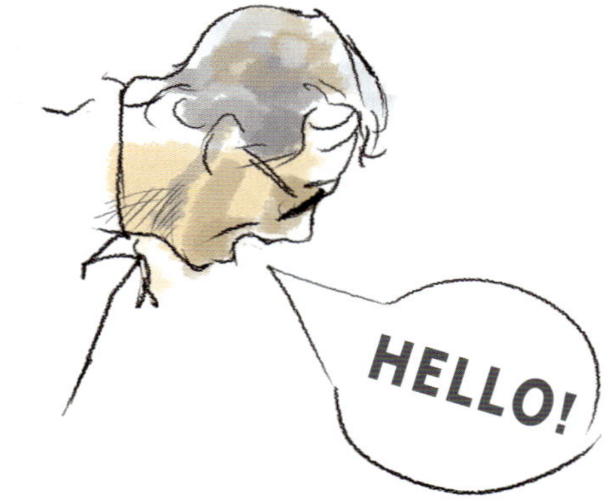

Conscious or unconscious?

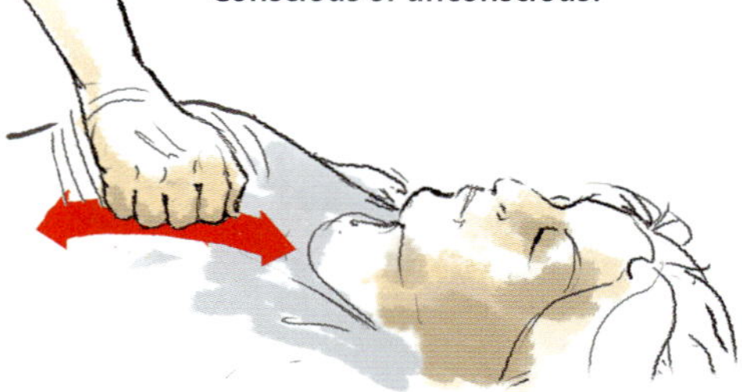

2. BREATHING: Check if the person is breathing, making sure airways are clear and free of obstructions. Chin lift = one hand on the forehead, two fingers under the chin, tilt the head backwards. See, listen, feel! Place your ear near the person's mouth and look down at the chest – can you hear breathing, feel the airflow, see and feel chest movements? Breathing is normally almost inaudible. The breathing is abnormal if it is irregular, shallow, or has strange sounds.

3. UNCONSCIOUS PLUS NO OR ABNORMAL BREATHING = Start CPR! If the person is unconscious and not breathing, or breathing abnormally, start CPR immediately. There is no need to check for a pulse. Call for help. Locate a defibrillator (AED, heart starter) if possible.

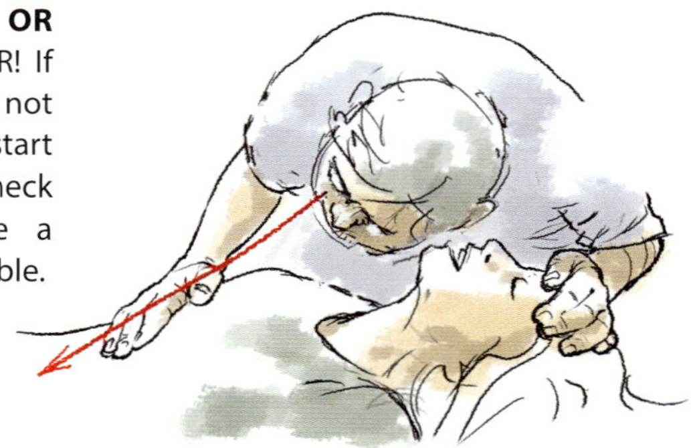

Breathing or not breathing?

> **IMPORTANT**
>
> If, for any reason, you cannot or do not want to provide rescue breaths, chest compressions alone are still valuable.

CPR technique

- Hand placement during CPR: Place the heel of one hand on the centre of the chest, between the nipples, and place the other hand on top and interlock the fingers.
- Perform 30 forceful compressions at a rapid pace, 100–120 compressions per minute (a helpful rhythm is to hum 'Staying Alive'), with a compression depth of 5–6 centimetres, followed by two rescue breaths.
- To give rescue breaths, tilt the head back with one hand on the forehead and two fingers under the chin. This is allowed in this life-threatening situation even when a neck injury cannot be excluded. Note that the recommended procedure may differ slightly from country to country.
- Place your mouth over the casualty's mouth and pinch the nose to close it – or use a mask (see image), give a normal breath until the chest rises. Repeat and give two rescue breaths, and check that the chest rises.
- Continue CPR until help arrives. Rotate rescuers every two minutes to maintain effective compressions. The effect of CPR performed by the same person diminishes rapidly after two minutes, which is why this task is best shared by at least two people.

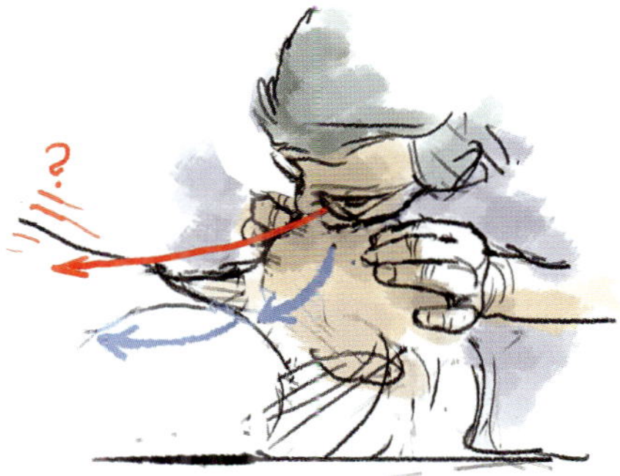

Rescue breath technique. Pinch the nose, give a breath mouth-to-mouth. Check that the chest rises.

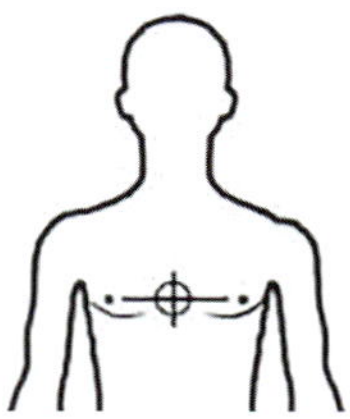

Body position and hand placement in CPR. Note – straight arms and stay on a firm surface!

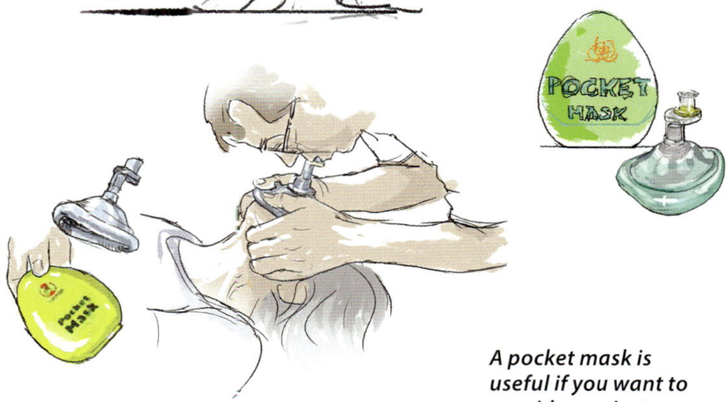

A pocket mask is useful if you want to provide respiratory support to a person. It provides a tight seal, with a filter that offers good protection for the rescuer. Practise keeping it airtight.

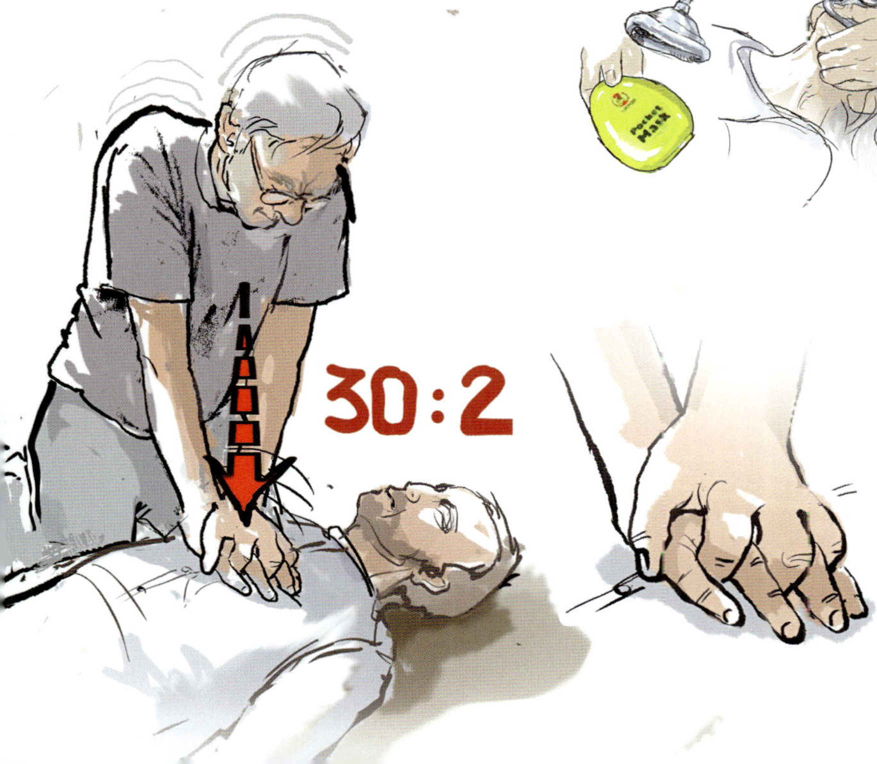

Automated External Defibrillators (AEDs)

AEDs are increasingly available in many public places, such as guest harbours, marinas, and even on some boats. They are user-friendly and provide clear voice prompts about where to put the electrodes, how to give chest compressions, and when to stand back for an electrical pulse. But consider taking a course in CPR to be prepared in an emergency. Using an AED within three to five minutes of cardiac arrest can double or triple survival rates. Chances of survival decrease by approximately 10 per cent per minute thereafter without defibrillation.

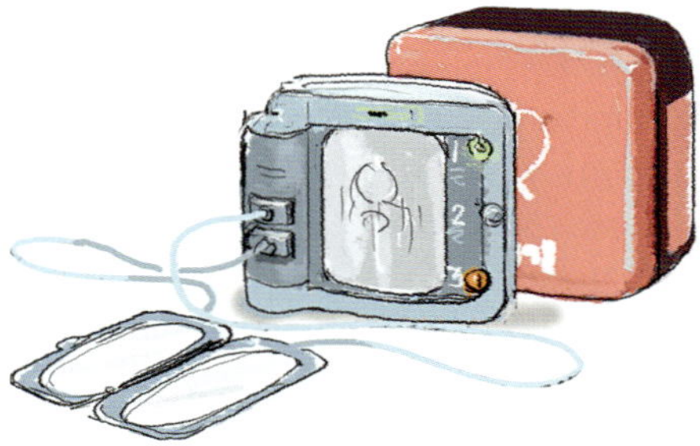

An AED.

RECOVERY POSITION

- Lift and rotate the nearest arm outwards.
- Bend the knee in the opposite leg 90 degrees and lock the foot under the nearest knee.
- Grab the far knee and far hand and tilt the person towards yourself.
- Put the person's far hand under their cheek.
- Position the upper leg in a way that stabilises the recovery position.

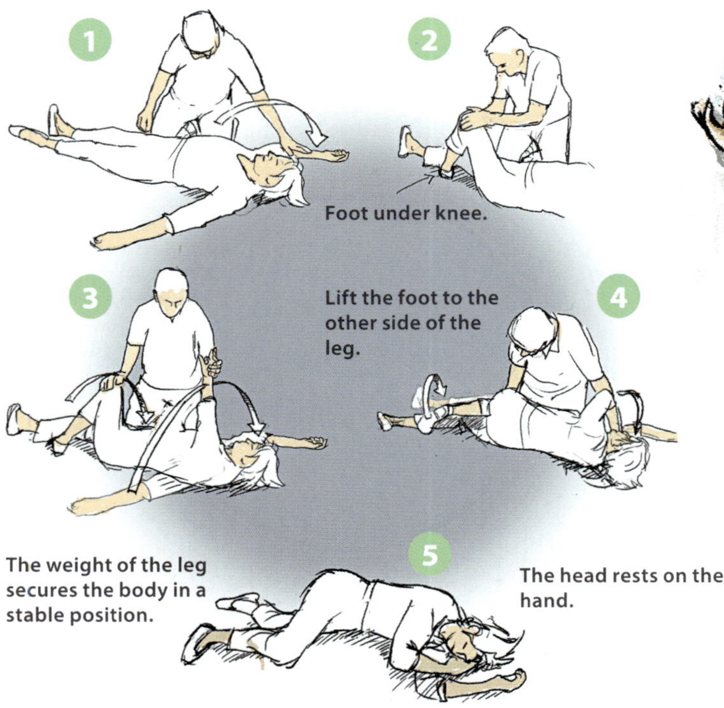

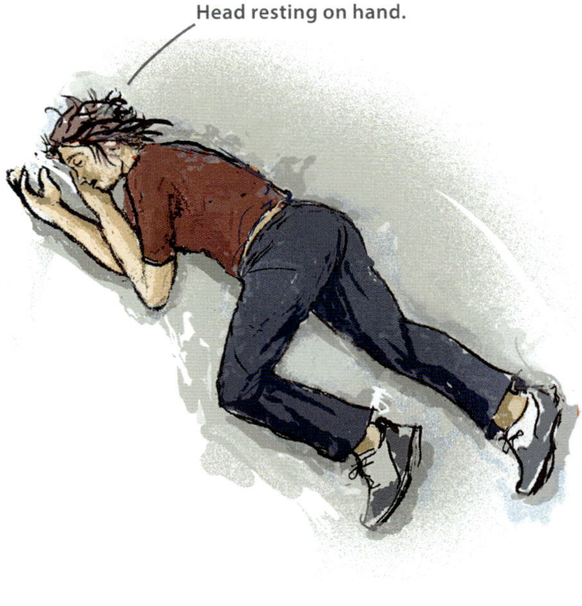

If a person is unconscious but breathing, put them in recovery position.

HANDLING FAINTING

'Ordinary fainting' (vasovagal syncope) can mimic a cardiac arrest but is usually a harmless disturbance in circulation. Often triggered by standing up quickly, prolonged standing, fluid depletion (hypovolaemia), or a low tolerance for pain. The person collapses, becomes pale, sweaty, loses consciousness, and may have seizures. To revive a fainting person:

- Differentiate from cardiac arrest. A person who has fainted will be breathing, and responds to voice and/or painful stimuli.
- Raise the legs to quickly restore blood flow to the brain.
- Place them in the recovery position if vomiting is likely.

A drop in blood pressure is normally accompanied by an increased heart rate, but in ordinary fainting the pulse instead decreases. It is recommended to seek medical control and evaluation to rule out other more serious causes.

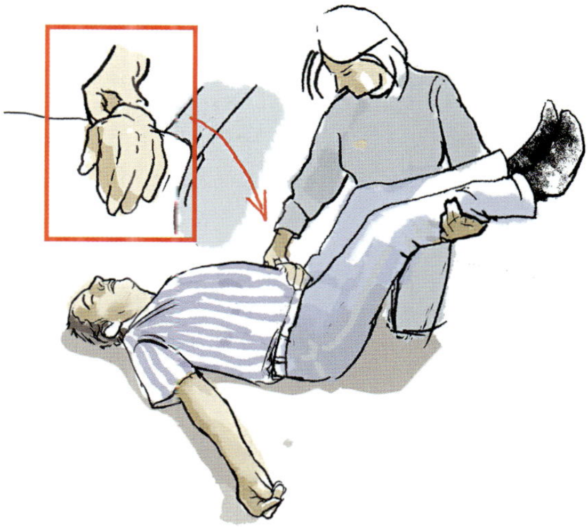

Someone who has fainted is breathing and can be woken up. Raise the legs. Pulse is usually low.

Raise legs to get blood into the head. Fan person if hot, for comfort.

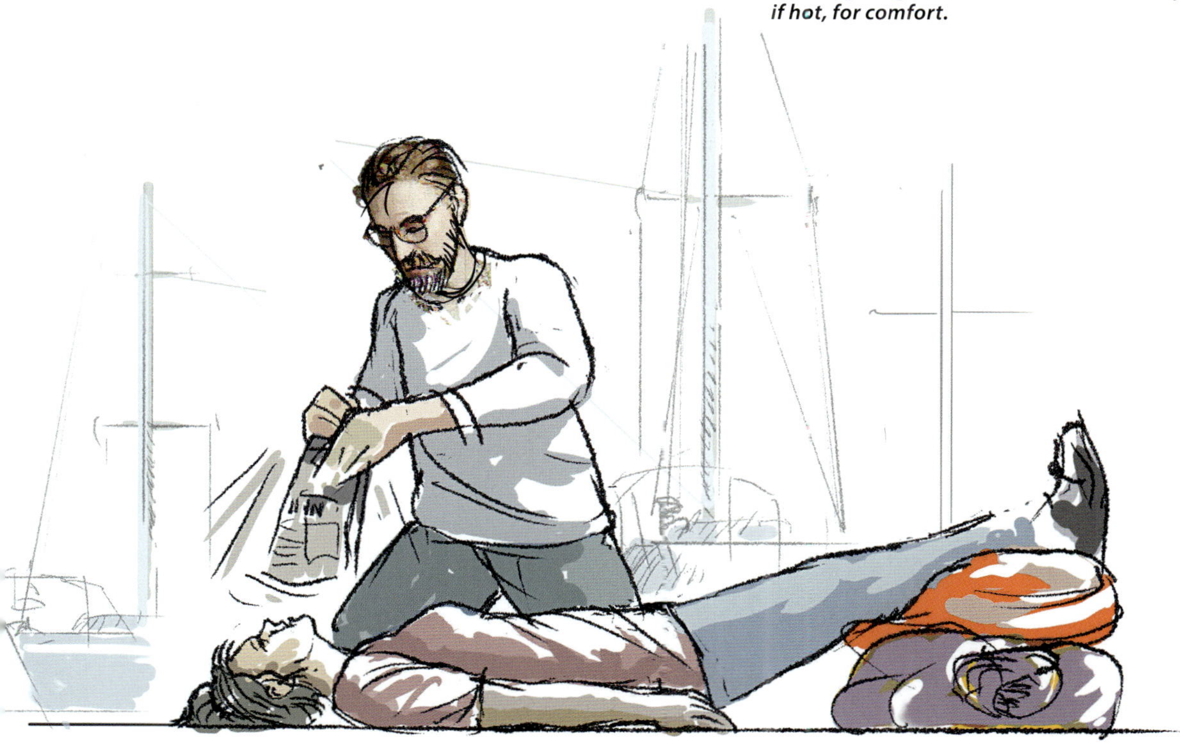

CPR IN CHILDREN

In children, cardiac arrest is rare but, on the other hand, extremely dramatic. It is important to be aware of the special conditions in children. The cause of cardiac arrest in children is usually a respiratory problem. This can be due to a foreign object in the airways, drowning or vomiting. It can also be part of an allergic reaction, with swelling of the tongue and upper respiratory tract.

Immediate action

1 Ensure an open airway. Always start with five breaths. Oxygen supply is most important for a child with cardiac arrest. Adjust the volume of blown air to the child's size.
2 Perform 30 compressions, 4–5cm deep, at a rate of 100–120 compressions per minute, followed by two rescue breaths.
3 For children under one year old, use two fingers for compressions. For slightly bigger children, use one hand. See below.
4 Seek professional assistance as soon as possible.

If a child is experiencing an acute mechanical airway obstruction:

1 Place the child on their stomach across your lap with their head hanging downwards.
2 Deliver five back blows with the palm of your hand between the child's shoulder blades.
3 If this does not work, turn the child over and perform five abdominal compressions.

For slightly older children, you can use the Heimlich manoeuvre.

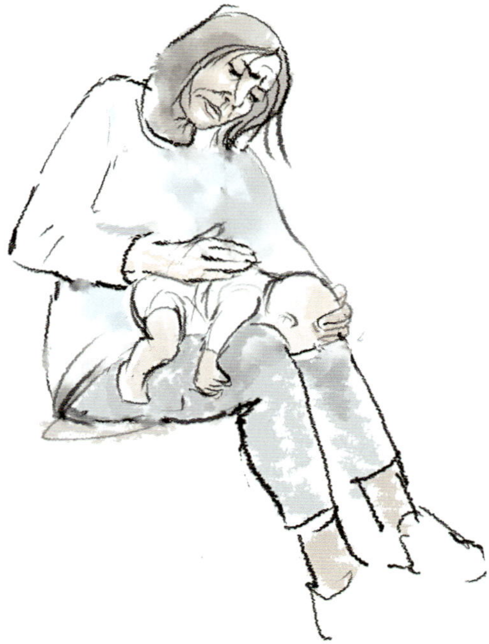

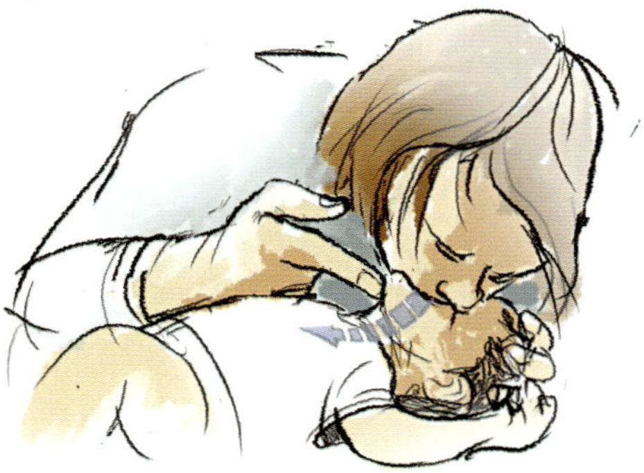

When performing mouth-to-mouth resuscitation on very small children, it is necessary to cover both the child's mouth and nose. Blow in an amount of air roughly equal to what you can hold in your own mouth, as children have small lungs.

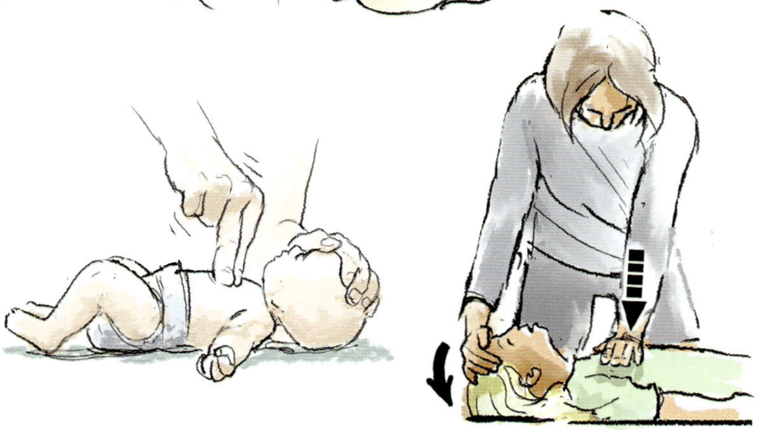

For children under one year old, use two fingers for compressions. For slightly bigger children, use one hand.

Normal breathing rate in children	
< 1 year	40–50 / min
–5 years	30–40 / min
> 6 years	*c.* 25 / min

Pulse rate	
< 1 year	120–160
1–2 years	100–120
> 2 years	as in an adult 50–100

Pulse rate in small children varies easily and is not as safe a parameter as in adults. Children have a strong cardiac function with a high compensatory capacity for shock. Their capacity to compensate blood loss by increasing heart rate is large. It is important to detect if a too low pulse < 50 – bradycardia – is developing.

ACUTE AIRWAY OBSTRUCTION

Airway obstruction caused by a foreign object typically occurs while eating and simultaneously talking or laughing. Even if the object does not completely block the airway, it can trigger severe spasms, worsening the situation.The person may clutch their throat, cough, become anxious, and attempt to breathe with forceful movements of the throat and chest. Their skin may turn pale, blue and sweaty.

Immediate action

Assess the severity. What can you do? Immediate action is dependent on whether the person can breathe or not.

- Can breathe, the person has difficulty breathing but can cough and speak. Encourage them to continue coughing, try to remove the foreign object, and ensure the mouth is clear. Do not allow the person to go to the bathroom and lock themselves in. The person may deteriorate and require assistance and must be reachable for help.
- Cannot breathe, cannot cough or speak, and there is a suspected complete airway obstruction due to a foreign object. Act quickly to remove the foreign object. If there is no result and the problem persists, the person may lose consciousness within a couple of minutes. Be prepared to lay the person down to prevent injury when falling. Check the mouth and remove foreign objects and initiate CPR. Call for help!

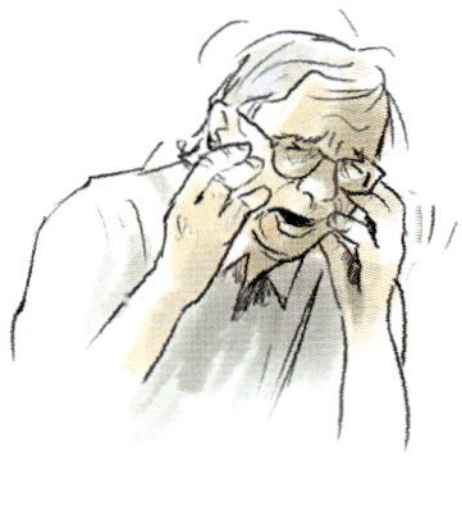

Symptoms in acute airway obstruction: anxiety, clutching the face, difficulty inhaling air, bending forward.

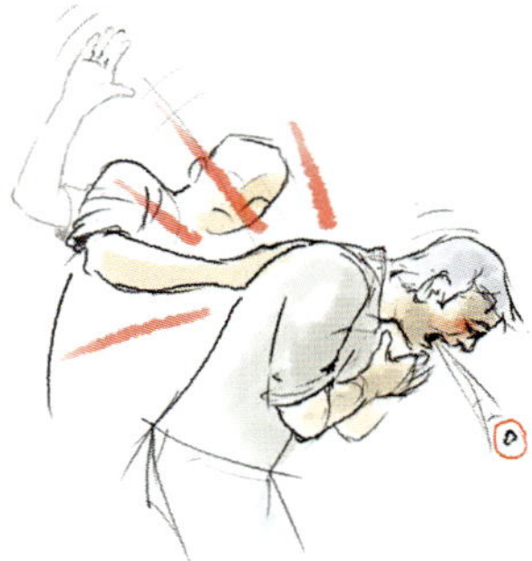

Bend the person forward and give five blows on the back, between the shoulder blades.

Follow the illustrations:

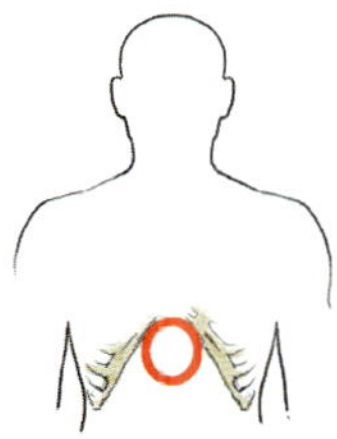

Correct position of the fist in the Heimlich manoeuvre.

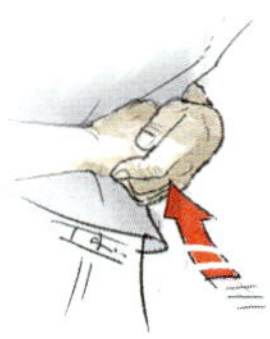

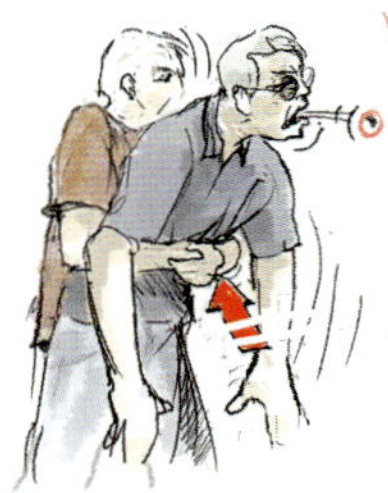

If there is no effect, immediately start the Heimlich manoeuvre. Stand behind the person and wrap your arms around their waist. Place a fist with the thumb facing inwards at the base of the ribcage and cover it with your other hand. Deliver forceful, upward thrusts in a diagonal direction. The goal is to create a strong airflow from the trachea to expel the foreign object.

If you are alone and no help is available, try this alternative.

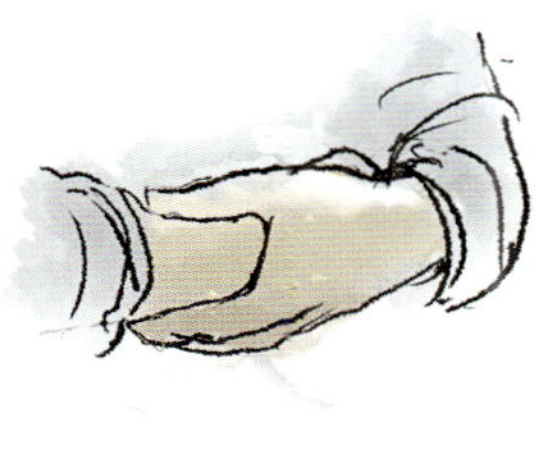

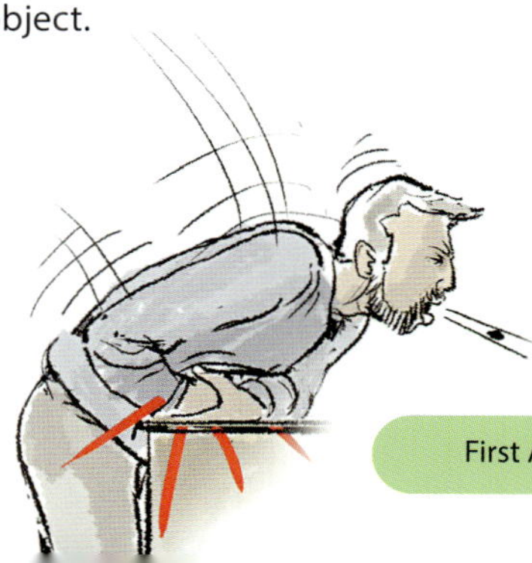

CIRCULATION / SHOCK

The word 'shock' is used to describe various psychological reactions, such as joy, sorrow, panic or surprise. However, 'real' circulatory shock refers to life threatening acute circulatory failure with inadequate oxygen delivery to the body.

There are many causes of circulatory failure and shock. Significant bleeding (page 21), septicaemia (page 38), anaphylaxis (page 58) or a major burn injury (page 34) can lead to fluid and blood loss, reducing the blood volume available to oxygenate the heart and brain. A heart attack (page 76) can impair the heart's ability to pump oxygenated blood throughout the body.

Signs and symptoms

- Pale, cold and sweaty skin
- Cyanosis (bluish discoloration of, for example, the lips and fingers) due to poor circulation
- Mental effects: agitation, restlessness, apathy or coma
- Rapid or very slow, shallow breathing
- Rapid weak pulse

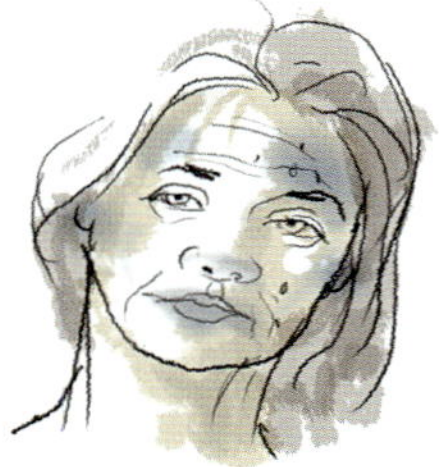

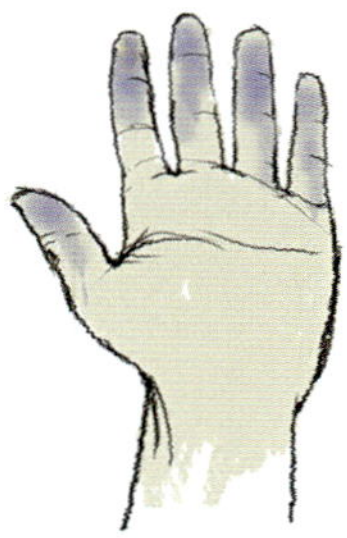

Cyanosis – a sign and symptom of shock.

Immediate action

Who requires urgent transport to a hospital due to suspected shock?

An adult with one or more of the above symptoms and:

- a pulse exceeding 120 beats per minute
- a breathing rate below 10 or above 30 breaths per minute

Such a person is in shock and should be transported to the hospital immediately.

The pulse at the wrist is the easiest to locate. Place your fingers a couple of centimetres below the base of the thumb, between the tendon and the bone. The carotid pulse may be easier to find if the person has low blood pressure or a weak pulse. To locate it, place your fingers between the larynx (Adam's apple) and the straight neck muscle, high up in line with the jawbone.

The radial pulse is usually palpable when blood pressure is greater than 70 mmHg, the femoral pulse at > 60 mmHg, and the carotid pulse at > 50 mmHg. A normal pulse rate is 60–100 beats per minute. To quickly check, count the number of beats in 15 seconds and multiply by four. Practise this skill regularly.

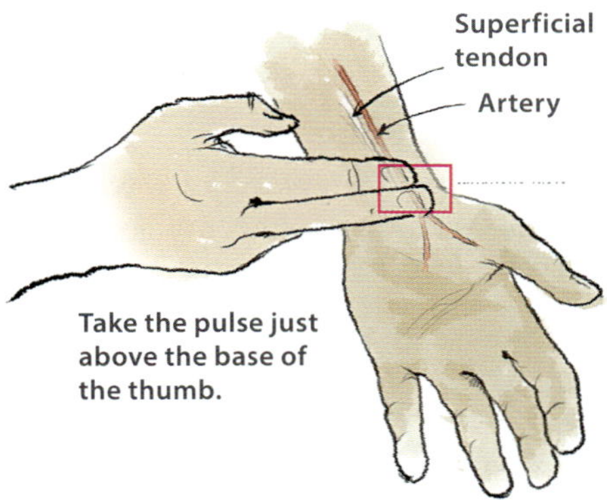

How to locate the wrist and carotid pulses, respectively.

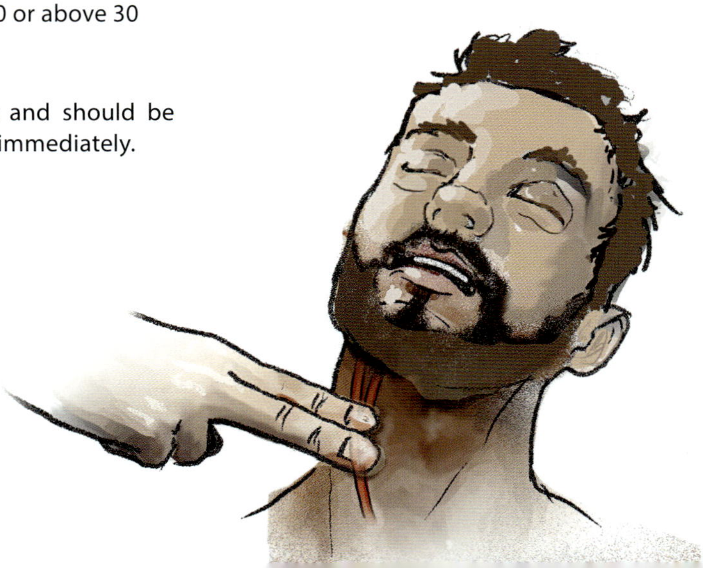

EXTERNAL BLEED

Most wound injuries result in bleeding. If the wound is small, the bleeding usually stops spontaneously after a short time. However, bleeding may be prolonged if the person is taking anticoagulant or antiplatelet medications, such as warfarin, aspirin, NSAIDs (Non-Steroidal Anti-Inflammatory Drugs, including ibuprofen and diclofenac) or apixaban.

In cases of large or deep wounds, bleeding can be significant, potentially leading to substantial blood loss and haemorrhagic shock. Spurting, pulsating bright-red blood indicates an arterial bleed, while venous bleeding is typically slower, oozing, and darker in colour. Most bleeding can be controlled with the application of a pressure bandage.

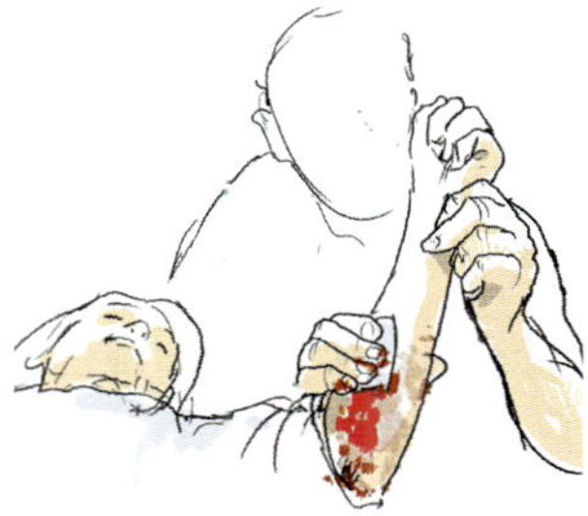

Stop the bleeding! Apply firm pressure over the wound using whatever is available. If needed, switch to a pressure bandage.

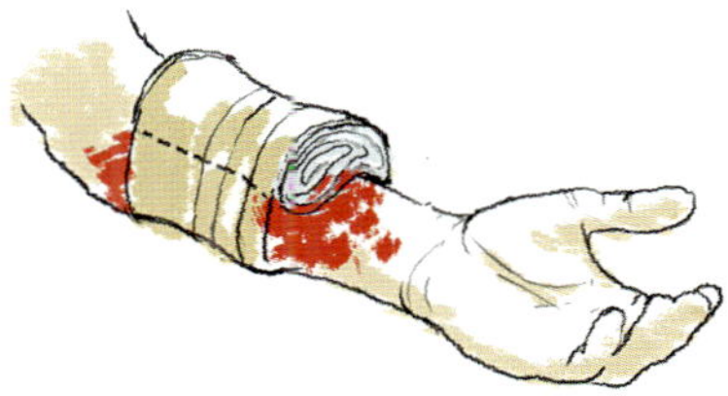

Immediate action

Apply firm pressure over the wound and create a pressure bandage. For significant bleeding, lay the injured person down, elevate the injured extremity, and press firmly over the wound and damaged blood vessel with whatever you have to hand, such as a clean towel or tightly rolled dressings, for at least 15 minutes. If the bleeding does not stop, add another layer and apply harder and longer pressure.

Five steps to make a pressure bandage.

1 Place a tightly rolled gauze or elastic bandage directly over the bleeding wound.
2 Secure it with an elastic bandage or a self-adhering wrap.
3 Wrap several layers of the stretched bandage to create firm, localised pressure over the bleeding site.
4 Ensure the wrap and pressure are effectively controlling the bleeding.
5 Complete the pressure bandage and secure it with tape.

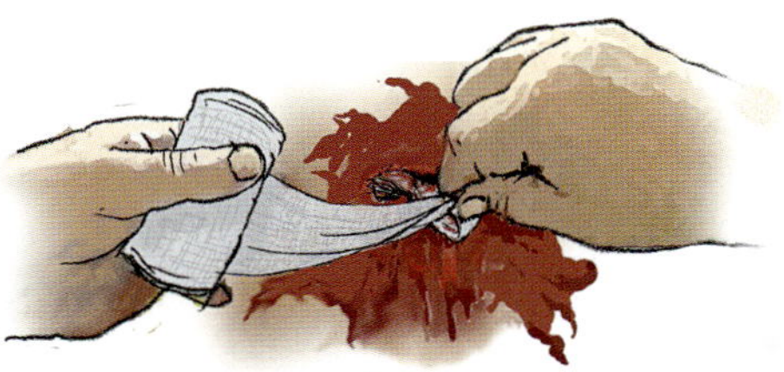

If the wound is deep and hollow, pack it hard with compresses or cloth– before applying pressure. Local pressure with fingers in the wound may be needed.

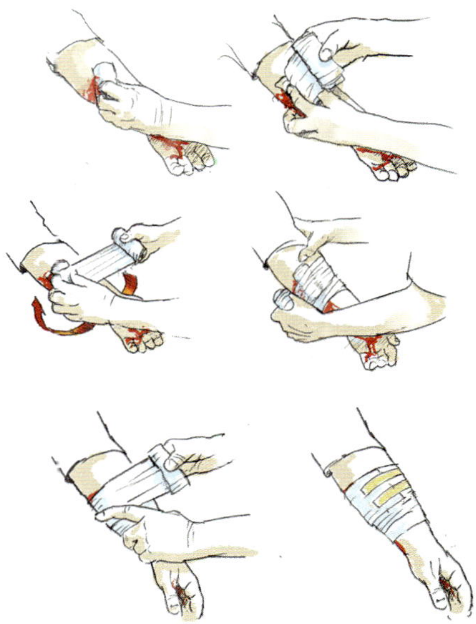

Tourniquet

A constricting bandage – a tourniquet – should be used in cases of life-threatening bleeding, such as amputation injuries or large lacerations (for example, shark bites), as it can be life-saving. A tourniquet completely cuts off circulation to the limb below the bandage. Severe pain typically develops within minutes of application and must be managed. Using narrow ropes or cords as a tourniquet carries a significant risk of damaging underlying structures, especially nerves.

Steps to apply a tourniquet:

1 Place a wide band around the limb, as close to the wound as possible, forming a half-loop.
2 Place a stick over the half-loop and secure it tightly with another half-loop.
3 Twist the stick until the bleeding decreases or stops.
4 Secure the stick in place with an additional loop.

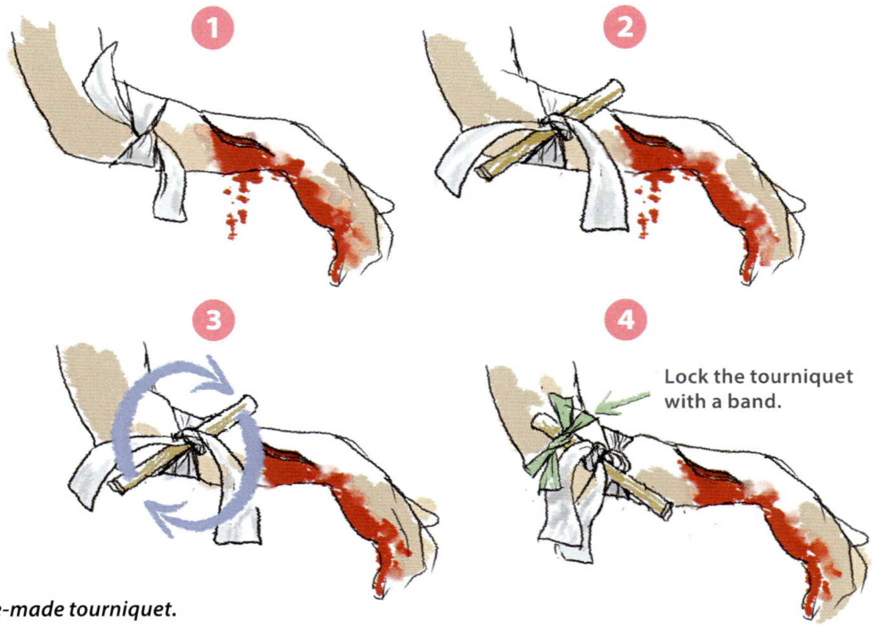

Home-made tourniquet.

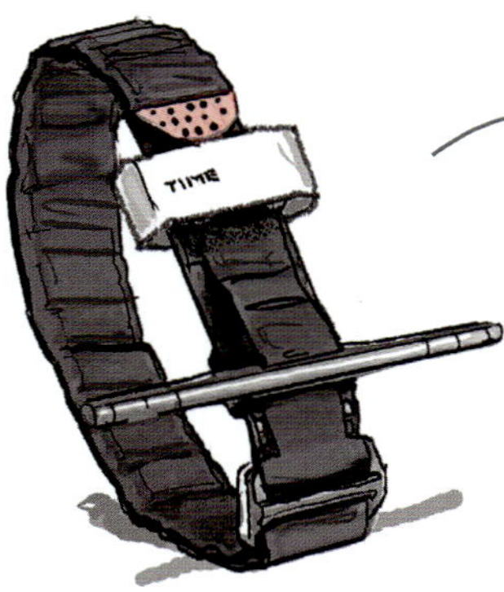

Professional tourniquet. If you buy one – practise!

There are pre-made professional tourniquets, used by police, military and paramedics, which carry less risk of damage and are available at a reasonable price. A tourniquet can save a life in cases of life-threatening bleeding, provided the hospital is not too far away.

Bleed	Symptom	Action
Up to 0.5–0.7 litre	Mild in a healthy person (blood donors give 0.3–0.4 litres)	Fluids, monitoring
0.7–1.5 litres	Pulse > 100 / min Breathing > 20 / min Anxiety, fear	Transport to hospital Intravenous fluids
1.5–2 litres	Pulse > 120 / min Breathing > 30 or < 20 /min Pale, dazed Cold sweat	Urgent need of hospital care Intravenous transfusions
> 2 litres	Pulse weak, not noticeable > 140 Cold and pale skin Consciousness diminished	Urgently life-threatening

This table summarises some parameters indicating the volume of loss of blood.

The blood volume in a 70kg person is approximately 5 litres.

Caution: It is very difficult to estimate blood loss when it is diluted with water. Haemoglobin is a strong dye – just a tablespoon of blood can turn 1–2 litres of water scarily red!

PENETRATING INJURY

Immediate action / Treatment

If someone has been impaled by a knife, screwdriver, tree branch or other sharp object directly into a body part, do not remove the object. Instead, stop the external bleeding and apply a bandage around the object. Removal should only be done in a hospital under careful surgical control. The object may have seriously damaged a blood vessel, but as long as it remains in place, it seals the injury and helps control the bleeding. Removing the object could result in sudden, severe bleeding. Call for an ambulance as soon as possible.

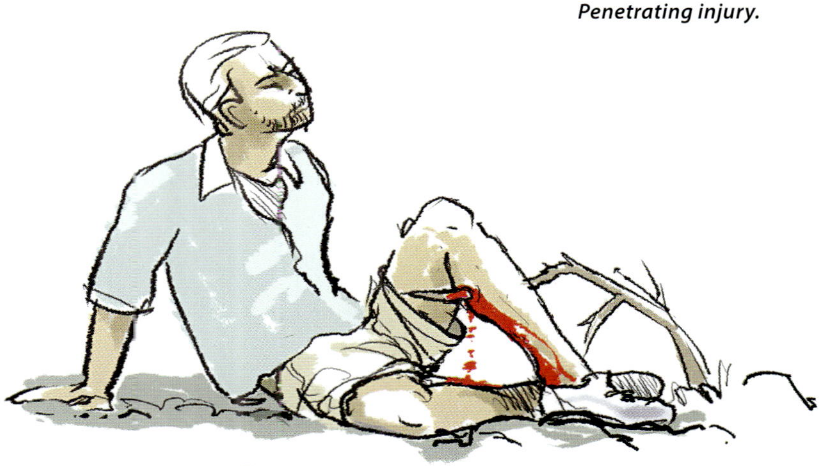

Penetrating injury.

Far from help

This can be a significant challenge, depending on the nature of the injury. Use communication equipment to seek advice on how to manage the specific situation. In cases like the one shown in the image, aim to follow the instructions above and arrange for assistance and rapid evacuation or transport to a hospital.

INTERNAL BLEED

Signs and symptoms

Internal bleeding is difficult to detect in a timely manner. Common causes include blunt force trauma to the abdomen, such as falls on to winches or handlebars (see Chest and Abdominal Trauma, page 152 onwards). The spleen, in particular, is fragile and prone to rupture even after moderate trauma if struck unfavourably. The liver is also vulnerable. Additionally, fractures of the femur and pelvis often lead to internal bleeding. Certain acute non-traumatic medical conditions, such as ectopic pregnancy (page 118) and ruptured aortic aneurysm (page 83), can also result in internal bleeding and pose a high risk of severe shock.

In addition to the signs of shock mentioned earlier (page 20), a person with abdominal bleeding may exhibit the following:

- Pain in the abdomen and back. For spleen injuries, pain often radiates to the left shoulder, while for liver injuries, pain typically radiates to the right shoulder.
- Distended abdomen
- Tender, 'board-like' abdomen
- Nausea and vomiting

Internal bleeding is also common with major fractures, such as femur fractures (page 213), pelvic fractures (page 209), or serious rib fractures that cause bleeding into the pleural cavity (page 154).

A person with suspected internal bleeding and shock should be transported to the hospital immediately.

Typical trauma with risk for internal bleeding.

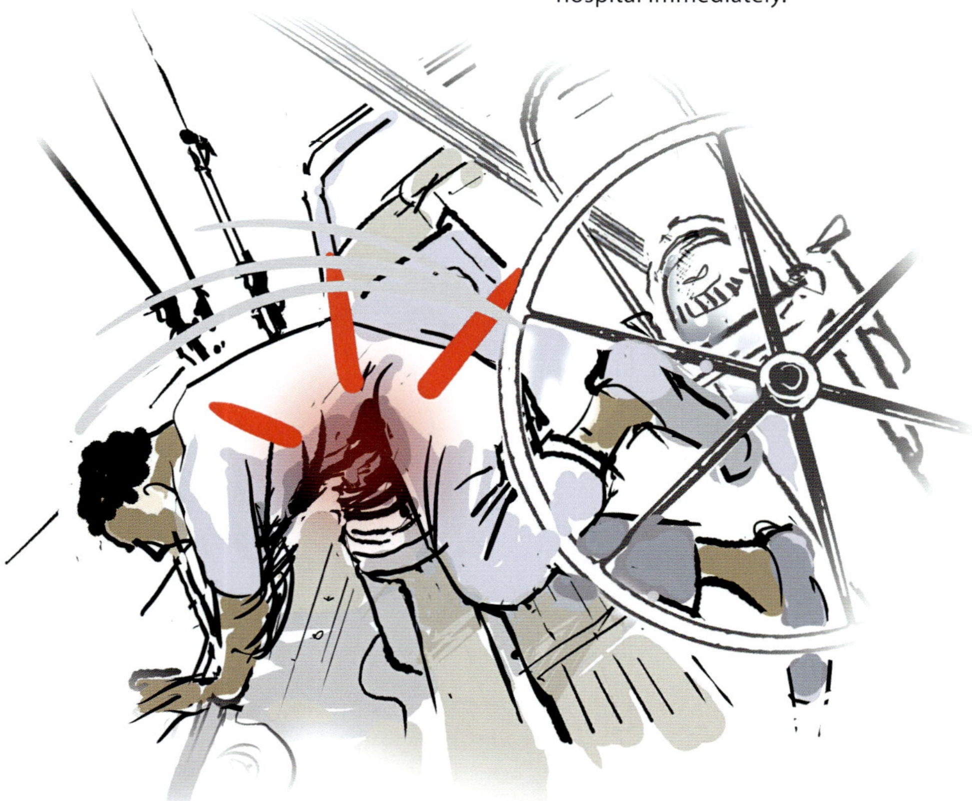

Immediate action

1 Lay the person down and elevate their legs.
2 Call for emergency evacuation.
3 Place the person in the recovery position if necessary (see page 16).

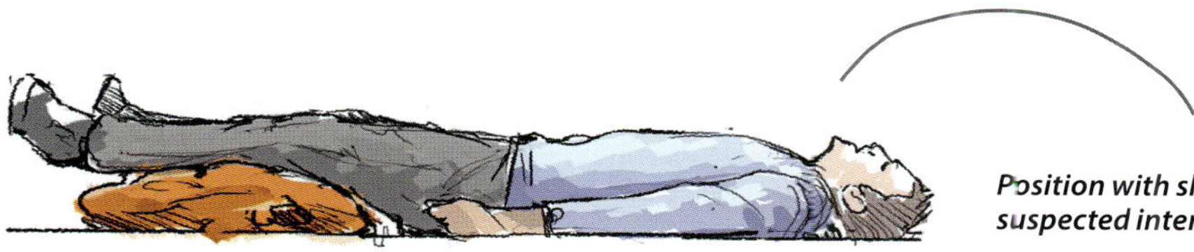

Position with slightly elevated legs if there is suspected internal bleeding in the abdomen.

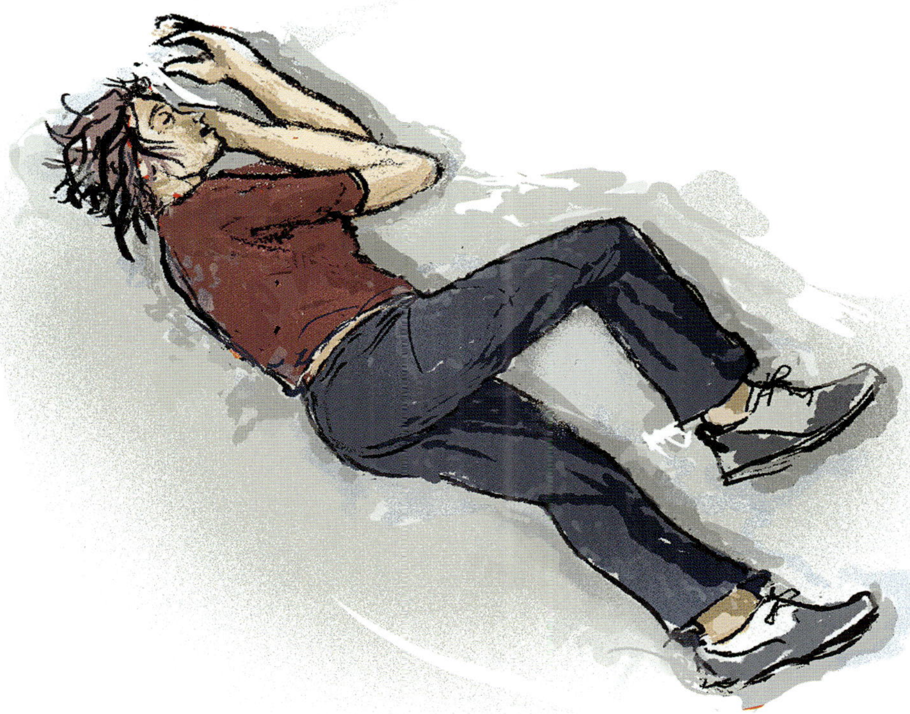

Recovery position (see page 16).

Far from help

A person with suspected or obvious circulatory shock presents a significant challenge, and the possibilities of saving them may be limited. Refer to 'Immediate action' above for guidance.

Prevention

The best approach is to prevent accidents that could lead to injuries with life-threatening consequences, such as severe internal bleeding. Women of childbearing age should be aware of bleeding complications related to pregnancy. Always plan ahead and assess risks!

3. WOUNDS

Be cautious when handling sharp knives. Always use a knife with a guard!

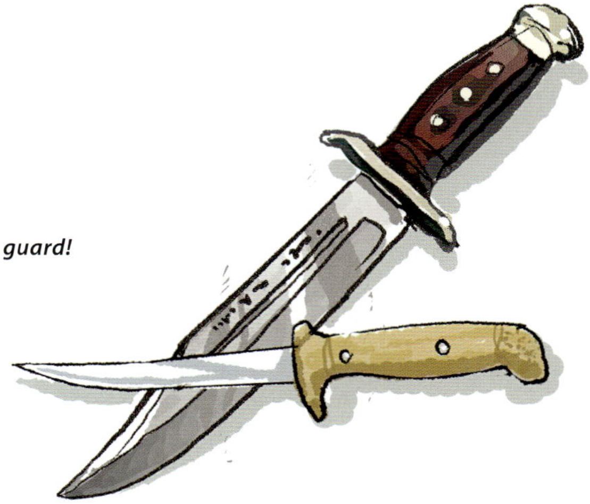

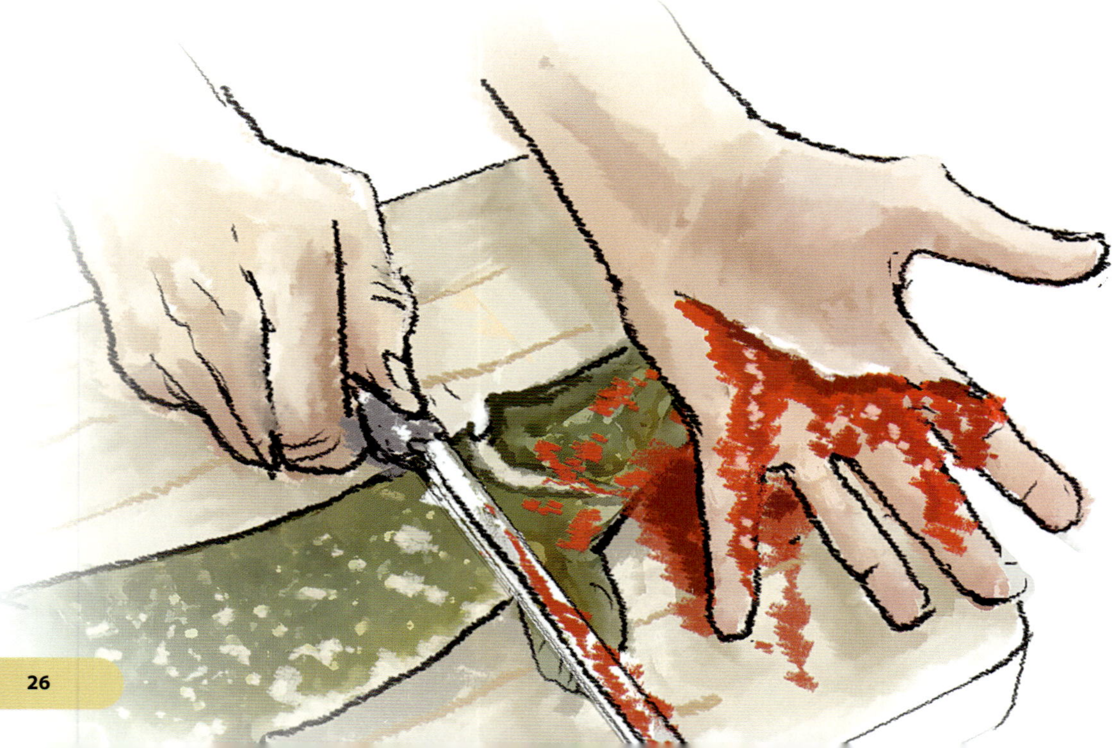

Wound injuries are a common medical issue on recreational boats. Everyone on board should know how to administer first aid for wound injuries. Also, ensure your tetanus vaccination is up to date!

Wound injuries have different causes, which affect the conditions for healing and the risk of complications. During longer voyages, the primary goal is to minimise the risk of serious infections.

WOUND CLASSIFICATION BY CAUSE

Incision wounds

Caused by knives or sharp glass. The depth, length and contamination vary, affecting the risk of infection. There is usually minor damage outside the incision, but there is a risk of blood vessel or nerve damage, especially in arm or hand injuries (see page 184).

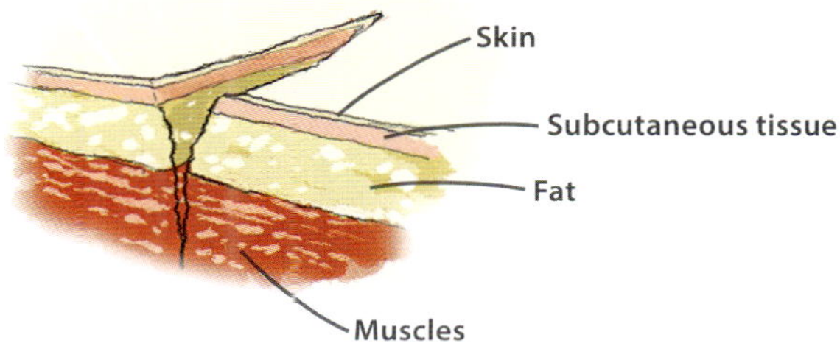

Incision wound.

Stab wounds

Caused by stepping on a nail, knife stabs, or bites from sharp teeth. Dirt can penetrate deep into the injured tissue. The puncture channel is narrow and difficult or impossible to clean, leading to a high risk of infection.

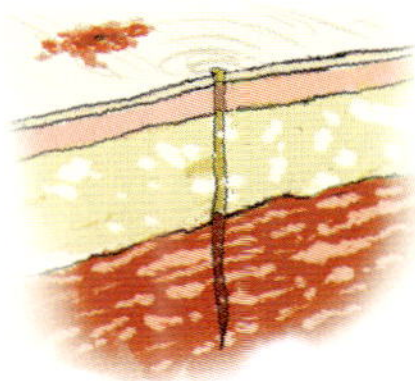

Stab or puncture wound.

Crush wounds

Caused by incidents such as a boom striking the head or a fall on to rocks. These injuries often have diffuse boundaries to undamaged tissue and vary in the degree of contamination. The presence of 'dead' tissue significantly increases the risk of infection.

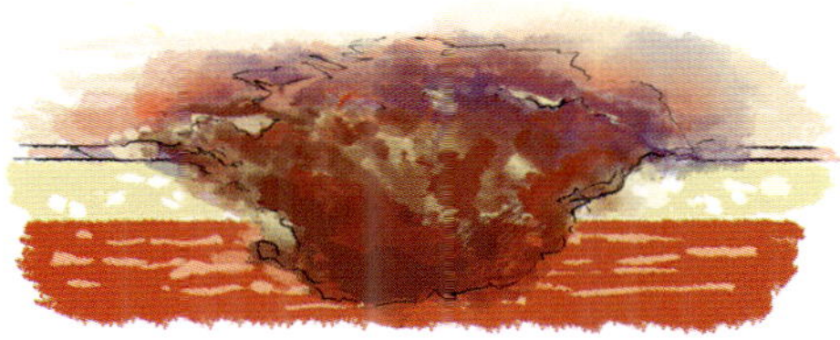

Crush injury.

Lacerations

Irregular wound edges, varying depth and contamination. Often 'pocket formations' under torn tissue that is difficult to clean. Risk of 'dead' tissue.

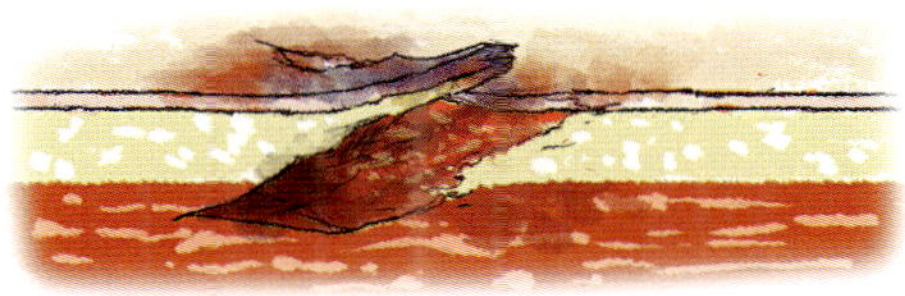

Laceration.

Abrasion wounds

Caused by a fall on to the ground or scraping against soil or rocks. These wounds are superficial but often heavily contaminated and may have elements of crushing injury.

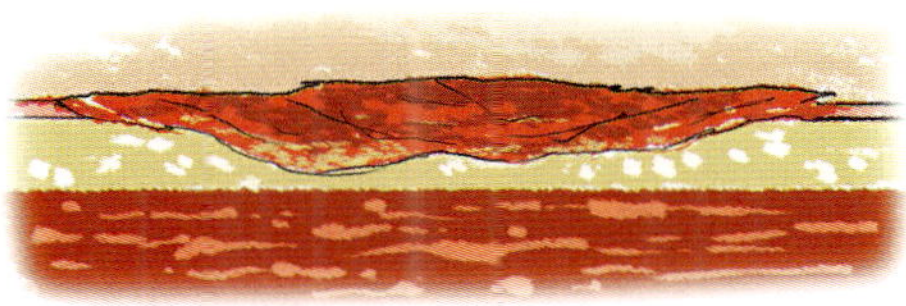

Abrasion.

Immediate action

1 Consider laying the person down to prevent fainting and the risk of secondary injuries from falls.
2 Control and stop external bleeding (see First Aid, page 21).

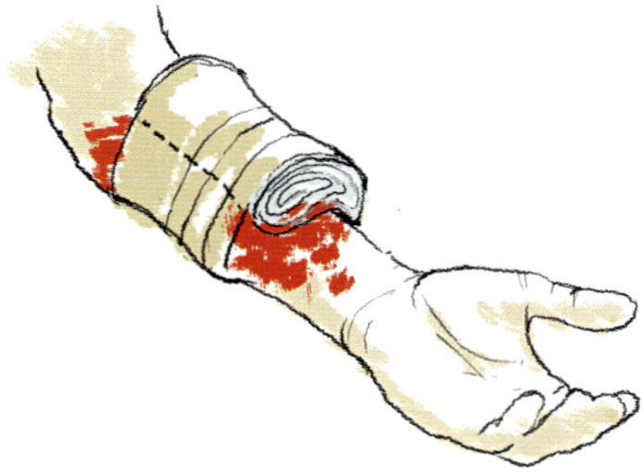

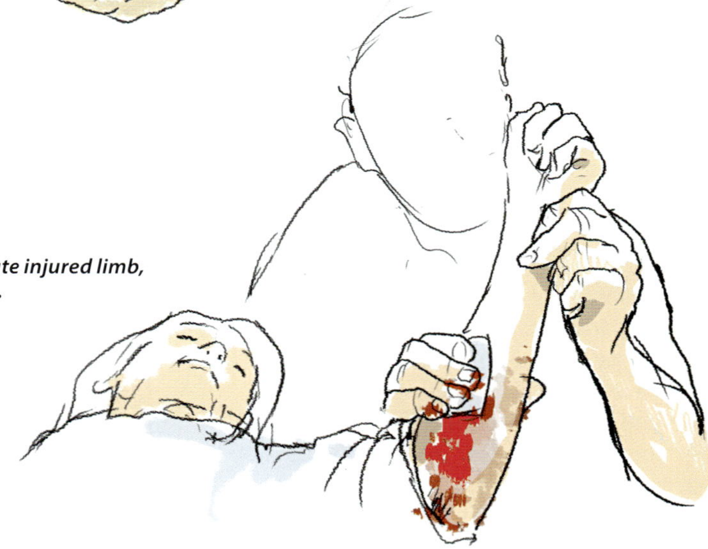

Lay the person down, elevate injured limb, tamponade, local pressure.

If deep injury with problematic bleeding, pack hard with cloth or compresses prior to applying pressure bandage.

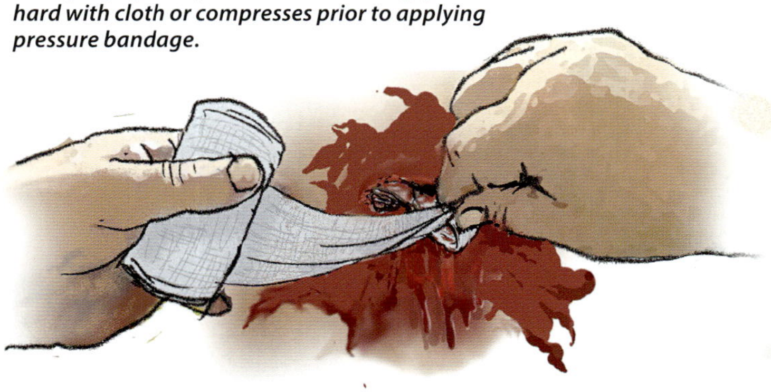

Treatment

All wounds from accidents are contaminated and carry a risk of infection and poor healing. Extensive cleaning (see below) is essential for all wound injuries.

- Minor wounds: Small wounds that can be managed with adhesive bandages, tape or simple dressings can be treated on board.
- Severe wounds: Wounds with significant tissue damage, heavy bleeding, or signs of tendon or nerve damage should be examined by a doctor the same day.

Far from help

When far from medical assistance, you must be prepared to handle even severe wound injuries on your own. The goal is to minimise the risk of serious infection and sepsis during long voyages.

- Consider the environment: Long journeys, particularly in tropical areas, often expose wounds to heat and humidity, increasing the risk of infection.
- Thorough cleaning: Extensive cleaning of the wound surface is crucial, even though it may be challenging without adequate anaesthesia.
- Pain management: For an adult, administer 1 g of paracetamol as a base. If needed, add ibuprofen or morphine. Painkillers take about 30 minutes to take full effect. See page 248, 'Ship's Dispensary'.
- Topical anaesthesia: If your ship's dispensary is well stocked, apply a layer of lidocaine gel or a compress soaked in a local anaesthetic alongside the painkillers. This type of topical anaesthesia is not perfect but is the best available option.
- Cleanliness: Remember, achieving sterility is impossible outside a hospital. On board, the focus should be on maintaining as clean an environment as possible.

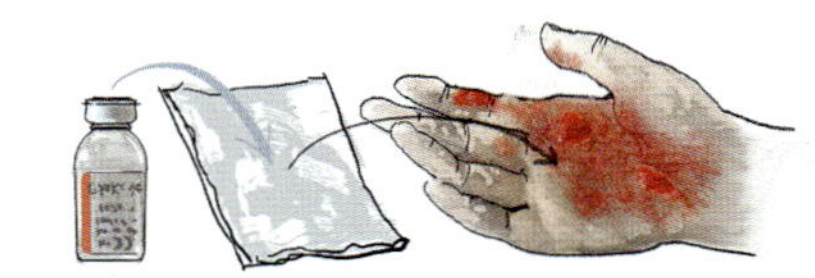

Xylocaine Cotton wad

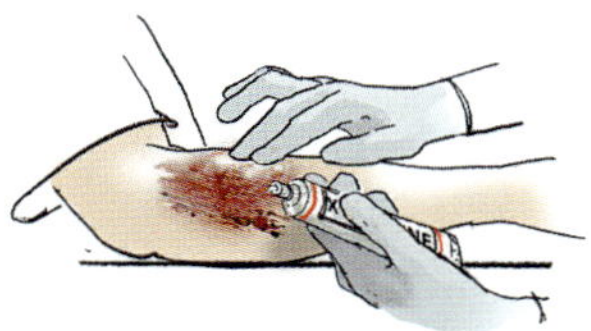

Topical anaesthesia. Soak a compress with lidocaine solution or gel and let it cover the wound closely. Wait for 20 minutes before attacking the wound.

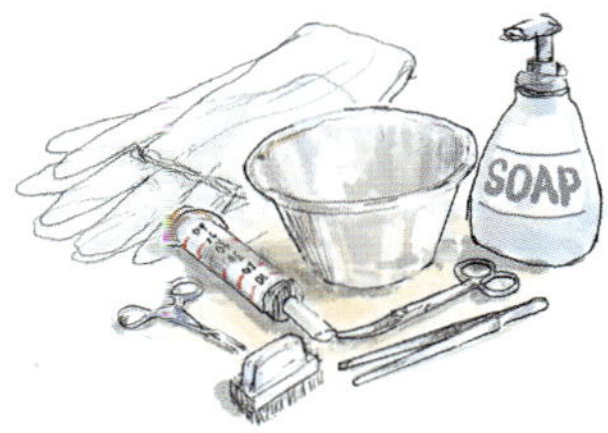

Equipment recommended for wound care.

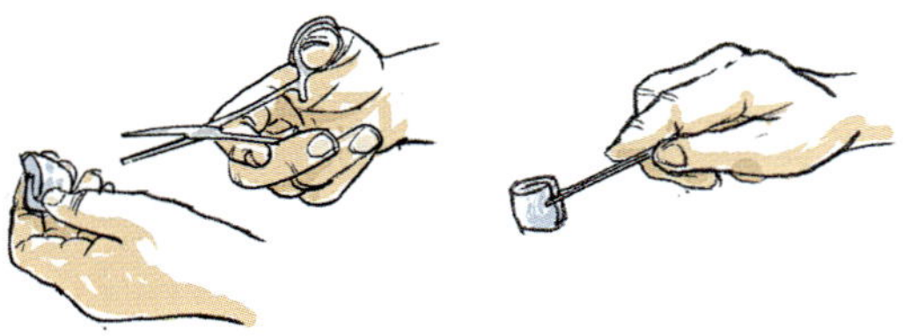

Fold and form a compress into a small ball and hold it in a clamp, a 'peanut' or a 'strawberry', depending on the size. An excellent tool for wound cleaning.

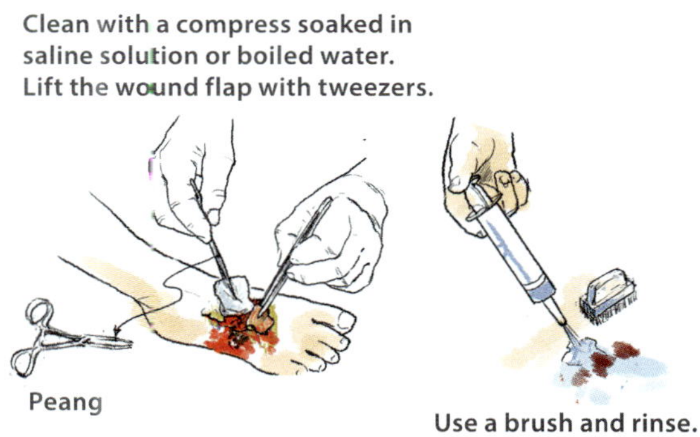

Use clean, disposable gloves. Swab the wound surface using gauze, a sponge or a soft brush. Flush or squirt the wound with clean water or saline solution. Lift the wound edges and remove all foreign particles. Repeat the process several times.

Important: Extensive cleaning is the most crucial step!

Do not use chlorhexidine or alcohol-based solutions to clean fresh traumatic wounds. Healing is optimal when wounds are cleaned with plain water and soap or, preferably, a physiological saline solution (see page 31).

Steps for proper cleaning

1. Use plenty of saline solution or clean, boiled (and cooled) water with soap (any can be used, but preferably a previously unused bar of soap or liquid soap).
2. Lift wound flaps carefully with tweezers.
3. Remove all visible dirt and debris using tweezers.
4. Rinse, squirt or flush the wound thoroughly with water.
5. Remove any coagulated blood.
6. Repeat the rinsing and flushing process to ensure cleanliness.
7. Dab or scrub the wound surface gently with a compress or soft brush.
8. Cut or trim away any obviously 'dead' tissue.
   - Wound edges that appear bluish-purple or black lack blood circulation, indicating 'dead' tissue, which can increase the risk of complications.
   - Carefully lift this tissue with tweezers and cut it away with scissors.
   - Rule of thumb: If it does not hurt, it is 'dead' and should be removed. If it causes pain, leave it intact.

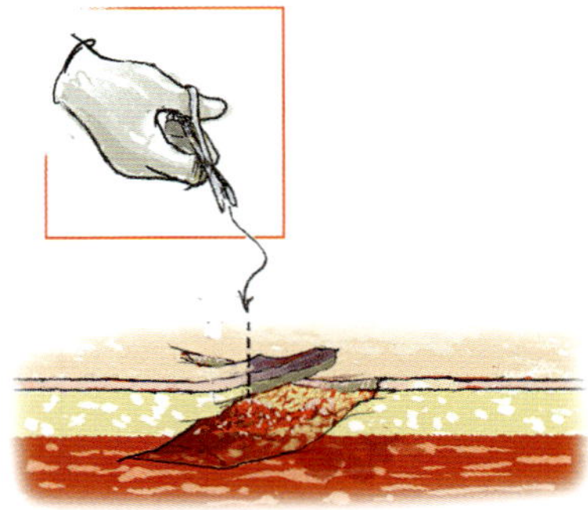

Dark or black thin skin edges. Possible dead tissue, increasing risk of infection. Try to cut it.

Does the wound need to be sutured?

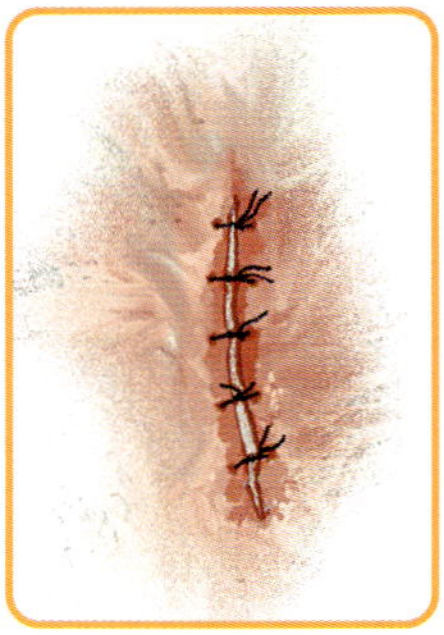

Closing a wound by bringing the edges together can be done using a needle and thread (suturing), tape, a stapler or an adhesive. This approach promotes faster healing and a neater result but comes with an increased risk of infection.

Leaving the wound open, as in war surgery, is a worthwhile alternative to consider when far from medical help. This involves not attempting to bring the wound edges together. Leaving the wound open minimises the risk of infection because fewer bacteria are trapped inside, as wounds provide an excellent environment for bacterial growth. After cleaning, apply a universal dressing (see next page).

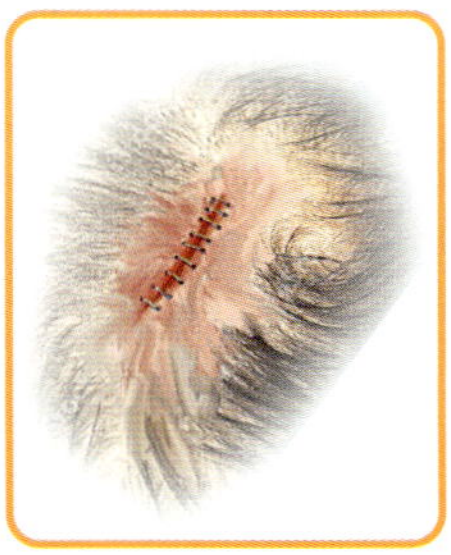

Wounds may be sutured at a later stage, such as after reaching port with an open but uninfected wound. Cosmetic adjustments can always be made later if necessary.

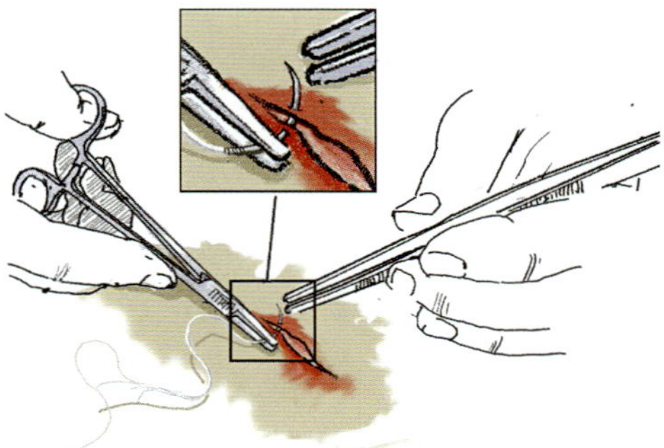

Suturing requires sutures, a needle holder, forceps and appropriate equipment. Simple sutures can be performed, but without anaesthesia, proper tools or experience, it may not always be the best choice.

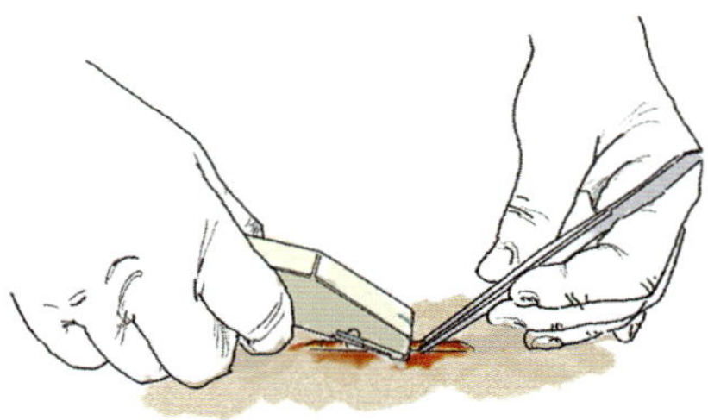

Disposable skin staplers are smart but expensive. Staplers require practice and a staple extractor for removal once the wound has healed.

Suture tape – the best alternative?

Fresh, clean wounds can often be closed with suture tape. After cleaning the wound and ensuring the skin is dry, the wound edges are gently brought closer together (though they do not need to touch completely). Use specialised suture tape when possible.

Advantages of suture tape:

- works best for fresh, clean and dry wounds
- suitable for cut wounds or those with straight edges
- less durable near major joints unless complemented with a splint to reduce mobility
- ideal for minor facial wounds, offering the best cosmetic result (see page 142).

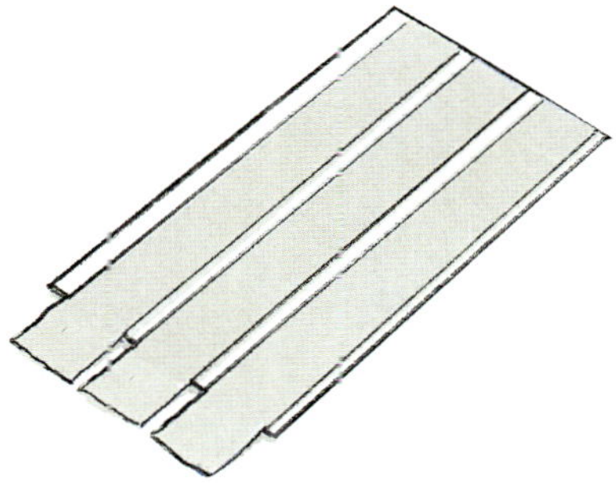

Suture tape comes in different widths from 3mm to 10mm, packed in small envelopes.

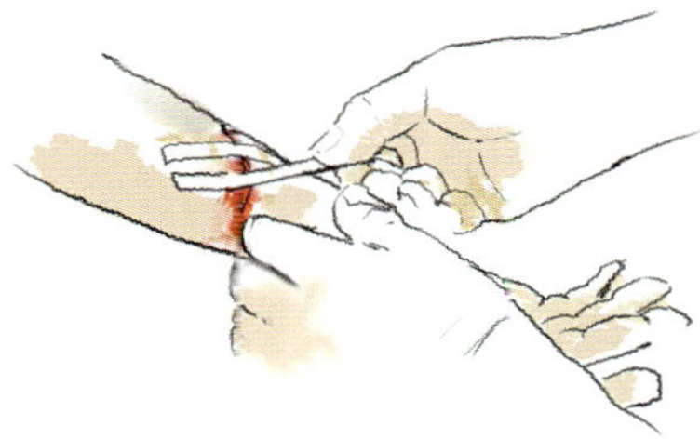

Attach the tape to one side of the wound. Pull the edges together and secure the tape on the opposite side. For larger wounds, use wider suture tape and, if possible, supplementary 'locks'.

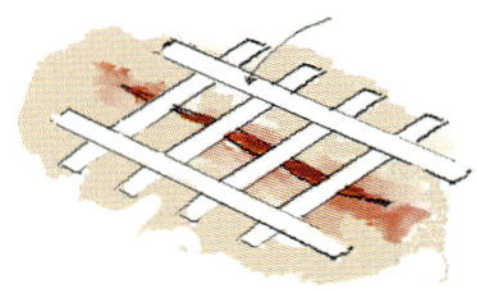

> **FACT**
>
> **What is physiological saline solution?**
>
> Physiological saline solution (sodium chloride, NaCl) is essentially regular salt water but at the same concentration of sodium chloride as found in the human body. This makes it 'friendly' for cleaning wounds and promoting healing.

Universal dressing

Dressings protect the wound during the healing process. For small wounds that have stopped bleeding, a Band-Aid or dry dressing is usually sufficient to secure the wound. For larger, moist surfaces, such as abrasions, burns, crush wounds or wounds that are still bleeding, a universal dressing should be used.

Infection – when to suspect?

How often should the dressing be changed?

The availability of dressing materials on board is likely to be limited. If no signs of infection appear, the dressing can remain in place for several days. However, if signs of infection are present, the dressing must be removed, sutures or tape taken off, and the wound reopened, inspected and thoroughly cleaned. Ideally, the wound should be aired out – left uncovered in fresh air for one to two hours – before applying a new dressing. Certain bacteria thrive in oxygen-poor environments, and airing the wound prevents them from multiplying.

Signs of infection (typically within two to three days):

- Wound secretion, pus and/or blood seep through the dressing
- The patient experiences increased pain in the wound area
- Fever
- Redness and swelling around the wound
- The wound remains 'messy'
- The dressing has a foul odour
- Tender lymph nodes in the groin or armpit

1 *Cover the wound with a compress impregnated with Vaseline to prevent the dressing from sticking to the wound.*

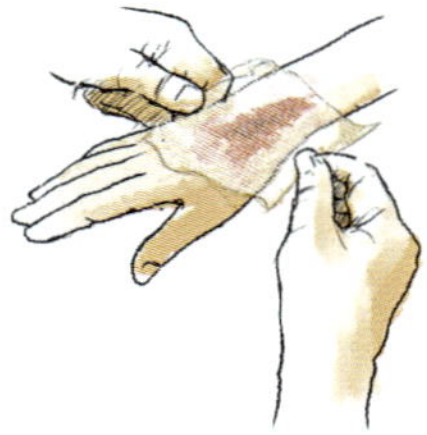

2 *Soak a woven compress with isotonic saline and place it on top of the impregnated compress.*

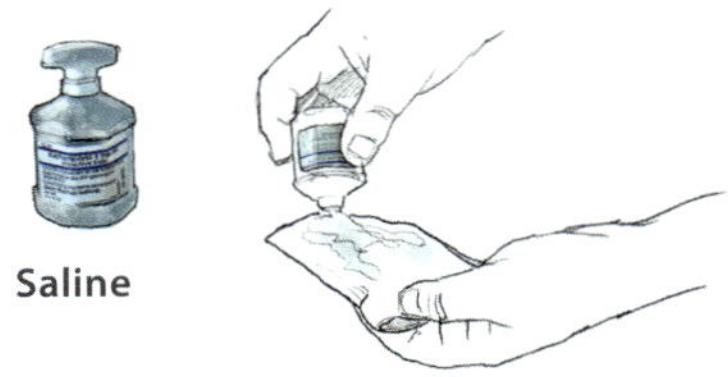

3 *Add a dry, fluffed-up compress over the saline compress to provide protection.*

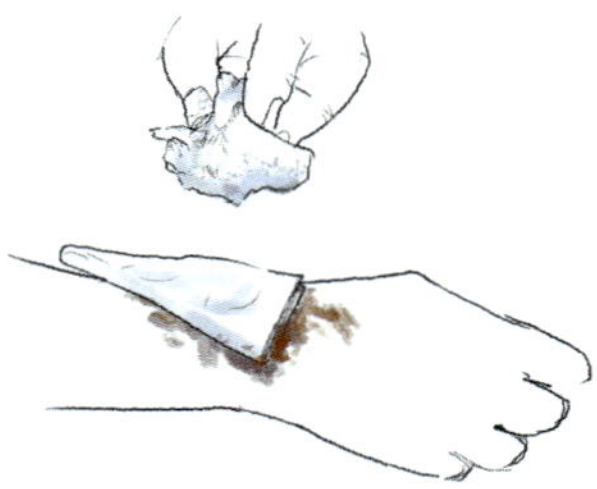

4 *Secure the dressing with an elastic bandage, gauze bandage or self-adhesive dressing.*

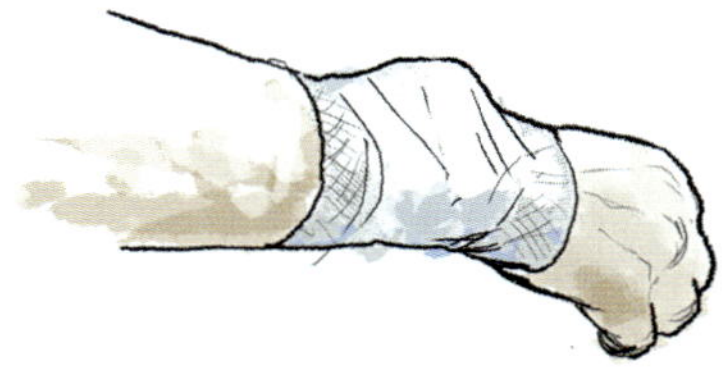

5 *Note: Remember to check the odour of the dressing at the start so you have a reference for comparison if you begin to suspect a wound infection.*

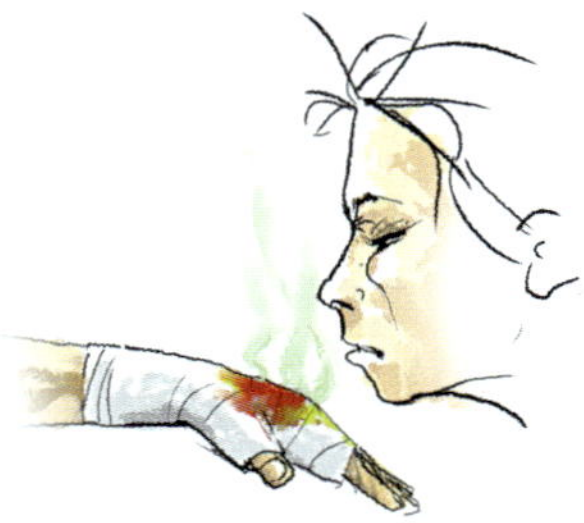

THE IMPORTANCE OF ODOUR

The smell of the bandage is a helpful indicator when determining if a wound is infected. Assess the odour immediately after the bandage is applied to establish a baseline. Then, repeat this assessment daily. If a sweet, slightly musty smell develops, it may indicate an infection.

BASIC TYPES OF INFECTION

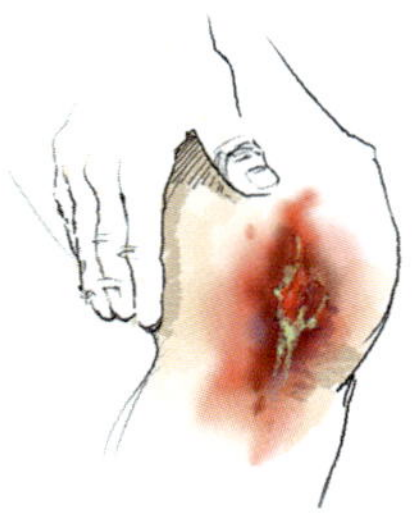

Purulent infection: A crush wound on the knee with pus, stickiness, redness and swelling, along with purulent secretions, is often caused by staphylococci or other bacteria. Clean the wound thoroughly and administer antibiotics, such as flucloxacillin (see table on page 249).

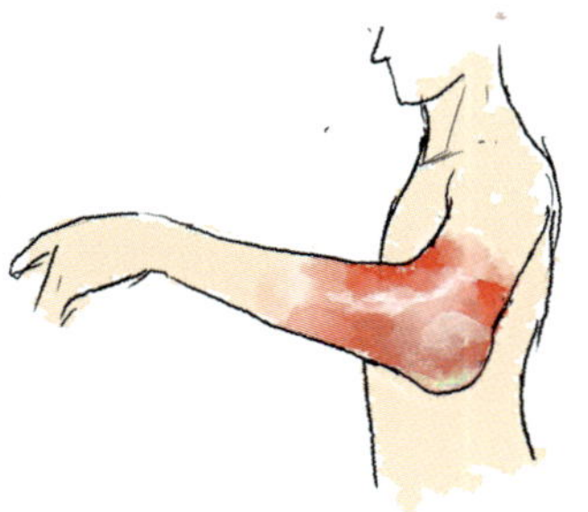

Erysipelas infection: An infection of the skin without a visible wound but presenting a strong reaction, including sharply demarcated redness, tenderness, pain, swelling and high fever, is usually caused by streptococci. Treat with antibiotics, such as phenoxymethylpenicillin (see table on page 249).

Special cases

Wounds with complicated tendon or nerve damage

This type of injury is most common in the arms, hands and wrists and typically involves cut wounds. Always check the distal status for such injuries (see page 165). Ideally, the injured person should see a hand surgeon or orthopaedic specialist as soon as possible. However, it is not uncommon for a doctor to delay nerve and tendon repair for one to two weeks until the wound has healed without infection. At sea or far from a doctor, follow the recommended wound care instructions and immobilise the injury using a plaster or mouldable aluminium splint. Administer antibiotics, such as flucloxacillin (see table on page 249), and seek medical attention at the next port.

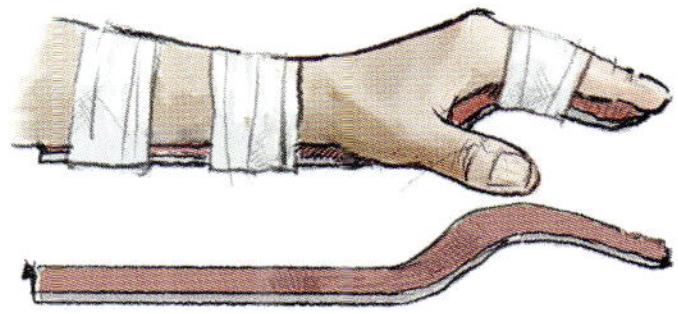

For suspected extensor tendon injury: Immobilise the hand using a mouldable aluminium splint, keeping the fingers extended and straight.

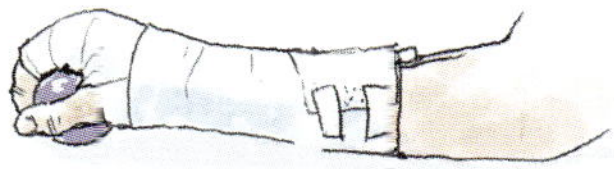

For suspected flexor tendon injury: Immobilise the hand with a straight wrist and the fingers slightly flexed.

Finger injury with the ring stuck

Warning! Remove the ring immediately, as the finger can swell quickly and cut off blood circulation. If it is difficult to remove the ring, refer to the 'string trick' on page 207.

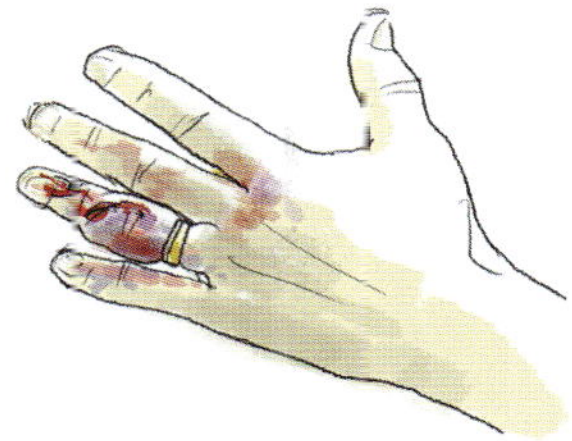

To prevent this, always remove rings before leaving your mooring.

Fishhook in skin

Fishing is a common activity while on a boat, but occasionally, you may hook yourself. To remove the hook, use pliers to push it through until the barb emerges on the other side. Then cut off the barbed part and back out the remaining hook. Apply a spirit dressing by wetting a compress with chlorhexidine or an antibacterial alcohol solution and placing it directly on the wound. Secure it with a gauze bandage or self-adhesive dressing. Change the dressing daily for two to three days. Watch for signs of infection over the following days. If pain and swelling worsen, consider starting a course of antibiotics.

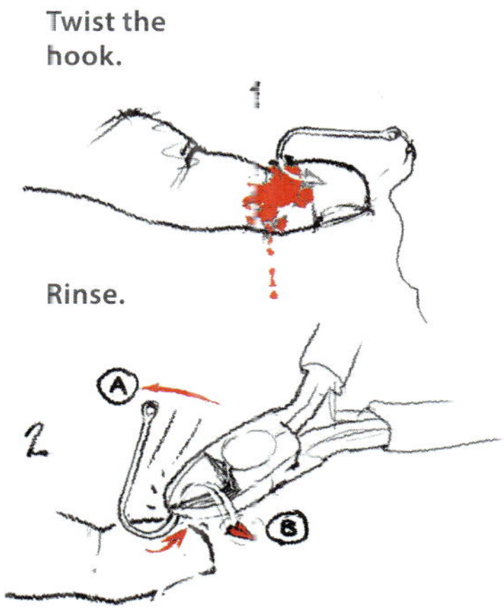

The barb must be cut off to remove the fishhook.

Ingrown nail infection

A common issue is small, often invisible, sores in the nail bed that become infected. While not dangerous, they can cause significant discomfort, including throbbing pain, swelling and tenderness.

If far from medical assistance, apply a dressing soaked in an antiseptic liquid or spirit for a couple of days to relieve symptoms.

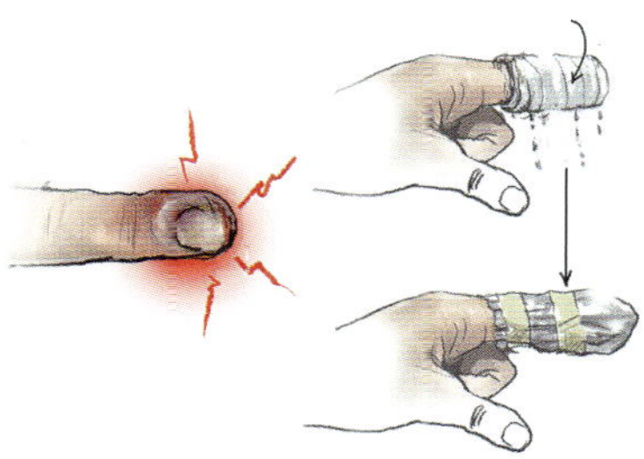

For paronychia, a small but bothersome infection in the nail bed, an alcohol-soaked bandage may help. Retain moisture by covering the dressing with a piece of plastic film.

4. BURN INJURIES

The galley – high-risk zone for burn injuries.

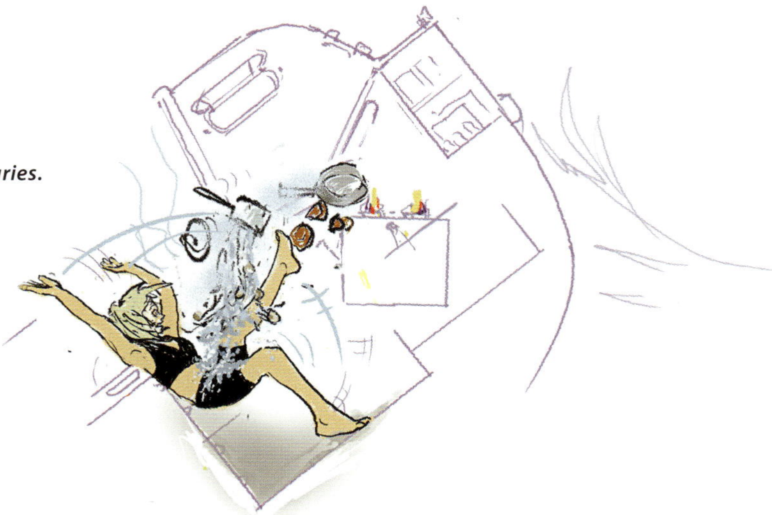

Follow DRABC (see page 12), and avoid getting burned yourself. Do not compromise your ability to provide first aid. Move the injured person away from the source, extinguish burning clothing, and assess the risk for explosions or open flames.

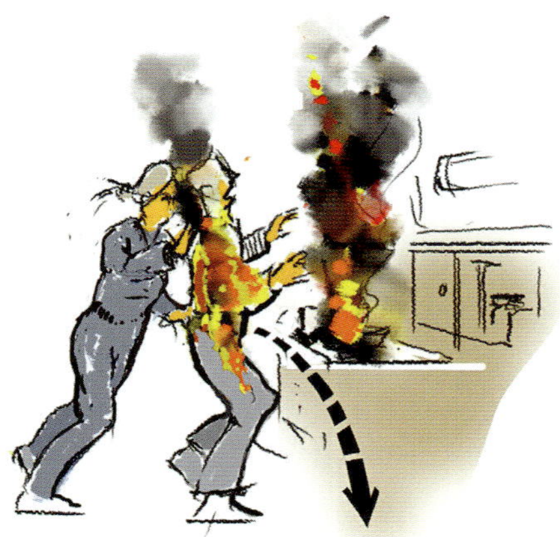

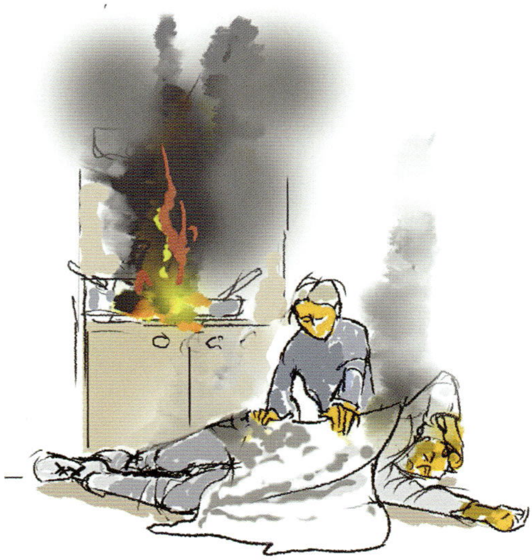

Burn injuries are common during sailing. They can vary significantly in depth and severity, ranging from minor skin redness to life-threatening injuries. Fortunately, milder degrees of burn injuries are the most common.

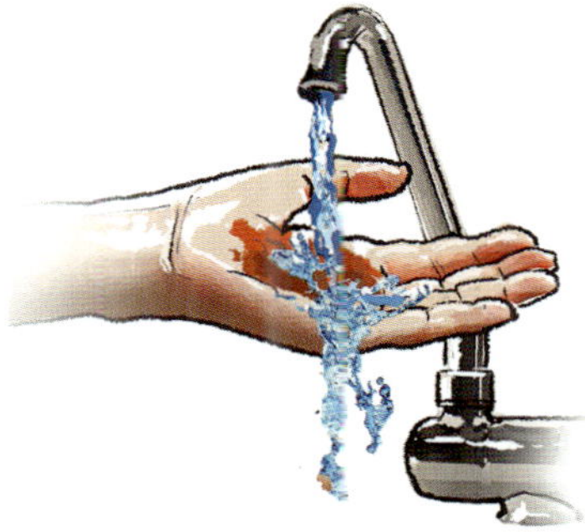

Burned hand cooled under the water tap at 15–20°C for 15–20 minutes.

Immediate action

Follow DRABC (see page 12).

Cooling

Begin cooling the burned body part by rinsing with water at a temperature between 15°C and 20°C to:

- stop further heat-related damage
- limit the spread of the injury
- provide pain relief

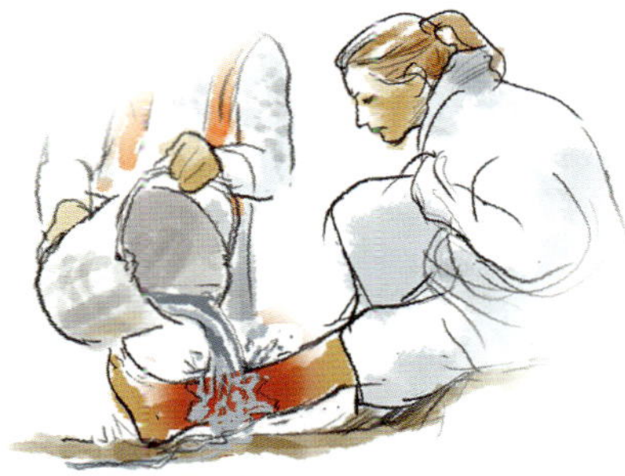

Cooling a burn injury on leg with sea water. Remember a warming blanket.

Continue to rinse with water for 15–20 minutes. Large amounts of water may be needed, so sea water can be used if the water in the fresh-water tank is insufficient. When a burned body part is effectively cooled, the entire body may become cooled and hypothermic. Keep the injured person warm with a blanket: cool the injury, not the entire person!

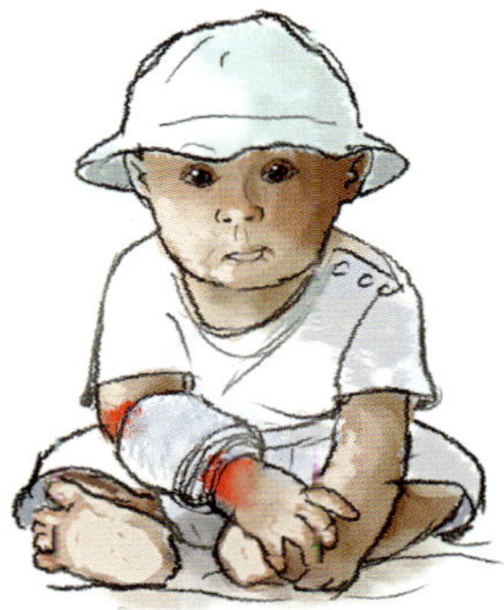

Cooling of burn on a small child.

For young children, there is a high risk of hypothermia during cooling. Instead, use compresses soaked with cool water to cover the injury. Ensure the compresses remain soaked.

INHALATION INJURIES

Inhalation of hot gases, steam or smoke – common in explosions and fires in enclosed spaces – can cause airway damage. Airway swelling may occur rapidly, so assess the risk of an injury early and arrange immediate transportation to a hospital. If far from medical care, consider evacuation if inhalation injury is suspected.

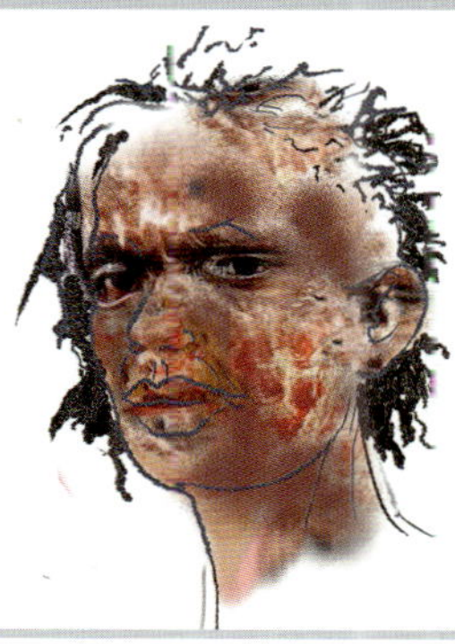

Signs of possible inhalation injury:

- *singed eyebrows and hair*
- *soot redness and swelling around mouth and nose*
- *anxiety and breathing problems*

ASSESSMENT OF BURN INJURY

The severity of a burn depends on the depth of the skin damage and the extent of the burn. This is essential information for the alarm call.

Depth of burn injury

Schematic presentation of the different layers of normal human skin and how they are damaged in different degrees of burns.

- *Epidermis*
- *Dermis*
- *Subcutaneous tissue*
- *Blood vessels/ capillaries*
- *Muscle/hypodermis*

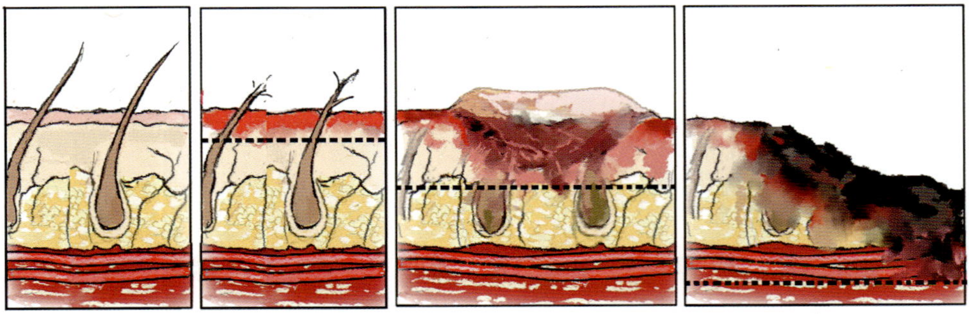

Normal *Superficial* *Partial thickness* *Full thickness*

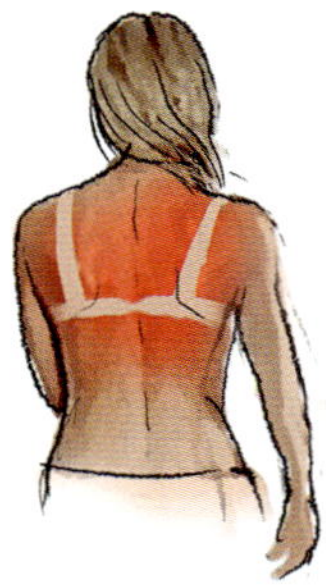

Superficial burn

Affects only the outermost skin cells, typically due to sunburn. Causes redness and pain; heals on its own. Use aloe vera gel placed in the fridge or hydrocortisone 1% cream.

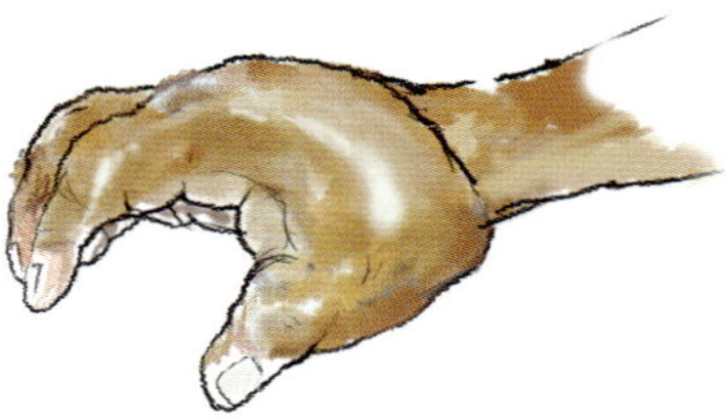

Partial thickness burn

Affects deeper layers, reaching hair follicles and blood capillaries. Often caused by scalding from hot water or oil. Blisters may be intact initially, with a red, moist wound surface, and are extremely painful due to intact sensation.

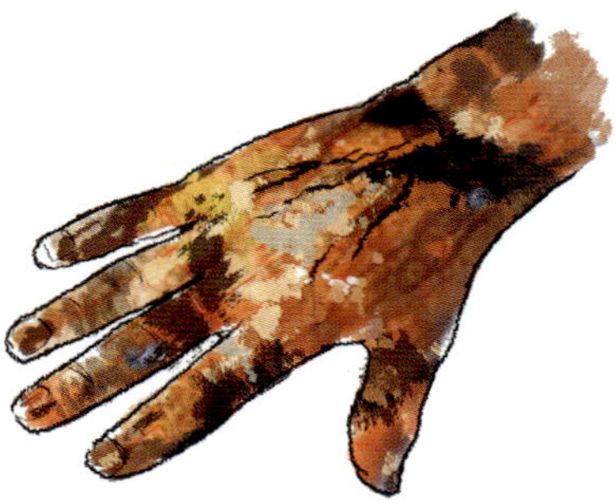

Full thickness burn

Burns all layers of the skin, including blood vessels and nerves. Typically caused by open flames or explosions. The wound base may appear white, dark red/brown or black, is dry, lacks sensation, and has no circulation. Deep burns often have broken blisters, reduced sensation and circulation, and a pale and dry wound surface. Most require surgical treatment.

HOW TO DIFFERENTIATE BETWEEN A PARTIAL OR FULL-THICKNESS BURN

The key factor is whether sensation (to touch) and blood circulation are preserved. Touch the wound surface with a gloved hand or with a gauze. Or prick the wound surface with a clean needle – if there is no sensation or bleeding, it indicates a full thickness burn. Press with a fingertip; if circulation is intact, a white spot will turn red again when pressure is released. If circulation is impaired, there will be no colour change when pressing with the fingertip.

Extent of burn injury

Estimate the burn as a percentage of the body surface. Each region accounts for roughly 9 per cent. A general guide: the palm corresponds to 1 per cent of the total body area, while an entire arm is 9 per cent. Note: This rule does not apply to children!

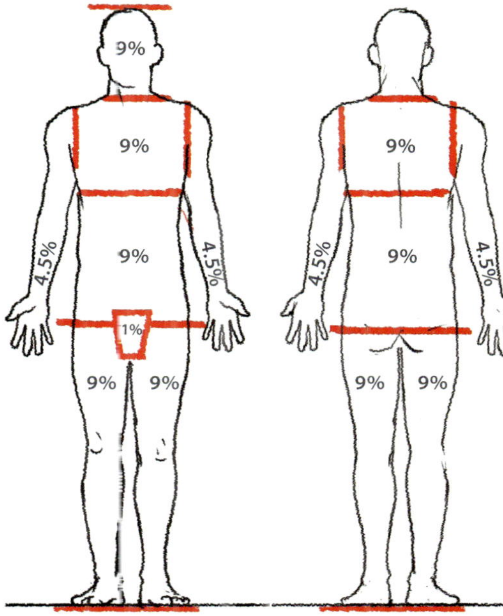

Body map for rule of nines. A whole arm is 9 per cent of total body surface area.

Treatment

- Provide pain relief promptly; pain from burns is often intense. Cooling itself can help relieve the pain. For adults, 1g of paracetamol is recommended. Escalate pain relief up to morphine if necessary, see page 248.
- Assess burn depth and extent to determine the next steps regarding subsequent action and treatment, see below. Small injuries can be managed on board; others require a doctor or even emergency hospital care. When in doubt, consult medical advice via radio.
- Clean the burn with water or saline solution, removing broken blisters. Use a protective dressing: for small injuries, a Band-Aid or gauze pad fixed with tape works well, while for larger, moist wounds, universal dressings (as described on page 31) can be used.
- Cooling burn gel or dressings specifically for burns can be used for minor burn injuries.

If a burn affects the hand, remove any rings immediately. A fresh plastic bag taped around the wrist is a good temporary dressing for hand burns, allowing movement and inspection while protecting the wound.

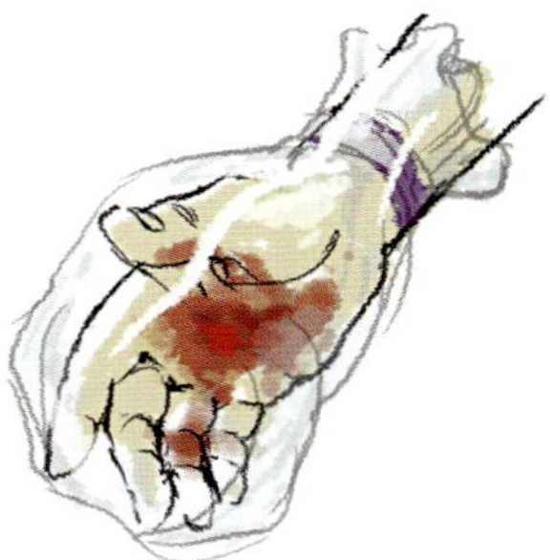

A plastic bag as a temporary dressing for a hand burn.

Self-care or hospital?

Most minor burn injuries can be managed with on-board medical supplies and common medications. However, a severe burn injury is one of the worst injuries when far from help. When calling for support on the radio or satellite phone, relay an estimate of the extent (percentage of body surface) and depth (superficial to full thickness).

- Superficial: Self-care with cooling and a mild hydrocortisone cream 1% can relieve discomfort.
- Partial: If the burn is more than 10 per cent surface area, immediate transport to a hospital may be necessary for assessment due to the risk of dehydration and shock and hard-to-treat pain. Professional consultation is

FACT

Certain areas require specialist care and should be handled by a hospital as soon as possible, regardless of extent:

- face/head
- throat
- hands and feet
- over joints
- genitals

Small children under five years: Seek out professional medical advice promptly.

recommended if the injury is larger than the size of a palm. Leave intact blisters and remove broken ones. Use dressings according to 'universal dressings', see page 31. For minor burn injuries, pre-made burn dressings are available.

- Full thickness: Immediate hospital transportation is required if the burn exceeds more than 1 per cent of body surface.

Far from help

Major concerns to be addressed:

- dehydration
- pain
- infection

A larger partial thickness or a full thickness burn injury is one of the worst things that can happen at sea. It is crucial to maintain hydration. If a partial thickness injury is more than 10 per cent, the person needs to consume significant amounts of fluid (more than 4–5 litres per day) with corresponding salts (see 'Treatment' under 'Dehydration', page 95). This may be difficult or impossible to achieve by drinking alone and will require access to IV fluids. It is important to seek medical advice in such a challenging situation and prepare for evacuation.

An approximate estimation of fluid requirement in a burn injury is: 4ml × body weight kg × extent of burn in % of body surface.

For pain management, morphine may be required. The risk of a complicating infection and septicaemia is significant, and early antibiotic treatment might be necessary. It is important to seek decision support via radio/satellite phone if possible. A larger burn injury is a case for emergency evacuation.

Infection? Smell the dressing.

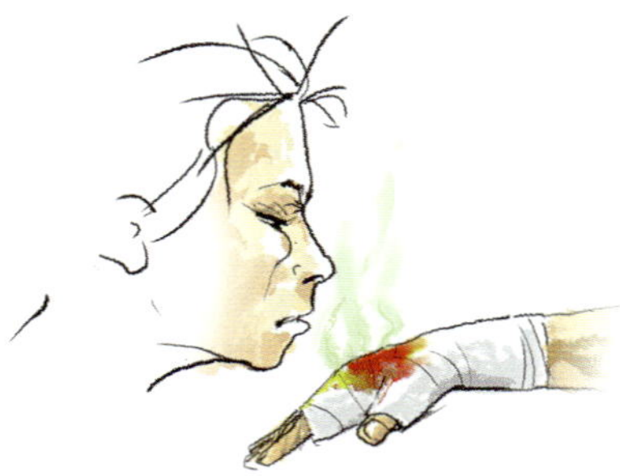

When to suspect an infection? See under 'Wounds', page 32. The smell of the dressing is a simple and useful parameter for determining infection. Immediately after applying the dressing, smell it. Then repeat this daily. If a sweet, slightly musty smell develops, it is a sign that could indicate an infection. If antibiotics are indicated, first choice is phenoxymethylpenicillin.

How often should the dressing be changed? Daily or every second day is ideal but the availability of dressing materials on board is likely not unlimited. If no signs of infection appear, the dressing can remain in place for several days. If signs of infection appear, the dressing must be removed, the wound inspected and cleaned again, and ideally 'aired out' by leaving it uncovered in fresh air for an hour or two before applying a new dressing.

Prevention

- Be cautious with sun exposure – use thick layers of sunscreen with SPF 30 or higher. Wear full-covering clothing; denim fabric offers excellent protection against UVB radiation.
- Handle explosive and flammable fluids/ fuels with care.
- Ensure the proper installation of gas equipment with a drained container for the gas cylinder.
- Be cautious with hot liquids in the galley. Use protective silicone gloves and full-covering aprons or sailing trousers and boots. Avoid sending anyone unfamiliar with galley work to cook or boil during rough weather.
- Do not walk on a sun-heated deck without shoes – burns on the soles of the feet are problematic.
- A special case for sailors is ropes that whip through a closed hand. This can lead to burns and abrasions of all degrees. Release the rope – nothing is more important than not damaging your hand! Gloves can offer some protection.

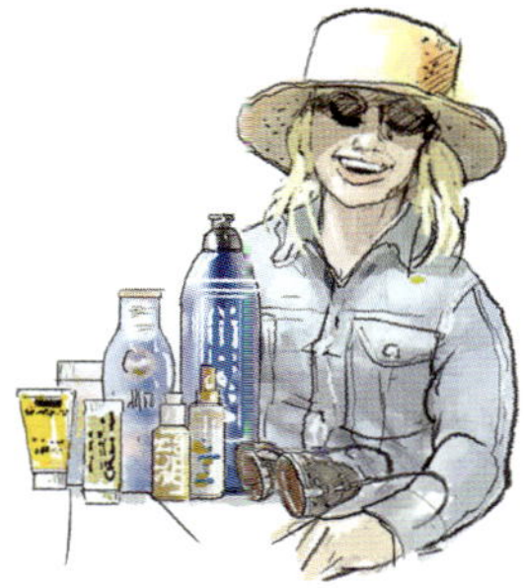

Dressed for heavy sun exposure.

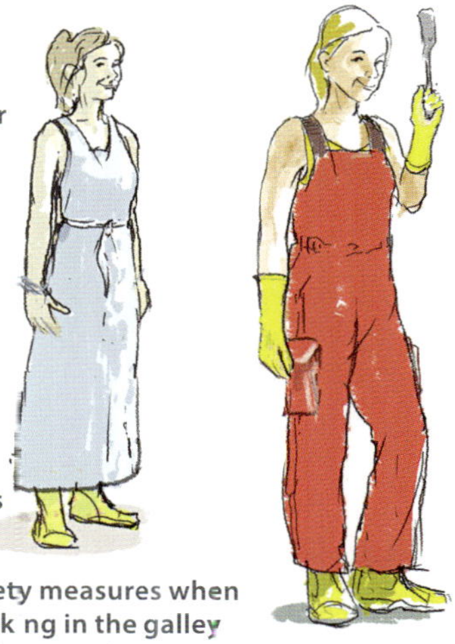

Safety measures when work ng in the galley during rough seas

The galley is a high-risk area for burn injuries – wear appropriate protective clothing. Sailing trousers or a long plastic apron, boots and silicone gloves.

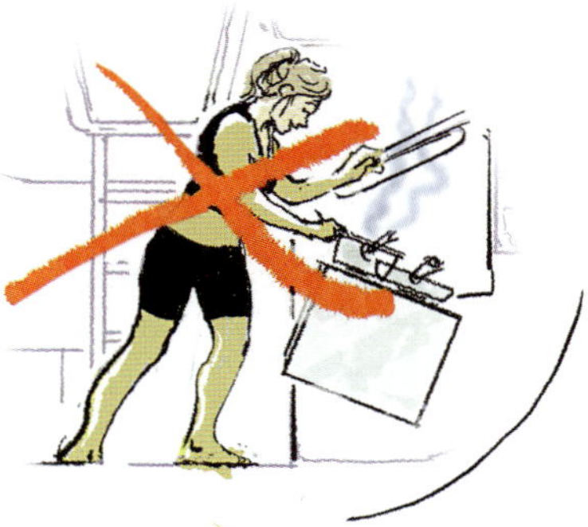

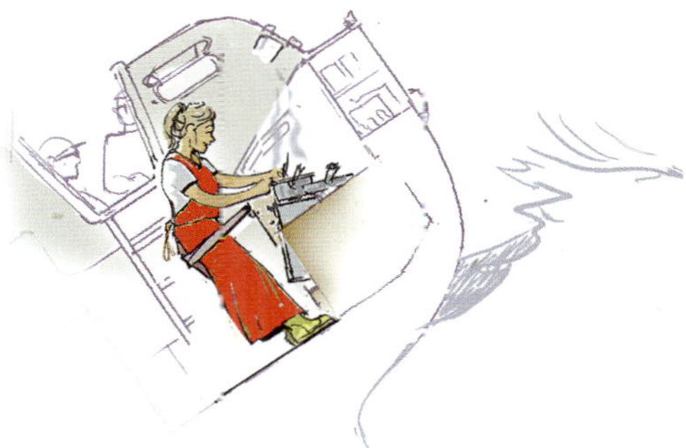

Using a safety strap in the galley protects from sudden body movements but excludes the possibility to jump away promptly if necessary.

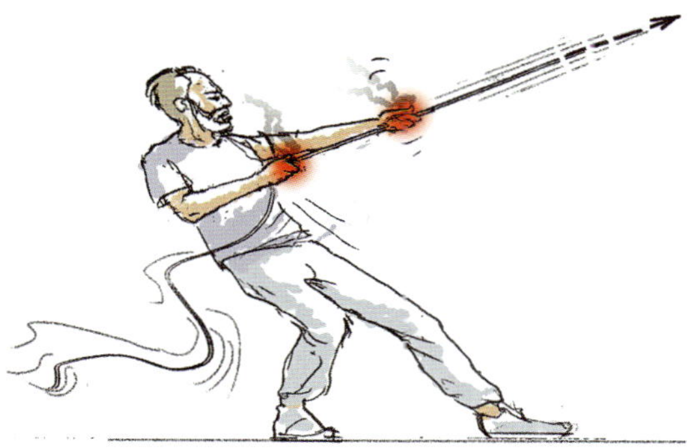

CAUTION! When handling ropes, avoid holding them too tightly; release the rope if necessary to protect your hands from burns and abrasions.

5. DROWNING

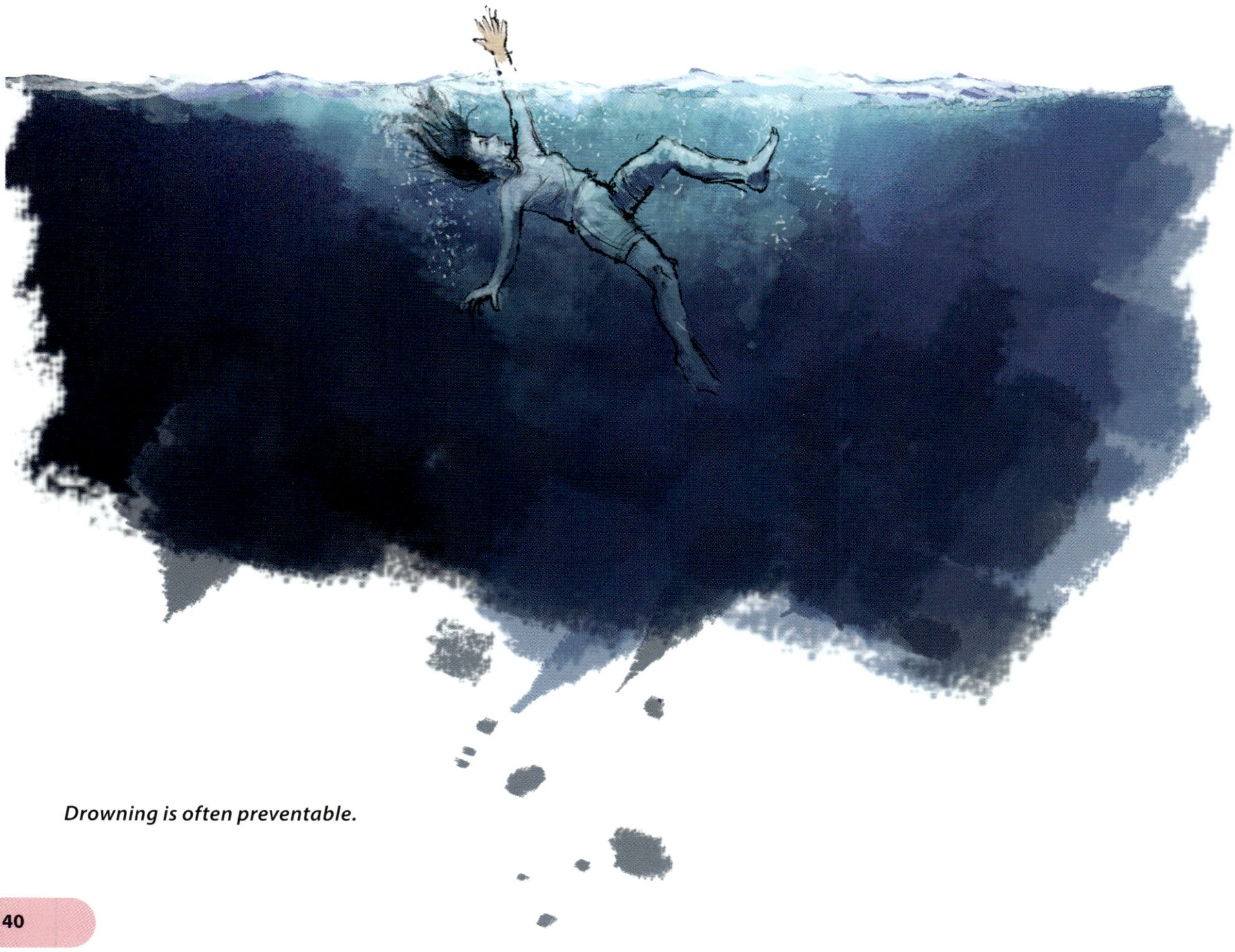

Drowning is often preventable.

Drowning is suffocation from inhaling fluid. If the inhaled volume is small, it may result in a severe coughing attack. However, in the worst cases, it can lead to serious lung complications.

A larger inhaled volume causes an immediate lack of oxygen, triggering a strong reflex to take deep breaths (lasting about one minute), which leads to even more water entering the lungs. Breathing then stops. Within three to four minutes, there is a risk of permanent brain damage and cardiac arrest. If submerged for more than 10 minutes, survival is rare, except in cases where the individual has also been severely hypothermic (see page 44).

Drowning can be classified as either observed or unobserved.

- Observed drowning: Another person sees someone struggling in the water.
- Unobserved drowning: Someone is found lifeless in the water, and the duration of submersion is unknown but is often too long.

The prognosis improves the shorter the time a person is underwater.

Drowning is a leading cause of death in children. Among adults, drowning victims are often intoxicated with alcohol.

Give rescue breath as soon as you can, in the water if possible. Hold one hand under the head and give five breaths.

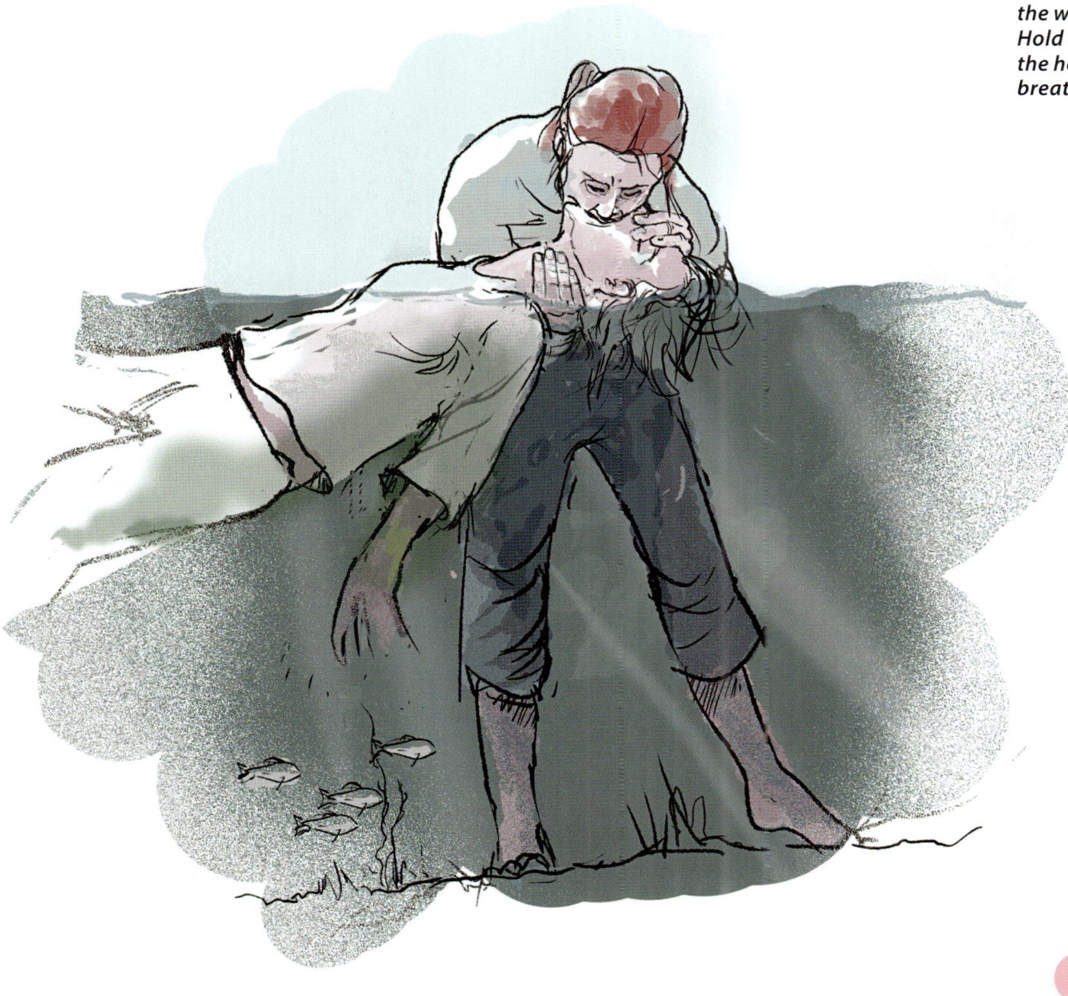

Immediate action

IMMEDIATE HELP is critical! Fast and heroic action is required to rescue the victim from the water, start CPR, and attempt to save their life. Follow the DRABC protocol to evaluate the situation but prioritise your own safety (see page 12).

Before attempting to reach the victim, consider the following key factors:

- wind
- water temperature
- currents
- access to a liferaft/boat
- flotation aids
- possibility of assistance from others
- the rescuer's mental and physical condition

In a drowning incident, it is crucial to give five rescue breaths as early as possible, ideally while still in the water. This should be done when the rescuer can stabilise themselves by touching the bottom or being supported.

Once on a firm surface (beach, jetty), immediately start CPR (see page 14). Clear the mouth of any foreign or loose objects. There is no need to evacuate water from the lungs.

Continue CPR until professional help or an ambulance arrives. If the person regains cardiac activity but remains unconscious, place them in the recovery position (see page 16). Remember to keep them warm with blankets. Note that children are particularly susceptible to hypothermia.

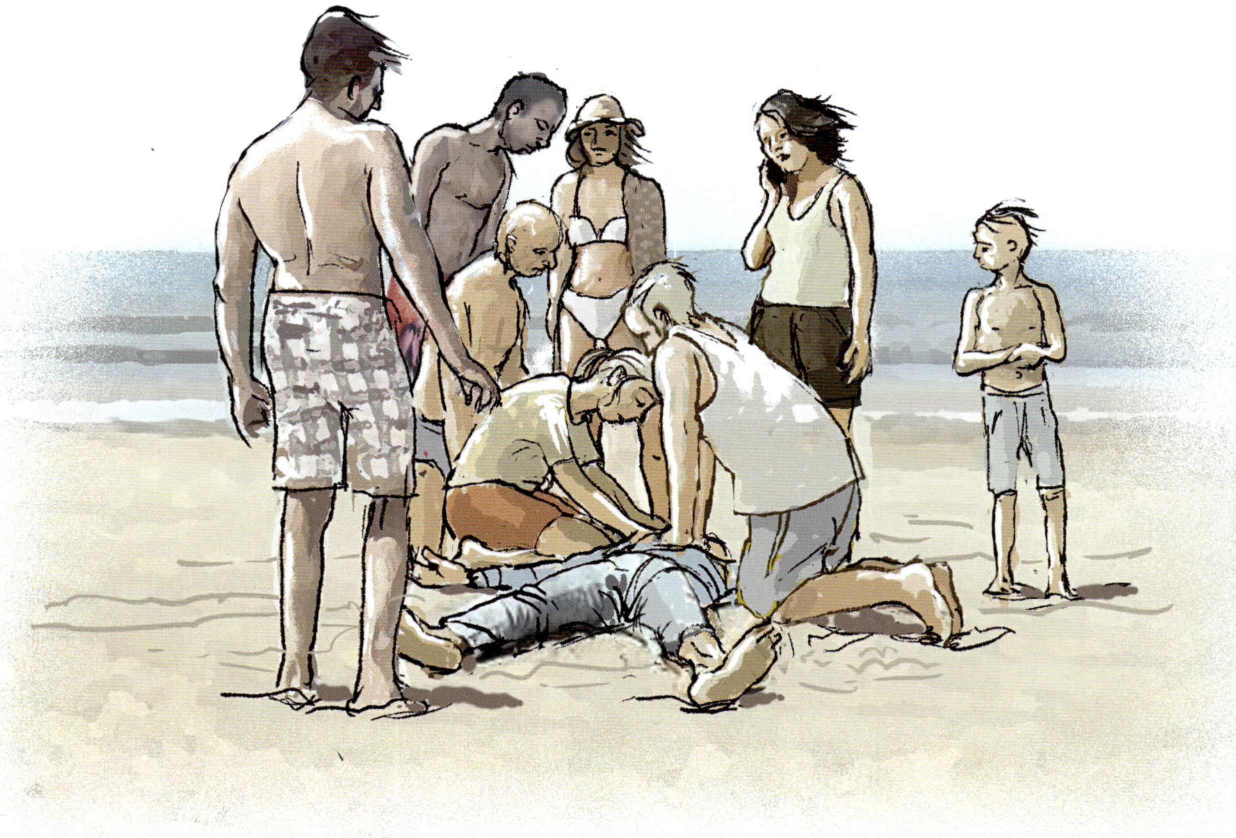

CPR – drowning. Lots of help is needed! It is hard work to do CPR for more than a couple of minutes.

Far from help

Always try to contact medical professionals for guidance. If far from professional help, your efforts will be limited to CPR. If there is no response, you may need to make the difficult decision to stop and discontinue resuscitation. Seek advice and emotional support when making this decision.

> **IMPORTANT NOTE**
>
> In cases where fluid aspiration is insufficient to cause acute respiratory arrest but large enough to damage lung tissue, chemical injury can lead to excessive fluid production (pulmonary oedema). This may result in acute breathing difficulties within hours or days. Always consult medical professionals to rule out lung damage in such situations.

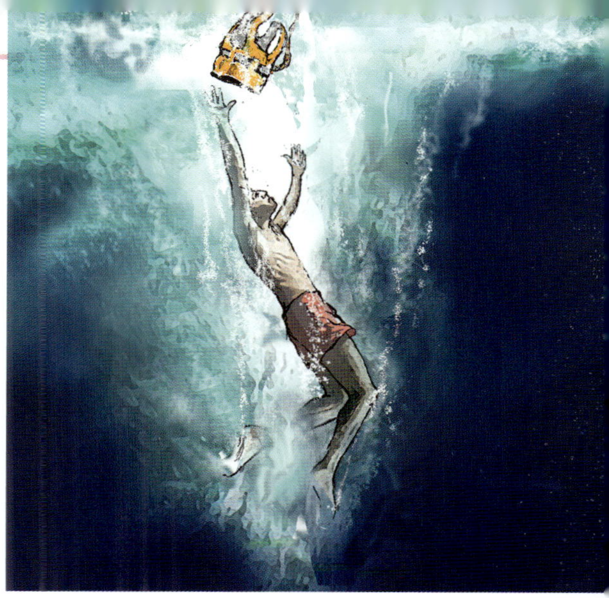

Always wear a lifejacket...

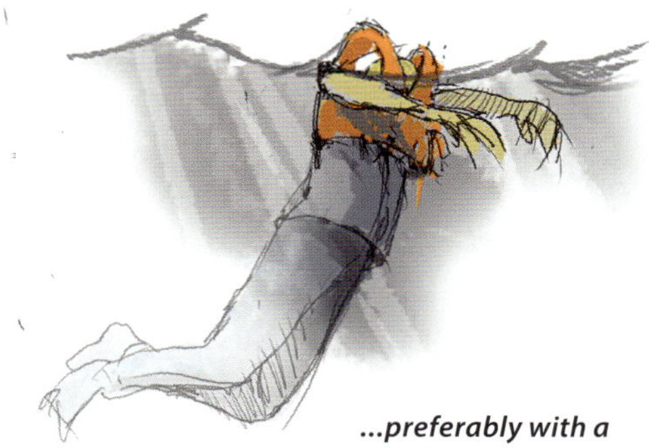

...preferably with a crotch strap.

Prevention

- Stay sober.
- Wear a lifejacket.
- Have company while swimming or boating.
- Avoid moving around in small boats.
- Carry man-overboard equipment.
- Ensure good communication equipment is available.
- Be cautious of swimming in areas with strong currents.
- Never allow children to swim without supervision.
- Assign someone as a 'lifeguard'.
- Avoid swimming too far from shore.

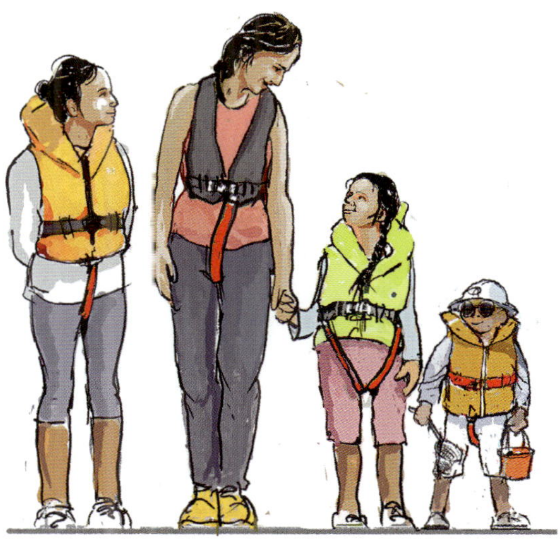

A lifejacket is useless – and even dangerous – if not worn correctly. Always secure the belt and crotch straps.

6. HYPOTHERMIA

Accidental immersion in the sea – preserve body temperature by remaining still.

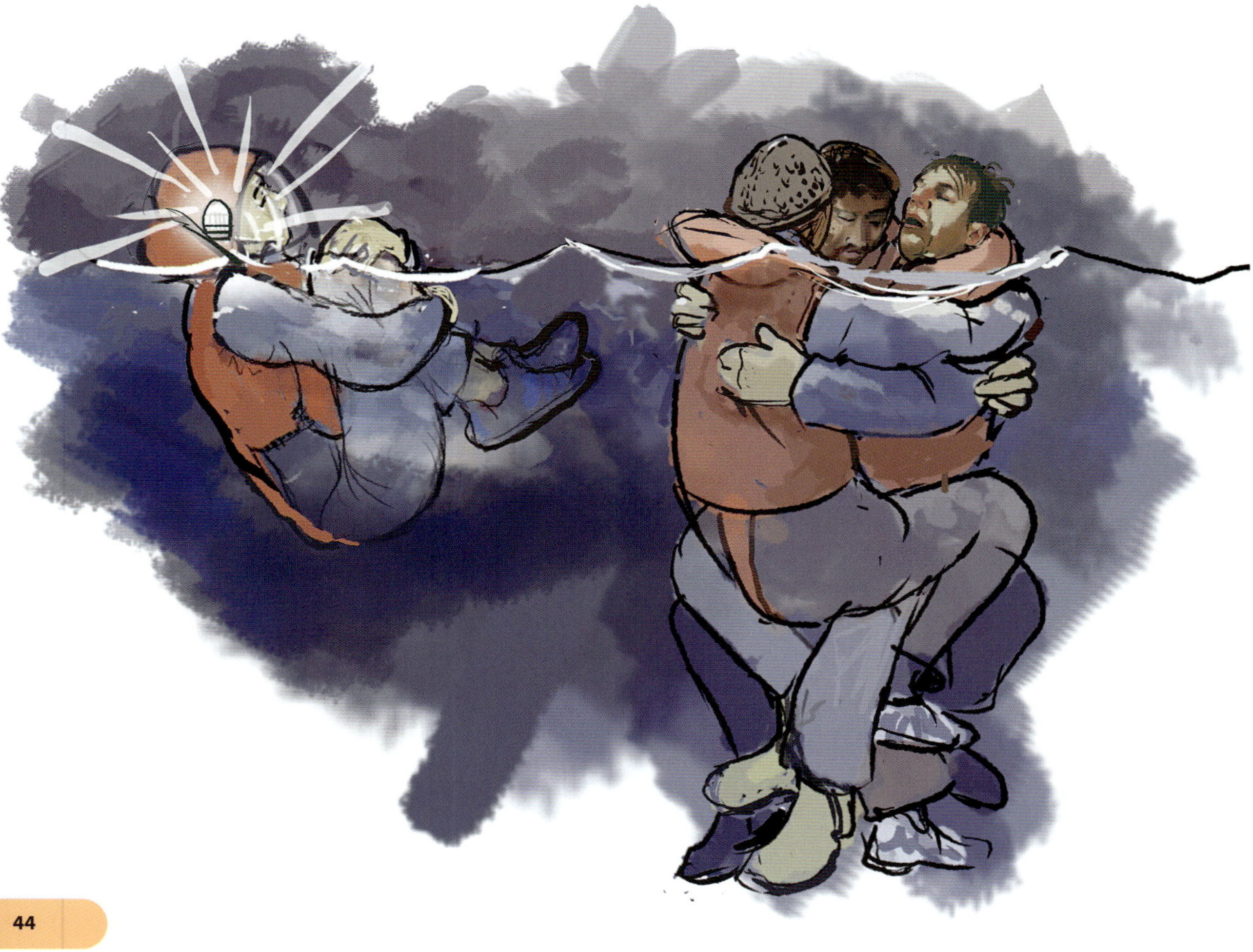

Hypothermia is often associated with outdoor activities such as sailing, water sports, mountaineering and skiing. Heat loss in water occurs 25 times faster than in air.

The risk of hypothermia and its severe effects is often underestimated. Hypothermia is a life-threatening condition that occurs when the body's core temperature drops by more than 2°C and falls below 35°C, impairing critical bodily functions.

When sailing in late autumn or winter, or in polar or Arctic regions, air and water temperatures can be dangerously low. If someone accidentally falls into the water while boating, the risk of severe hypothermia depends on the water temperature. This is summarised in the table below:

Water temperature °C	Unconscious – time to	Death – time to
0	< 15 min	< 45 min
0–10	15–60 min	30 min – 2 hours
10–15	1–2 hours	1–3 hours
15–21	2–7 hours	2–30 hours

INCREASED RISK OF HYPOTHERMIA

- Alcohol: Increases heat loss and eliminates shivering.
- Elderly and children: Reduced heat production.
- Trauma: Impaired temperature regulation.

Signs and symptoms

Body temperature	Symptoms
37°C	Normal temperature regulation
36°C	Increased metabolism
35°C	Severe chills and shivering, discomfort, fatigue, uncoordinated movements, confused, slurred speech, numbness
33°C	Shivering stops, muscle stiffness, slow heart rate
32°C	Extreme sluggishness, 'sleep-like' state, wide pupils but reactive reflexes, slow pulse
30°C	Decreased consciousness, shallow breathing 5–10 breaths/minute
28–26°C	Unconsciousness, pupils unresponsive to light

Immediate action

1 Rescue and shelter: Get the person out of the water and into shelter from the wind. Handle them gently to prevent additional heat loss.
2 Heat preservation: Use blankets to prevent further cooling. Evaluate the degree of hypothermia (see page 45).
3 Emergency contact: Call for help and prepare for emergency evacuation.

Attempt to lift the person in a supine, horizontal position, especially if they are unconscious. A sudden vertical lift, such as pulling them up by a lifejacket, can increase the risk of cardiac arrest due to cold blood redistribution.

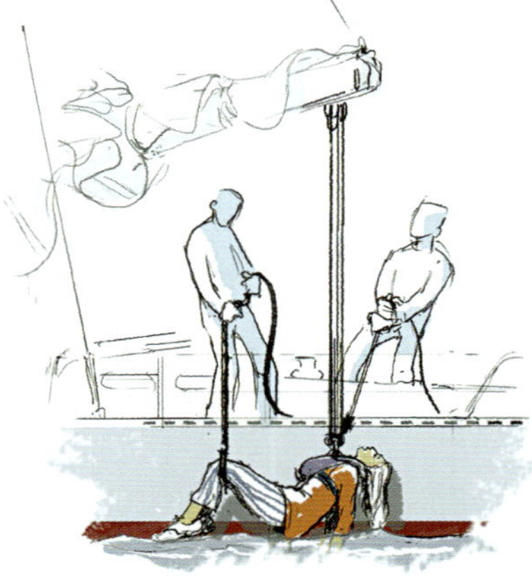

In suspected hypothermia, lift horizontally.

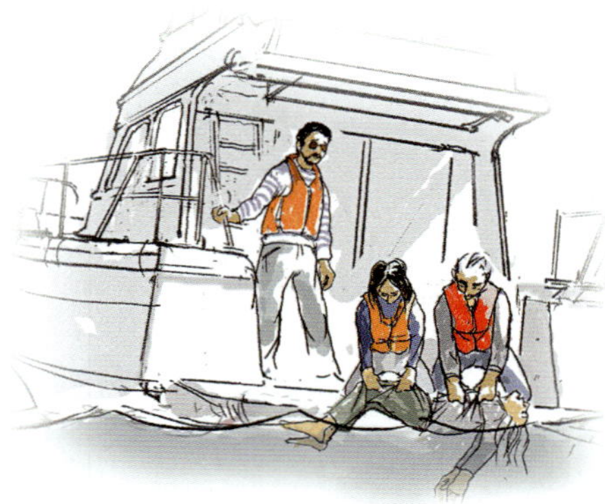

Suggestions for arranging a horizontal lift in severe hypothermia. Use the boom as a crane, or the dinghy as a platform.

Assess the degree of hypothermia using whether the person is shivering or not shivering.

Shivering is our body's way of trying to create more heat by letting the muscles work. Shivering can increase heat production by two to five times. If the person shivers, it indicates that hypothermia is still relatively mild. If the shivering has stopped, hypothermia is usually severe and the person's energy supply is depleted.

CAUTION: This common and effective lifting technique must be avoided in severe hypothermia since it may increase the risk of cardiac arrhythmias.

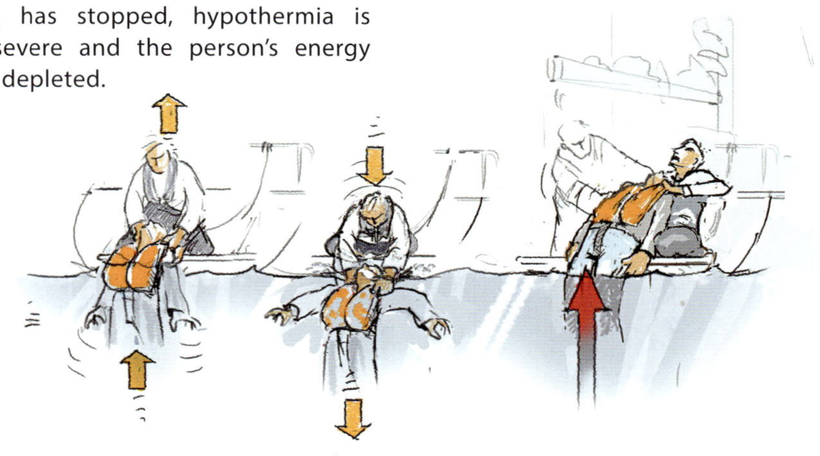

Treatment

Shivering is the body's natural way to generate heat through muscle activity.

- Mild hypothermia: If the person is shivering, hypothermia is still relatively mild. Encourage movement, provide hot drinks, change into dry clothing, and wrap them in blankets in a wind-sheltered area.
- Severe hypothermia: If shivering has stopped, the situation is critical. The body's energy reserves are depleted, and the risk of cardiac arrest is high. Focus on stopping further heat loss, cutting off wet clothing (if possible), and wrapping the person in dry blankets. Do not attempt to actively rewarm them. Keeping the person at ordinary room temperature is ideal until emergency services arrive.

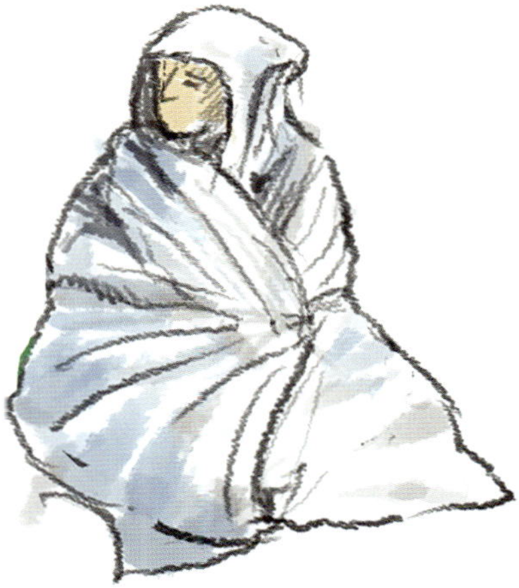

Mild hypothermia. Blankets, wind shelter and hot drinks - though only if the casualty is capable of holding the cup without help.

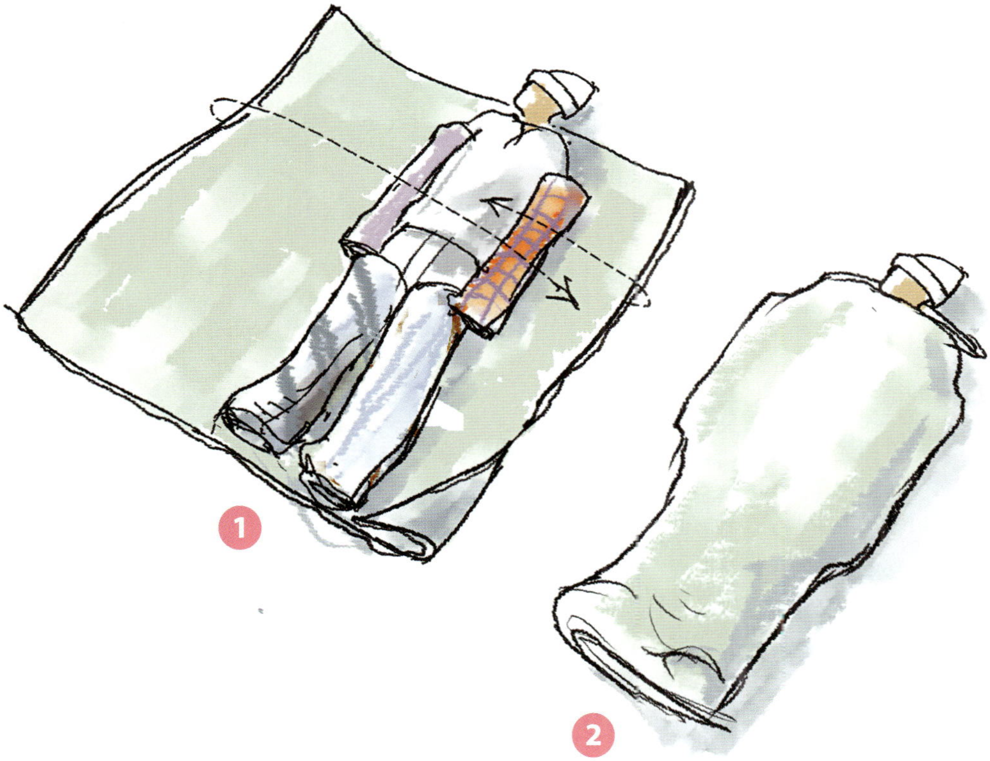

Severe hypothermia. Lay the person in a bunk or stretcher with dry, warm blankets underneath. Add a woollen hat and mittens to minimise heat loss from the head and wrists. Wrap body parts in separate blankets.

Far from help

Severe hypothermia presents a significant challenge, and outcomes may be poor despite appropriate action. Seek medical and psychological support via radio or phone.

NOTE

In cases of extreme hypothermia or suspected cardiac arrest, do not assume the person is dead. Continue CPR until professional help arrives. Determination of death should only be made by a doctor after the individual has been rewarmed. There are documented cases of survival at body temperatures as low as 13–14°C.

Prevention

- Wear layered weather-appropriate clothing, including a lifejacket with a life sling, strobe light and whistle.
- Be aware of the risk of hypothermia during long watches in cold or rainy conditions.
- In polar or Arctic waters, consider specialised neoprene undergarments or bodysuits.
- If accidentally immersed in water:
  - Avoid hyperventilation caused by sudden exposure to cold water. Do not swim; instead, huddle into a 'ball' position with knees and hips bent, and hold the position with your arms.
  - Stay calm and await rescue.

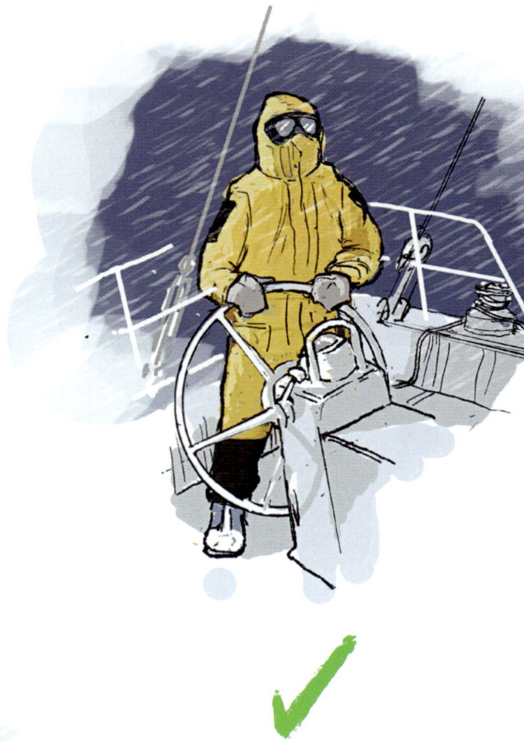

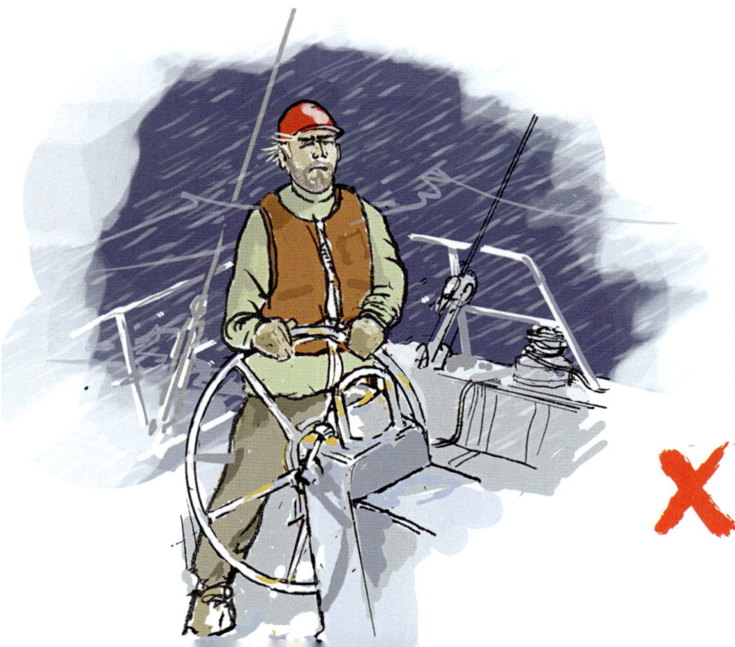

Dress appropriately for preventing hypothermia in foul weather conditions. The helmsman on the left will rapidly become wet, risk hypothermia, and then lose competence.

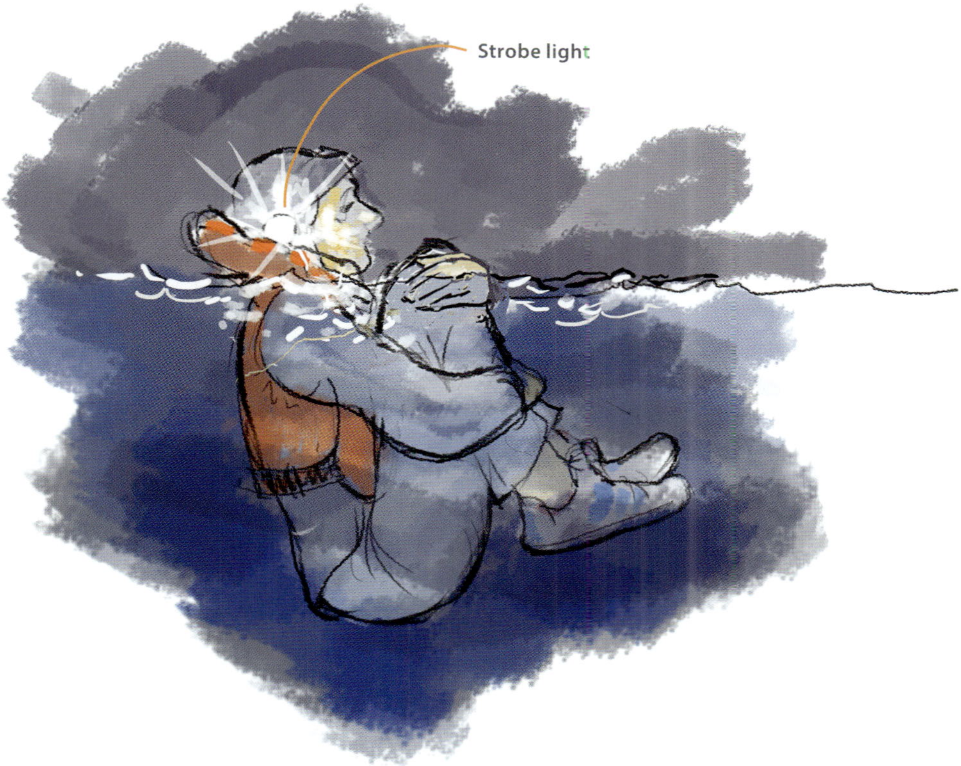

A person in the water can reduce heat loss by remaining still in a 'ball' position. Swimming accelerates heat loss.

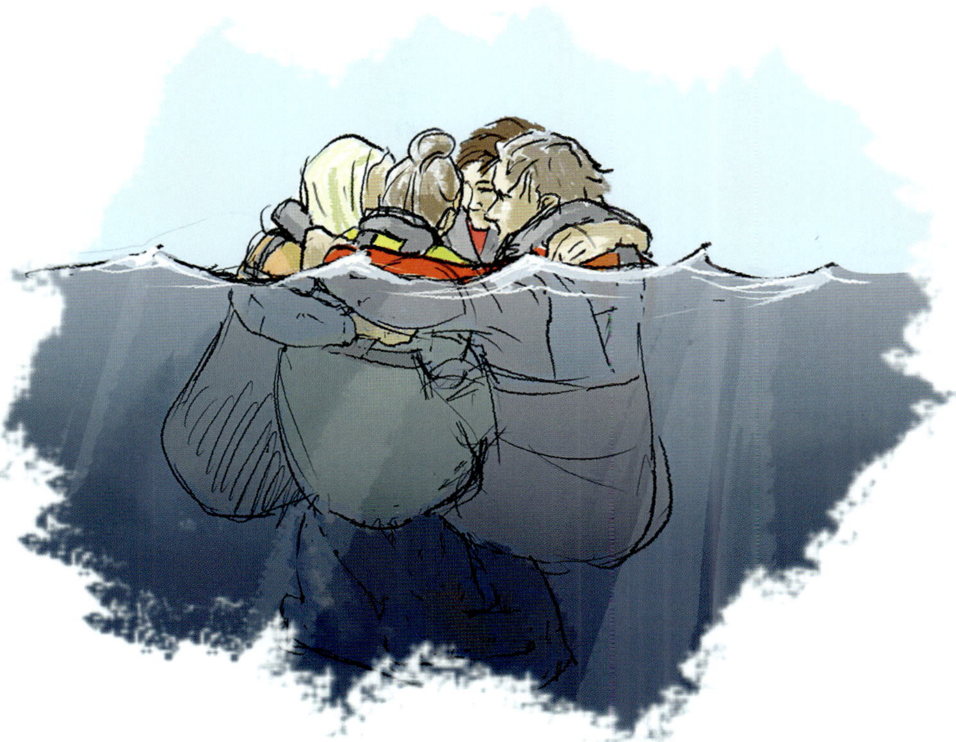

If more than one person is in the water, stay close together to conserve heat.

7. HYPERTHERMIA/ HEATSTROKE

Hyperthermia/heatstroke is a potentially very serious condition.

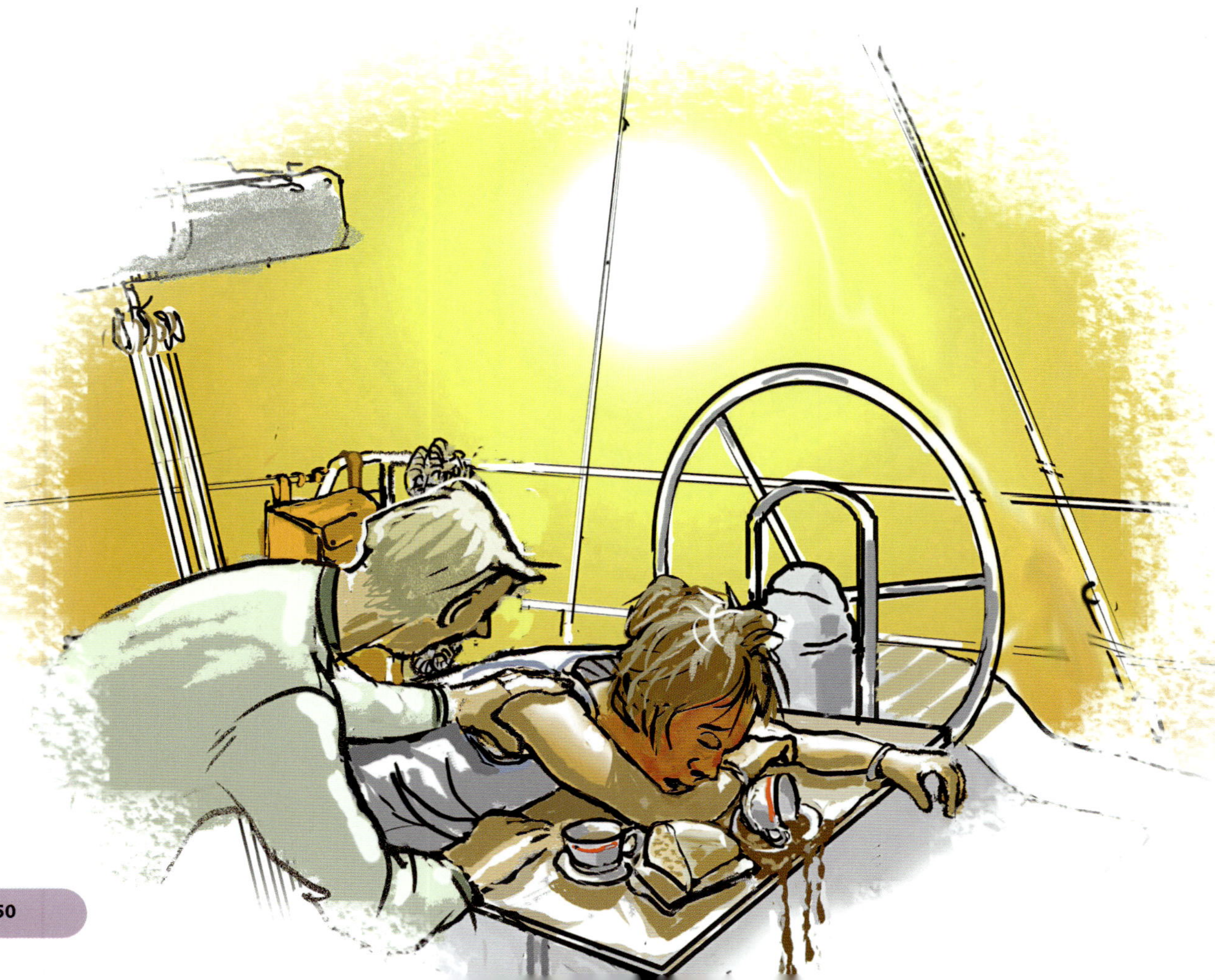

Heatstroke can be as dangerous as hypothermia! It typically takes about a week to acclimatise to a warmer climate. Sweating is the body's natural way of cooling itself when exposed to hot temperatures or during intense physical activity. However, in very humid and hot climates, the cooling effect of sweating can be reduced due to high moisture levels in the air.

Proper hydration is essential for effective sweating. Dehydration, fluid loss and alcohol consumption can reduce the body's ability to produce sweat, leading to overheating. Wearing overly warm clothing can also impair the body's capacity to cool down. Children and the elderly are at greater risk of heatstroke. One common cause is excessive physical exertion in hot climates while wearing too much clothing. Avoid working too hard in the heat.

Immediate action / Treatment

1. Stop physical activity immediately.
2. Seek shade or a breezy location, or use a fan.
3. Loosen or remove excess clothing.
4. Wet the skin with water or damp towels.
5. Provide cold drinks to rehydrate.
6. Place a couple of pillows under the feet to improve circulation to the upper body.
7. Regularly check the person's temperature.

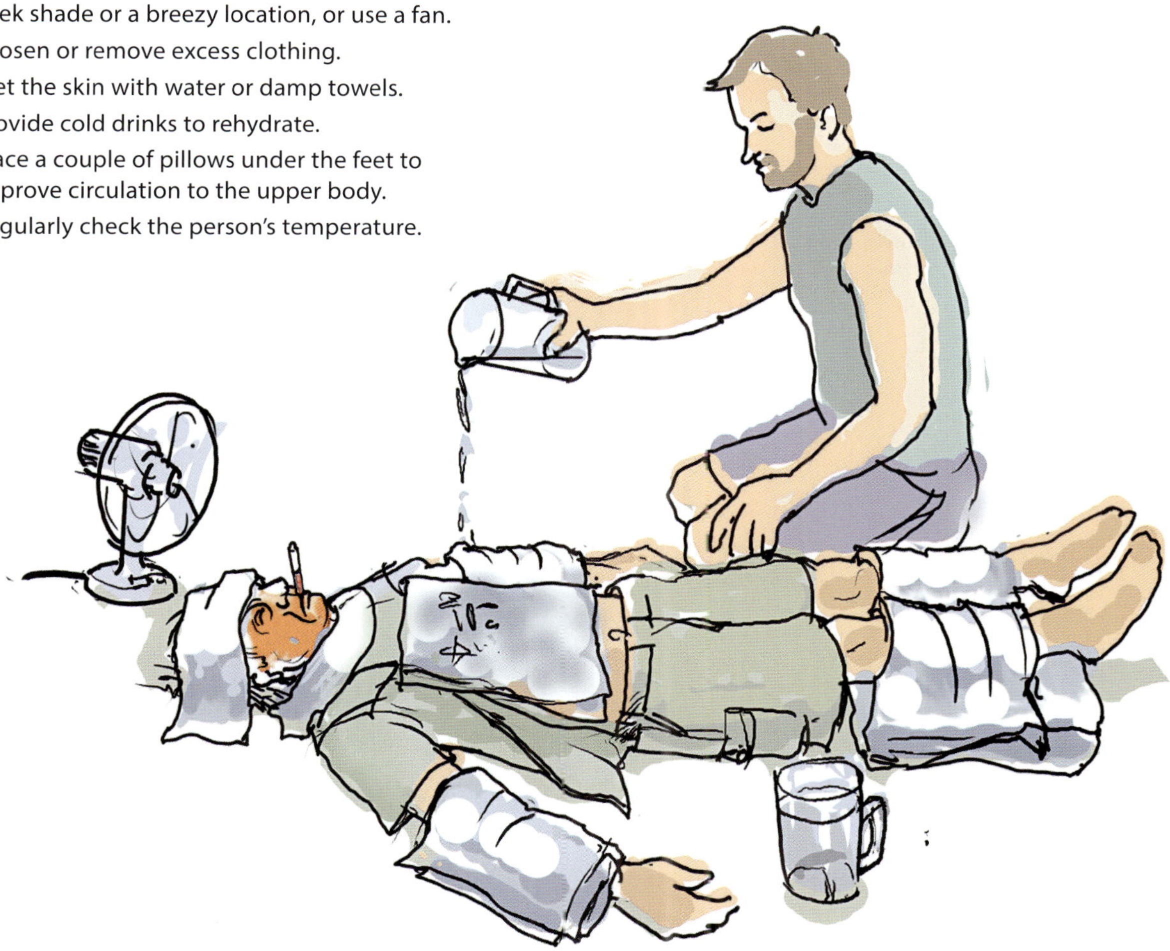

Heatstroke – correctly performed immediate actions can save lives. Seek shade!

Signs and symptoms

Heat exhaustion

The person may experience:

- headache
- nausea and vomiting
- visual disturbances
- dizziness, irritability and confusion

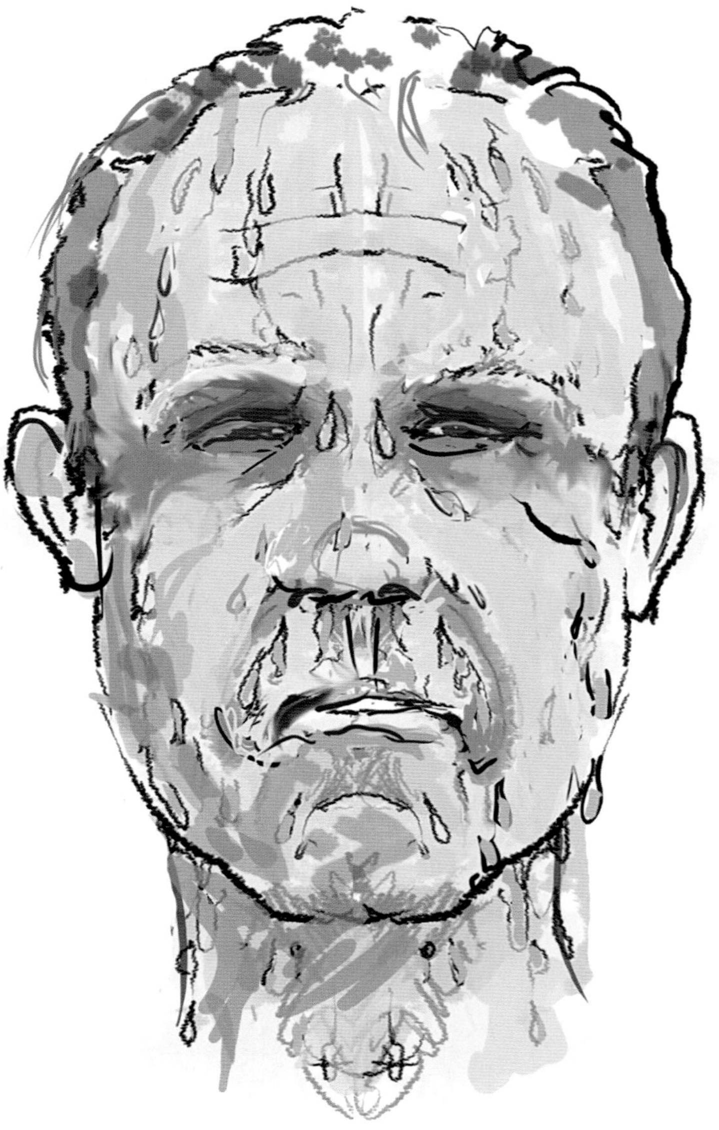

Heat exhaustion. The initial sign of overheating is often excessive sweating and pale, damp skin.

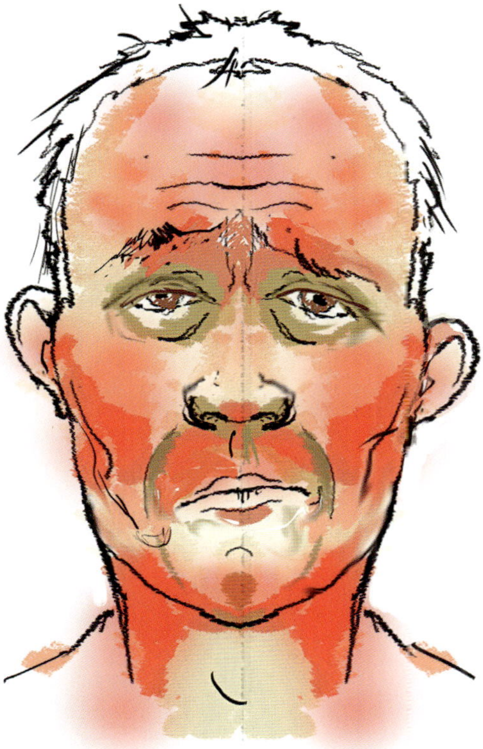

Heatstroke. In a fully developed heatstroke, the skin becomes warm, dry and red, and body temperature rises to 39–40°C.

Heatstroke

Heatstroke is a life-threatening condition requiring immediate action. The person may exhibit:

- rapid pulse
- accelerated breathing, indicating shock

If untreated, heatstroke can lead to severe complications and requires hospital care.

Prevention

- Avoid strenuous physical activity in hot and humid climates.
- Stay hydrated by drinking plenty of fluids.
- Avoid wearing excessive clothing.
- Refrain from consuming alcohol.
- Allow time to acclimatise to the climate.
- Wear loose-fitting, breathable clothing.

Temperature °C	Degree of severity	General treatment
38°C	Mild hyperthermia	Oral rehydration, keep cool, reduce work
40°C	Moderate hyperthermia	Oral rehydration, active cooling, candidate for hospital
42–45°C	Severe hyperthermia, life-threatening	Active cooling, IV fluids, need to be hospitalised

Recommended actions to counteract hyperthermia.

8. ALLERGY

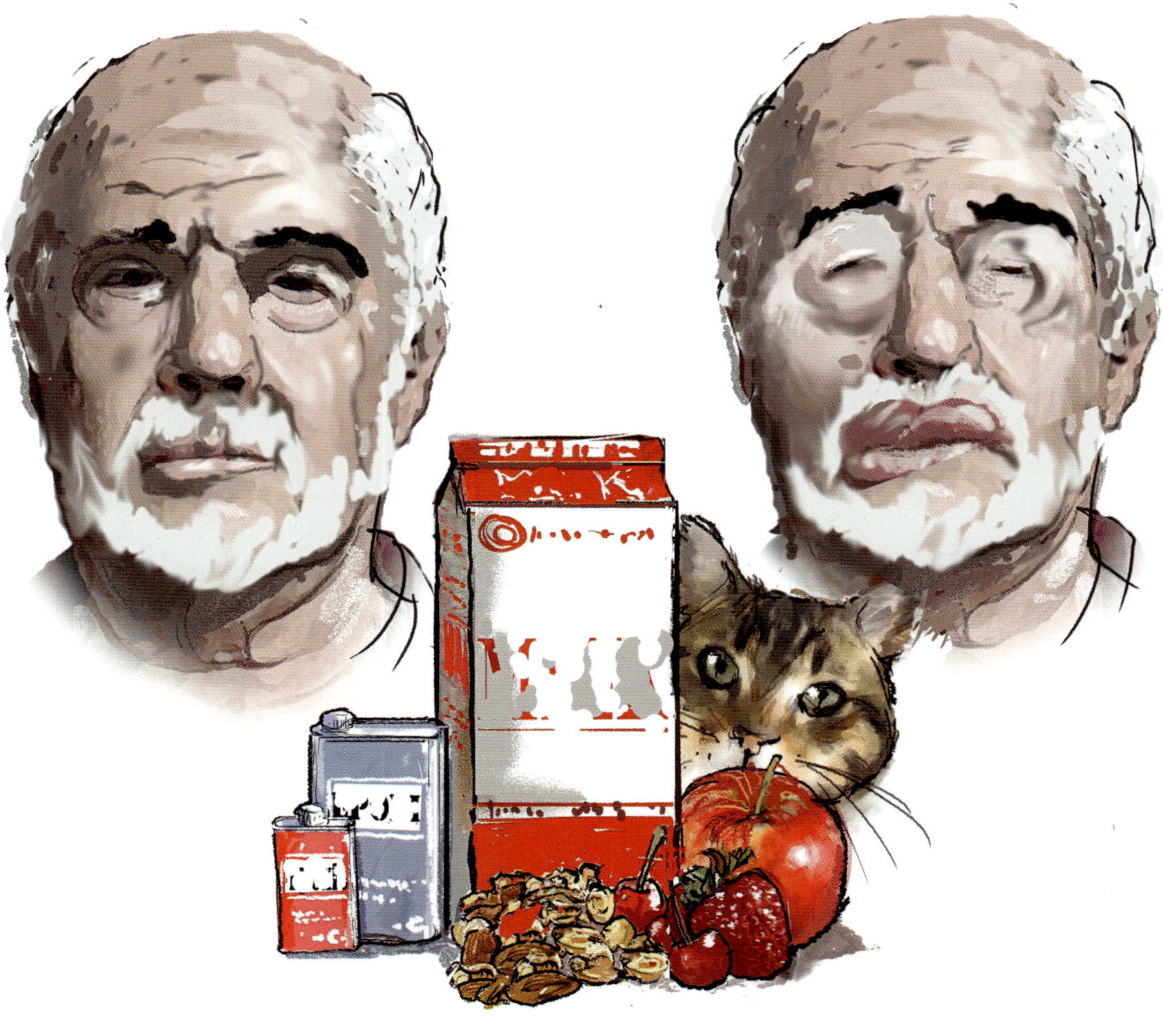

Common allergens. Facial oedema in allergic reaction.

Allergy is a major public health issue. Common allergens include pollen, pets, dust mites, food and medications. Regardless of the specific allergen, there is always potential for rapid progression to a severe anaphylactic reaction or shock.

In pollen allergies, cross-reactivity is common. This means the allergic reaction can also be triggered by food products, such as nuts and fruits, containing similar chemical compounds to those found in pollen. This can complicate the situation, as suddenly occurring allergic reactions may develop to previously tolerated foods.

Food allergies (for example, milk, eggs, nuts) are common in children and younger individuals. Among adults, allergies to medications and insect stings – especially wasps – are more prevalent. Allergy to chemicals, such as epoxy, is increasing and can be problematic for boat owners.

A skipper's responsibility includes knowing if any crew members have allergies and to which allergens. Avoid exposure to known allergens and ensure relevant medications are on board. Refer to page 247 'Ship's Dispensary', or confirm that allergic crew members bring their necessary medications. We recommend having two adrenaline injectors on board for anyone with severe allergies. Remember: it's too late to read instructions once an acute allergic reaction has started! Be prepared by familiarising yourself with the injector and its use before setting sail. This knowledge could save a life!

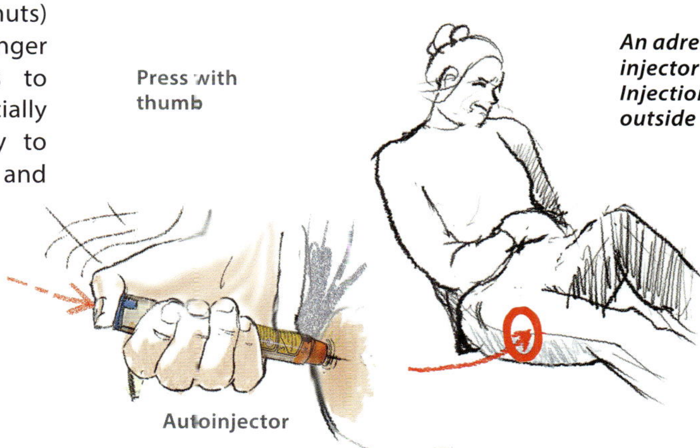

An adrenaline auto-injector (Epipen). Injection site is always outside of the thigh.

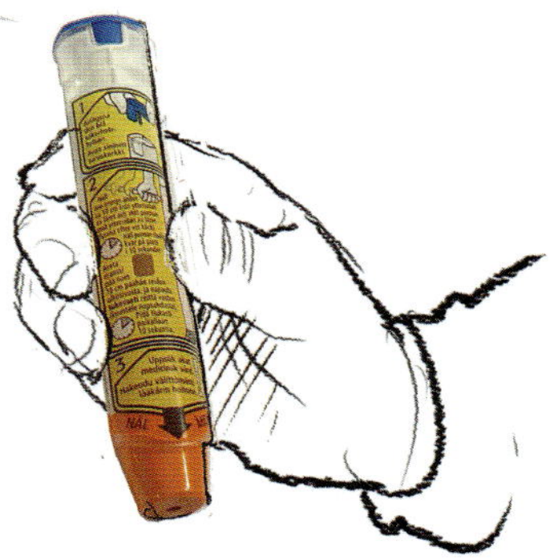

Small allergic children on board: Ensure medications are in a suitable form, such as syrup or mixture.

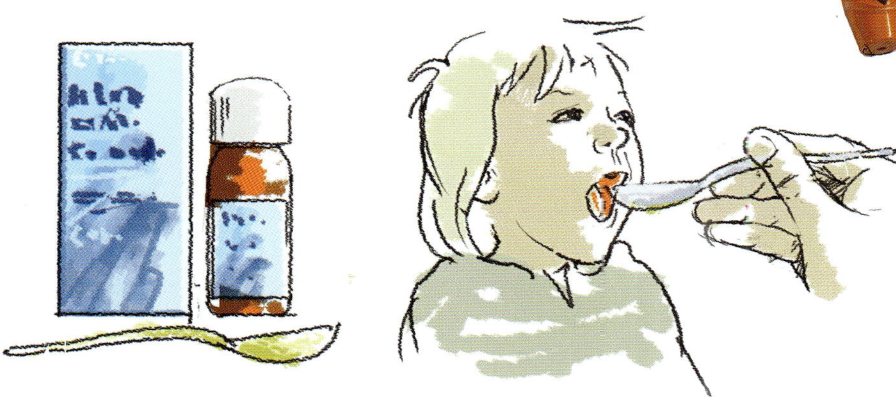

Syrup or fluid medication is best for children.

Whether sailing in coastal waters with easy access to medical help or on an extended voyage lasting several days far from medical assistance, the same emergency measures apply on board. Follow the three-step treatment plan below. NOTE that in some cases symptoms develop very rapidly, necessitating immediate administration of adrenaline followed by the rest of the medication.

The start and development of an acute allergy is a dynamic process with unpredictable speed and extent.

Continuous careful monitoring of the affected person is crucial in all steps. We recommend early contact with healthcare professionals for advice and support.

Acute allergic reaction

↓

Anaphylactic reaction

↓

Anaphylactic shock

STEP 1: ACUTE ALLERGIC REACTION

First symptoms are swollen face and itching rash – hives.

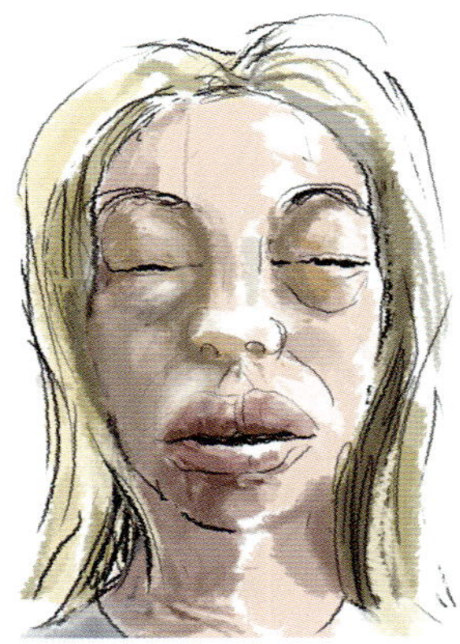

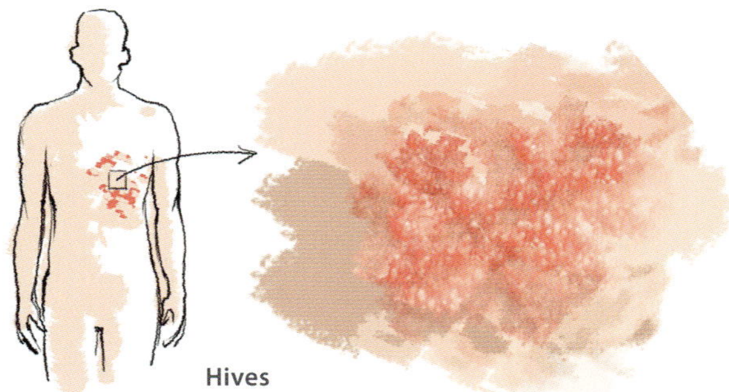

Signs and symptoms

Symptoms often start very quickly, within seconds, but can take hours:

- hives
- itchy rash
- watery, red eyes
- swelling of the face and lips
- nasal congestion
- sneezing
- itching in palms, soles of the feet, throat or mouth
- nausea

Immediate action

- Administer antihistamine and steroids simultaneously to alleviate symptoms and slow progression.
- Antihistamine, chlorphenamine tablet 4mg, effect within 30 to 60 minutes.
- Steroid, betamethasone tablet 0.5mg, 10 tablets, effect within 2 to 3 hours.
- Alternatively prednisolone 5mg, 8 tablets.

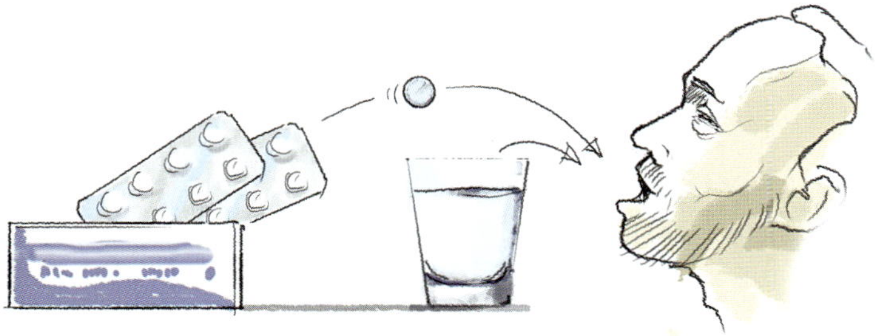

Antihistamines

Adults: 1 tablet chlorphenamine (Piriton) 4mg every 4–6 hours.

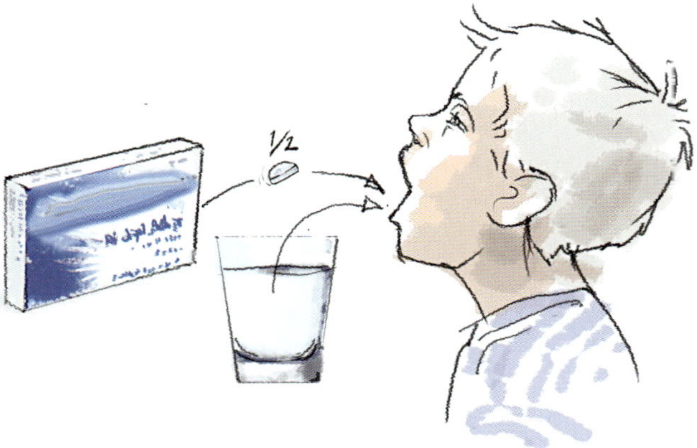

Ages 12 years and younger: 0.5 tablet or an equivalent amount of liquid form every 4–6 hours.

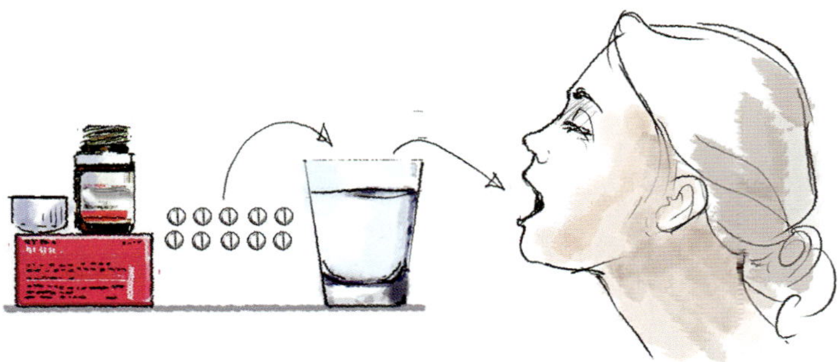

Steroids

Adults and children > 6 years: dissolve 10 betamethasone 0.5mg tablets in water.

6 tablets dissolved in water

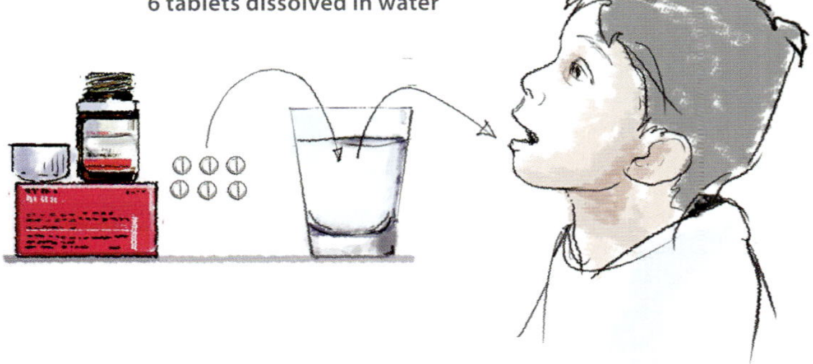

Children < 6 years: dissolve 6 betamethasone 0.5mg tablets in water or give an equivalent amount of mixture/ syrup.

STEP 2: ANAPHYLAXIS, SEVERE ALLERGIC REACTION

Shortness of breath and general skin rash are prominent in anaphylaxis.

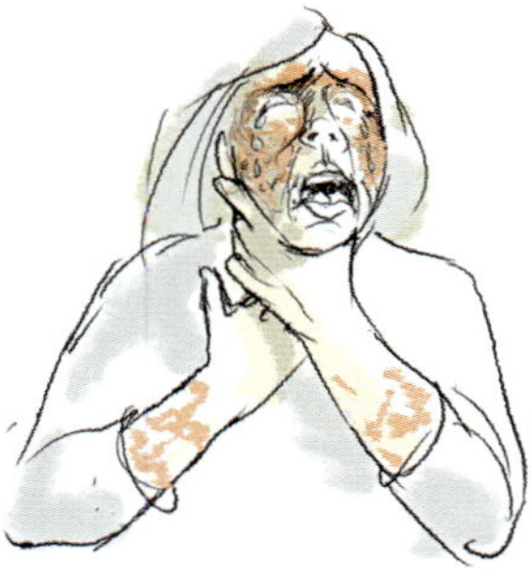

Risk factors for anaphylaxis

- Allergic asthma
- Allergic eczema (atopic eczema)
- Hay fever
- Hives (urticaria)
- Allergic rhinitis and 'red eyes'
- Family history of severe allergies
- Previous anaphylactic episodes

Auto-injection can be done through clothing but always on the outside of the thigh.

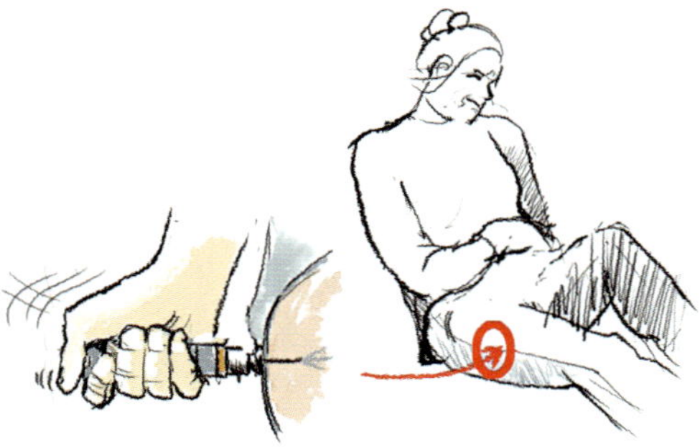

Inhalation of bronchodilator can help relieve breathing problems.

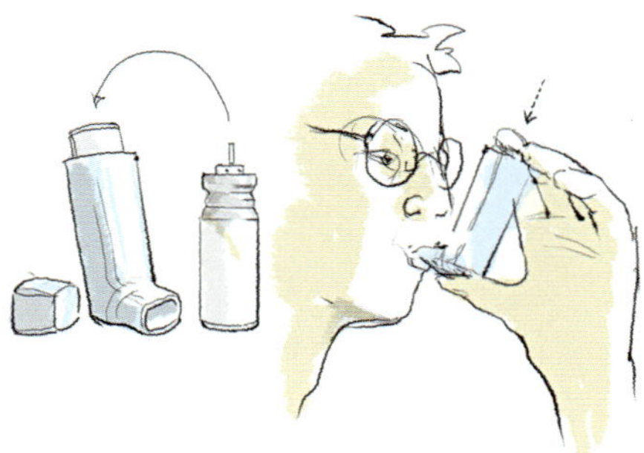

Positions preferred in anaphylaxis with respiratory and circulatory problems.

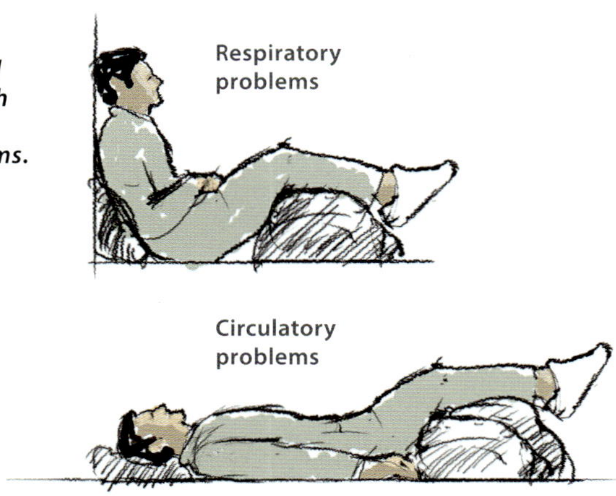

Signs and symptoms

- Breathing problems or shortness of breath, wheezing
- Abdominal pain
- Vomiting
- Diarrhoea
- Fatigue
- Anxiety or restlessness
- Coughing
- Difficulties swallowing

Immediate action

Call for an ambulance! A person with anaphylaxis needs urgent transport to the hospital. Treat as follows:

1 Injection adrenaline – auto-injector 300µg on the outer thigh.

Effect within 5 minutes. Repeat within 5 to 10 minutes if insufficient effect.

2 Give antihistamine and steroid as in step 1 above.

3 Inhalation bronchodilator – salbutamol, 4 puffs every 5 minutes, for breathing difficulties.

Effect within 5 minutes. Repeat every 10 minutes, up to six times.

4 Position – breathing problems often require a sitting position for relief. If circulation is affected, supine with elevated legs is best. Remember a blanket to keep the person warm!

Far from help

See above under Immediate Action. Disregard calling an ambulance and try to find medical support instead.

NOTE: Twenty per cent of anaphylaxis cases may experience a two-phase reaction, with recurrence within 1 to 24 hours.

STEP 3: ANAPHYLACTIC SHOCK (LIFE-THREATENING)

Anaphylactic shock is defined as symptoms in at least two of the following systems: skin, gastrointestinal, respiratory and cardiac, with mandatory involvement of the last two.

Signs and symptoms

- Cyanosis (lack of oxygen)
- Cardiac irregularities (low, high or erratic pulse)
- Severe breathing difficulties or respiratory arrest
- Involuntary urination and defecation
- Fainting – unconscious
- Cardiac arrest

Immediate action

1. Follow DRABC protocol (see page 12).
2. Give adrenaline.
3. Call for an ambulance for immediate transport to hospital.
4. Administer treatments from steps 1 and 2 above.
5. Position: Supine, with elevated legs.
6. Check airway and respiration. If unconscious but breathing, use the recovery position (see page 16). If not breathing, start CPR.
7. Keep the person warm.

Prevention

- Avoid allergenic food like nuts.
- Do not store allergenic products on board.
- Prevent wasp stings (they do not sting unless they feel provoked).
- Keep relevant medications in the ship's dispensary.
- Administer medication liberally when allergic reactions are suspected.
- Avoid alcohol, as it can worsen allergic reactions.

Far from help

Anaphylactic shock is an extremely challenging situation with a poor prognosis. If medical advice and medication are available, they may buy time to arrange transport to a hospital.

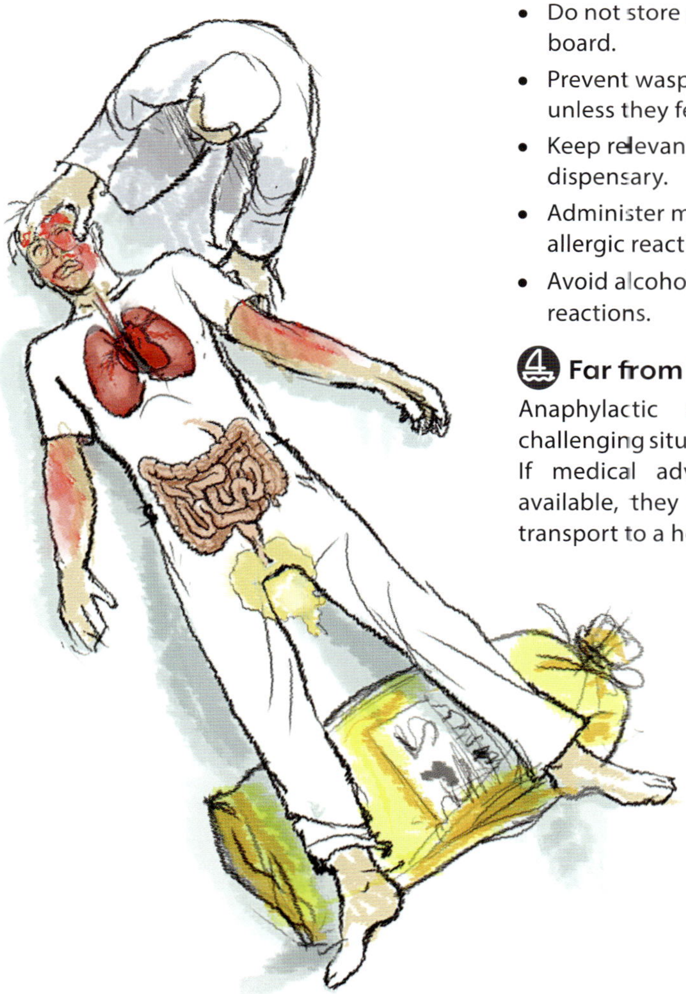

Anaphylactic shock – a life-threatening condition.

9. EAR PROBLEMS

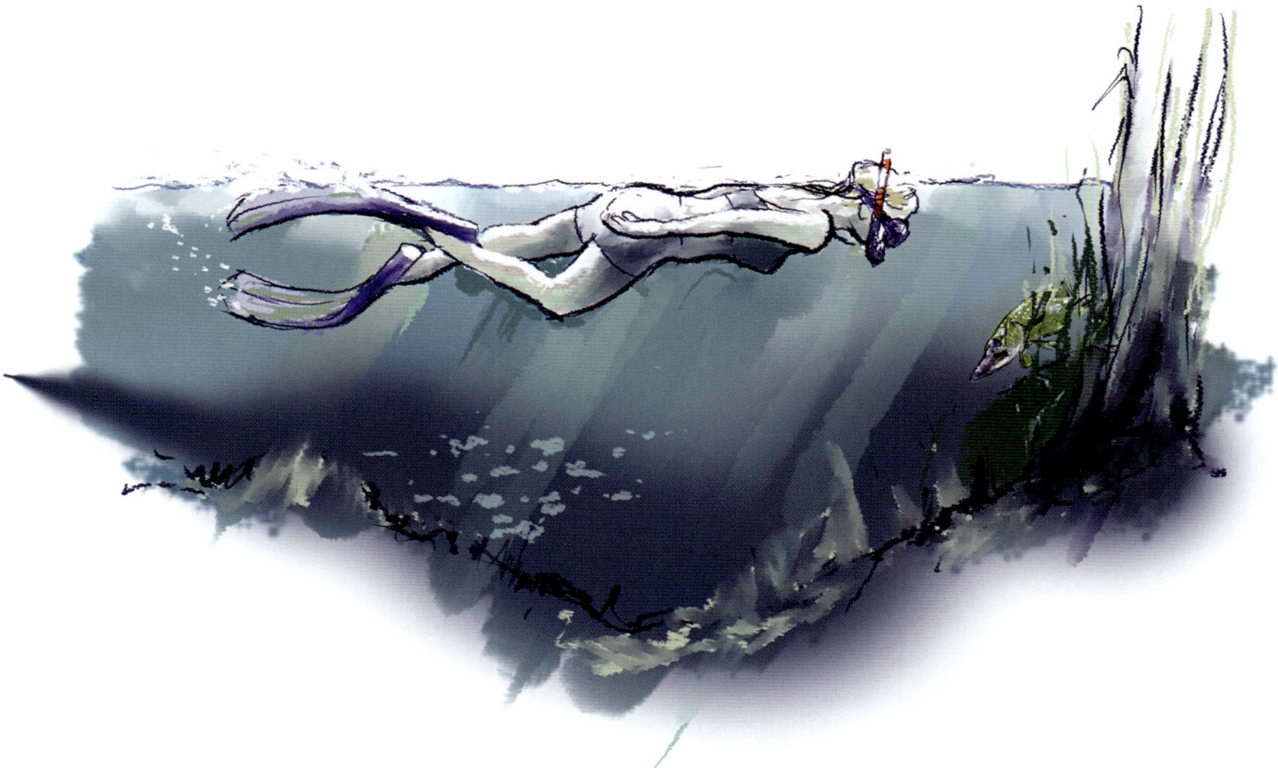

Snorkelling is a common cause of 'swimmer's ear'.

Our ears are crucial for hearing and balance – functions of great importance in our daily life, particularly in a sailing context.

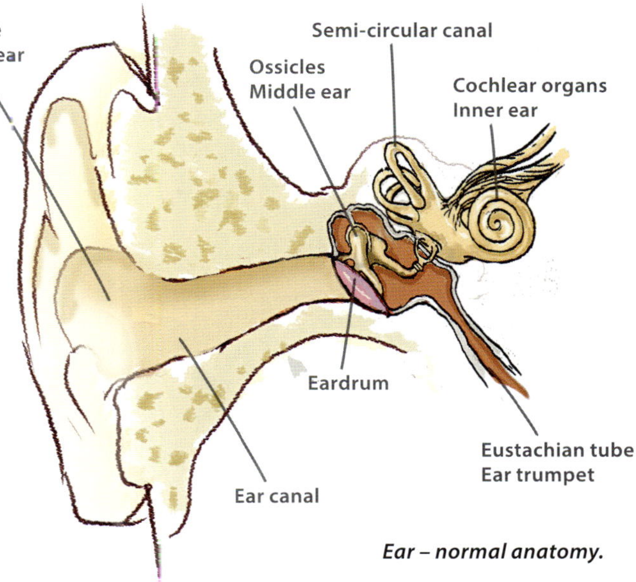

Ear – normal anatomy.

EARWAX BLOCKAGE

Earwax blockage and inflammation in the ear canal are common issues in a boating context and can become troublesome within a short period.

The ear canal has a self-cleaning mechanism, and earwax plays an essential role in this process. Specialised skin cells produce earwax, which helps to remove dead skin cells from the ear. Most people have experienced earwax blockage at some point.

Signs and symptoms

Common symptoms of earwax blockage include:

- reduced hearing in the affected ear
- pain or a feeling of pressure
- 'ear popping' sensations
- tinnitus (ringing in the ear)
- dizziness, which can impair balance while on a boat
- a cough reflex triggered by the blockage

Hearing loss can worsen suddenly after showering, swimming or diving if water becomes trapped between the earwax and the tympanic membrane and cannot drain.

Treatment

Try one or two drops of olive oil in the ear canal or use over-the-counter earwax-dissolving solutions for a few days, following the instructions. If the hearing loss persists, consult an ear specialist to rule out other causes and have the wax removed by suction.

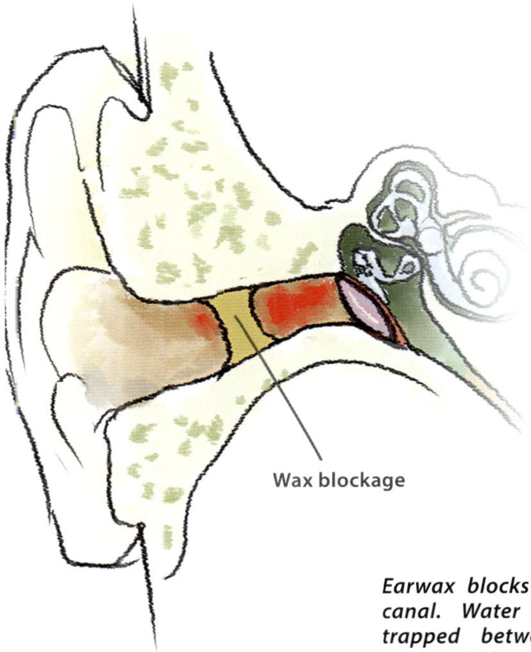

Earwax blocks the ear canal. Water can be trapped between the wax and the tympanic membrane.

Far from help

If symptoms persist and become a great problem, flushing the ear with a bulb syringe may be necessary. Use caution if a tympanic membrane injury cannot be ruled out (for example, purulent discharge, barotrauma after diving, or previous surgery). Seek medical advice when possible.

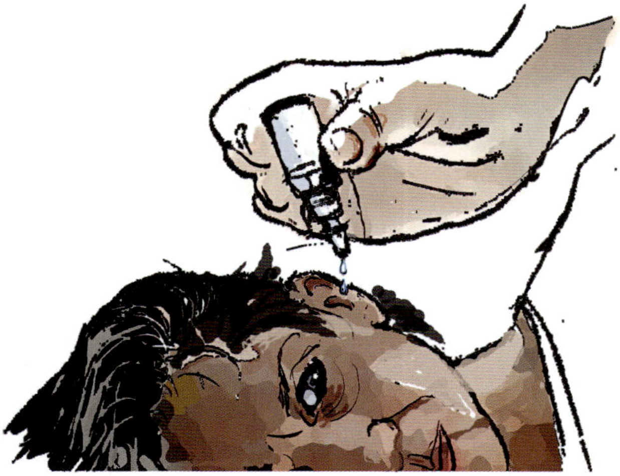

Unrefined cotton plug

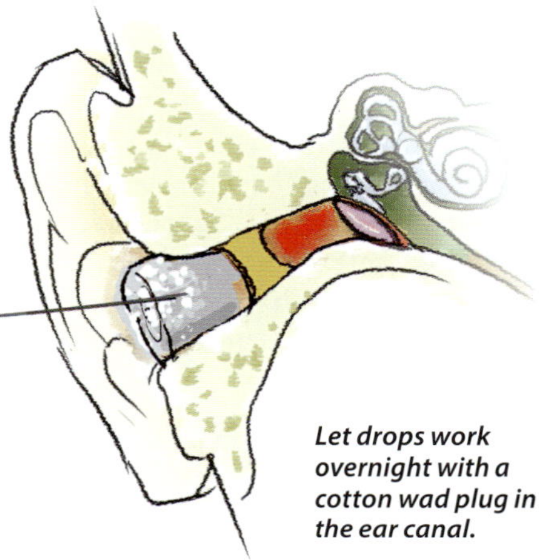

Let drops work overnight with a cotton wad plug in the ear canal.

Flush the ear canal. Turn your head to the side over a sink. Fill the bulb syringe with lukewarm water, place it near the ear canal opening and squeeze the bulb. Repeat as necessary. The warm water should break up the wax, allowing it to flow out.

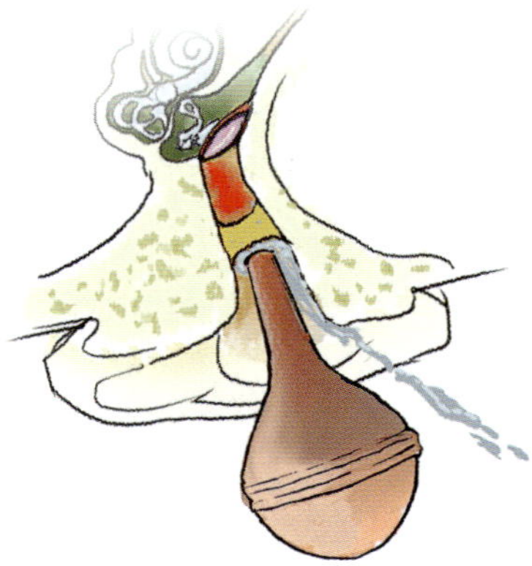

Prevention

- Avoid using earplugs for electronic devices that may damage the ear canal.
- If earwax build-up is a frequent problem, consider regular use of earwax-dissolving solutions.

CAUTION

Caution! Never insert cotton swabs, toothpicks or similar objects into the ear canal, as this can cause severe injuries and infections.

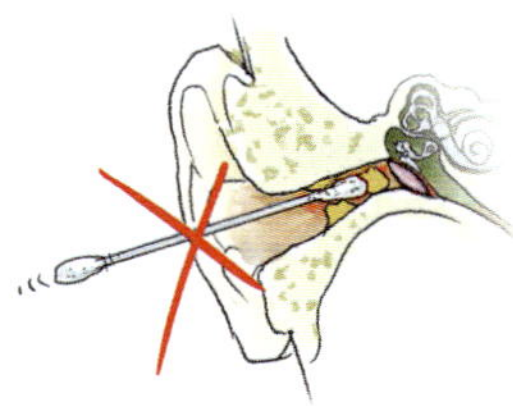

'SWIMMER'S EAR'

Swimming, snorkelling and diving are common activities on boats, often in salty sea water. Highly saline water can damage the ear canal, leading to eczema and infections. This condition, commonly known as 'swimmer's ear' or 'diver's ear', is technically referred to as otitis externa (external otitis).

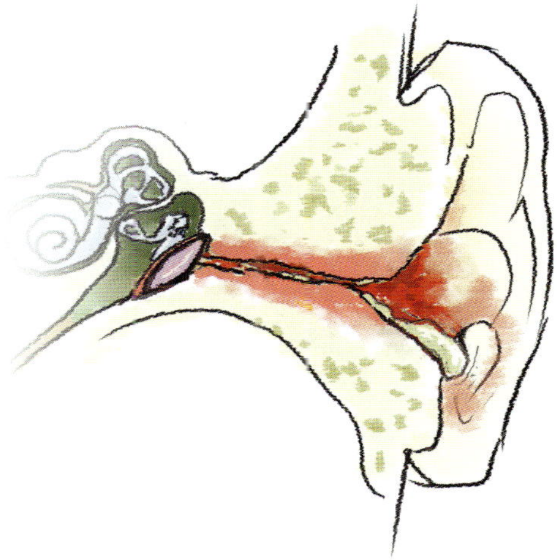

Swimmer's ear (otitis externa)

Symptoms

Symptoms include:

- itching, discharge and swelling in the ear canal
- pain, especially when pressing on the ear
- blocked ear canals, which may affect hearing

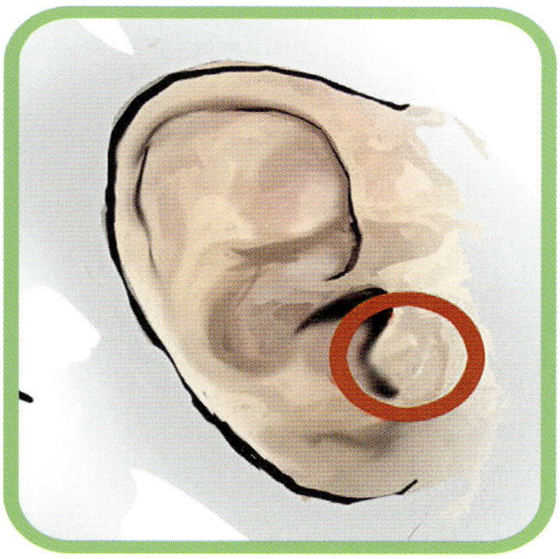

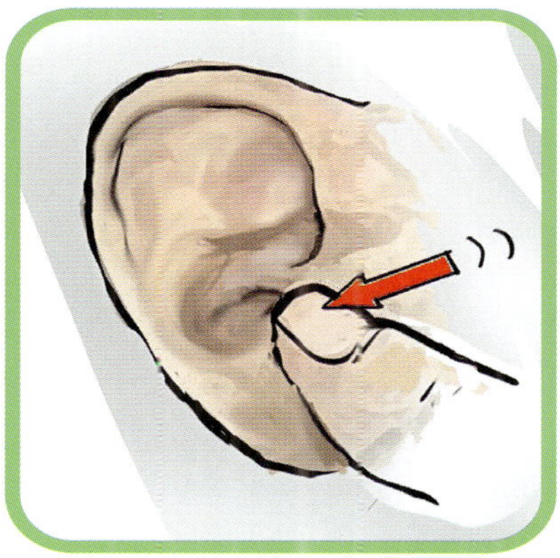

A clue on how to differentiate otitis externa from otitis media (medial otitis). Otitis externa causes pain when pressing on the ear. This test is usually negative for middle ear infections (otitis media).

Treatment

If the ear canal remains open, treatment with ear drops containing a steroid, antibiotics or antifungal agents is effective. Flushing with water is controversial, as dampness can worsen symptoms. If the canal is completely blocked, an ear specialist may need to remove the blockage.

Far from help

This condition is not an emergency and can wait until a medical evaluation is possible. However, if in doubt, seek advice.

Prevention

- Dry the ear canal after swimming.
- Some recommend flushing the ears with fresh water after swimming in salt water, while others prefer drying with warm air.
- Earplugs may help but must allow for pressure equalisation if used during diving.

INFECTION IN THE MIDDLE EAR (OTITIS MEDIA)

Middle ear infections often occur during colds caused by viral infections. These infections are most common in children up to 10 years of age but can also affect adults.

Signs and symptoms

Typical symptoms are:

- localised ear pain during a cold
- hearing loss
- fever and purulent discharge (indicating bacterial infection and possible eardrum perforation)

Treatment

Symptoms often subside in a few days with symptomatic treatment, such as nasal sprays. For bacterial infections, antibiotics (for example, phenoxymethylpenicillin) may be needed. Pain relief with paracetamol is often helpful.

Far from help

Follow the above treatment recommendations. If fever and pain persist, consider using antibiotics liberally. Seek medical advice when possible.

Prevention

Avoid catching colds, if possible. Children with cold symptoms in daycare are typically contagious.

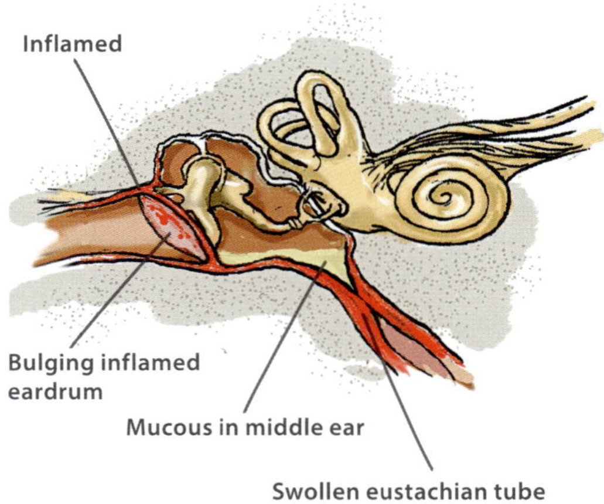

Otitis media: Red and swollen membranes. Fluid/pus. Occluded ear trumpet.

'CRYSTAL DISEASE'

Vertigo is a common problem with various causes. One of the most frequent is benign paroxysmal positional vertigo (BPPV), or 'crystal disease'. It is an ear disease occurring when a crystal from the inner ear becomes dislodged and moves into one of the semicircular canals, disrupting the balance system. It occurs at any age, but the incidence increases with age.

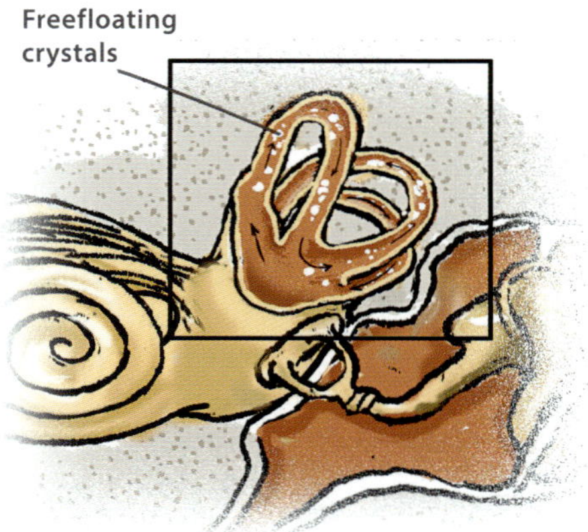

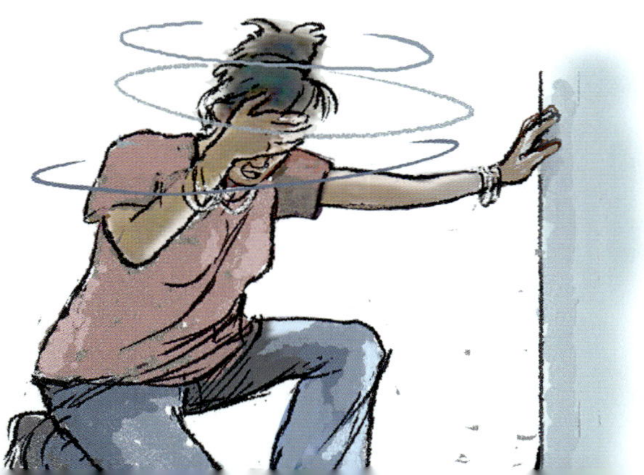

Vertigo – 'crystal disease'.

Signs and symptoms

- Sudden, severe spinning sensation triggered by head movements.
- Symptoms typically last less than a minute but can recur over weeks or months.
- Nausea and vomiting may occur.
- 'Dancing eyes' (nystagmus) may be observed, characterised by phases of slow and rapid eye movements.

Immediate action

Consider the risk of falling and getting secondary injuries. Give help and support.

Treatment

If near the coast, seek medical help within a day or two for diagnosis and treatment. On board, a series of head movements (see below) can be attempted to dislodge the crystal. These exercises are safe but may trigger vertigo during the process.

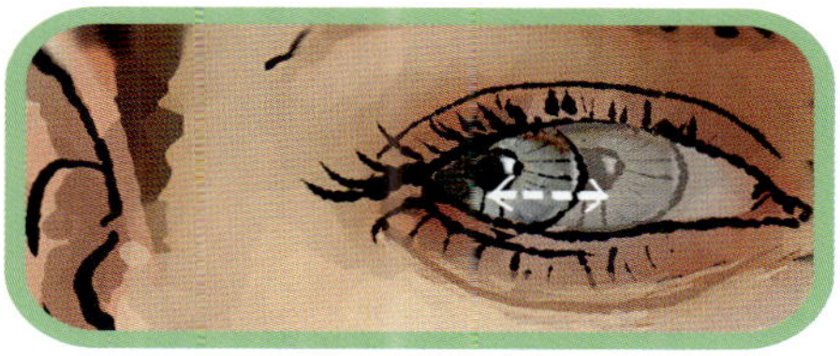

Nystagmus: rapid eye movement towards the affected side.

Far from help

Try exercises to move the crystal out of the semicircular canal. It is preferable to figure out which side is affected and adjust the pattern of head movements accordingly. This is difficult, however – try one direction and, if no effect, repeat but towards the opposite direction.

The exercises suggested below offer a good chance to achieve relief if performed properly and repeatedly. It is important to have assistance since the exercise might provoke symptoms. If possible, communicate to achieve medical advice and support before starting exercises.

1 Stay in the first position for 1–2 minutes.
2 Lie flat on your back.
3 Slowly, taking 1–2 minutes, turn your still hanging head over to the opposite side.
4 Finally, rise and sit on the opposite side of the bed and keep the head as shown for a couple of minutes.

If the exercise is successful, repeat daily. If there is no effect, a medication against seasickness (antiemetic or antihistamine) might give some relief. The crew member must try to avoid duties provoking vertigo. Seek medical attention when possible.

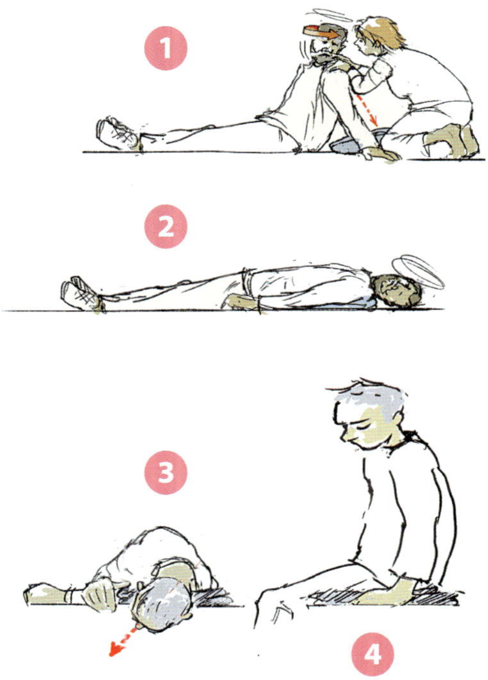

Sit on a bunk. Turn the head 45 degrees away from the affected side. Lie down on the affected side with the head hanging over the edge or over a pillow.

Prevention

Known BPPV episodes can be prevented by the above exercises. There is limited evidence for primary prevention, though vitamin D supplementation may help in some cases.

10. EYE PROBLEMS

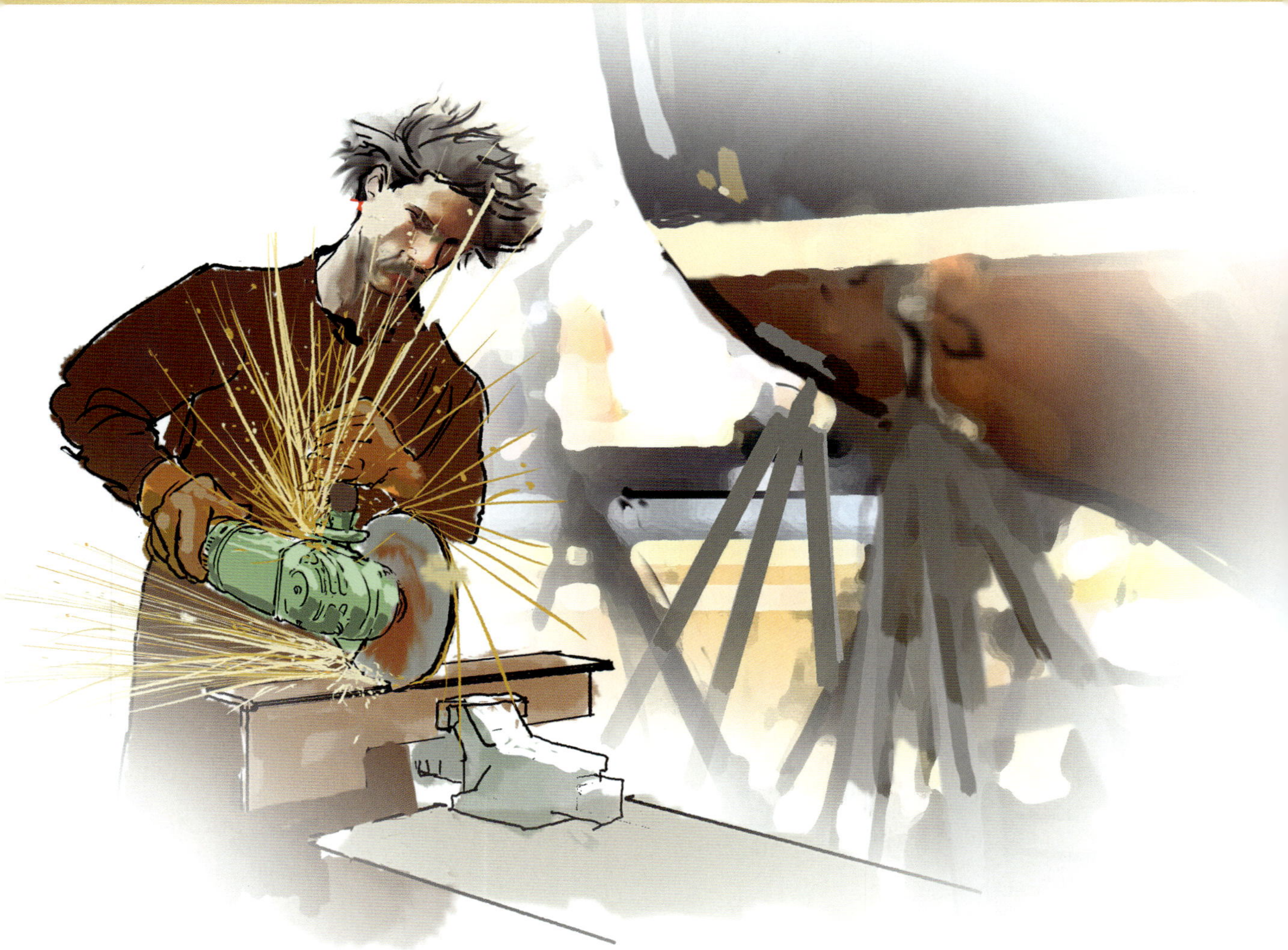

When performing repairs and other tasks related to mechanics, there's always a risk of damaging your eyes, so always wear protective lenses!

Vision is crucial for daily activities and quality of life. The eyes are sensitive and complex in structure. The optic nerve is a direct extension of the brain. This guide focuses on common, uncomplicated problems with unaffected vision that are manageable on board. For any visual impairment, always consult a specialist.

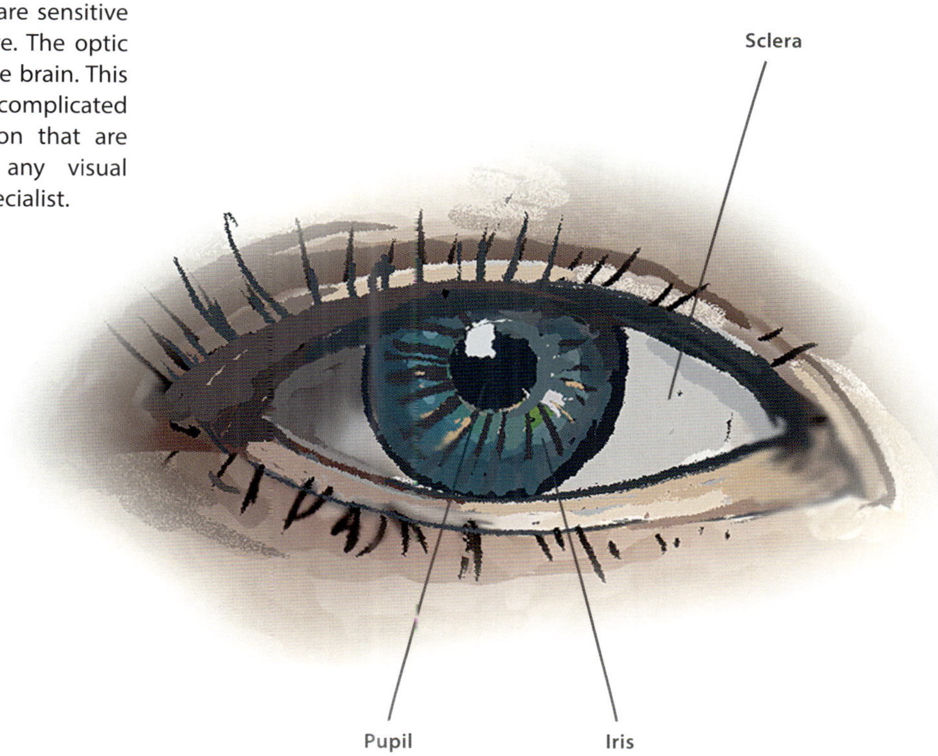

Human eye normal anatomy.

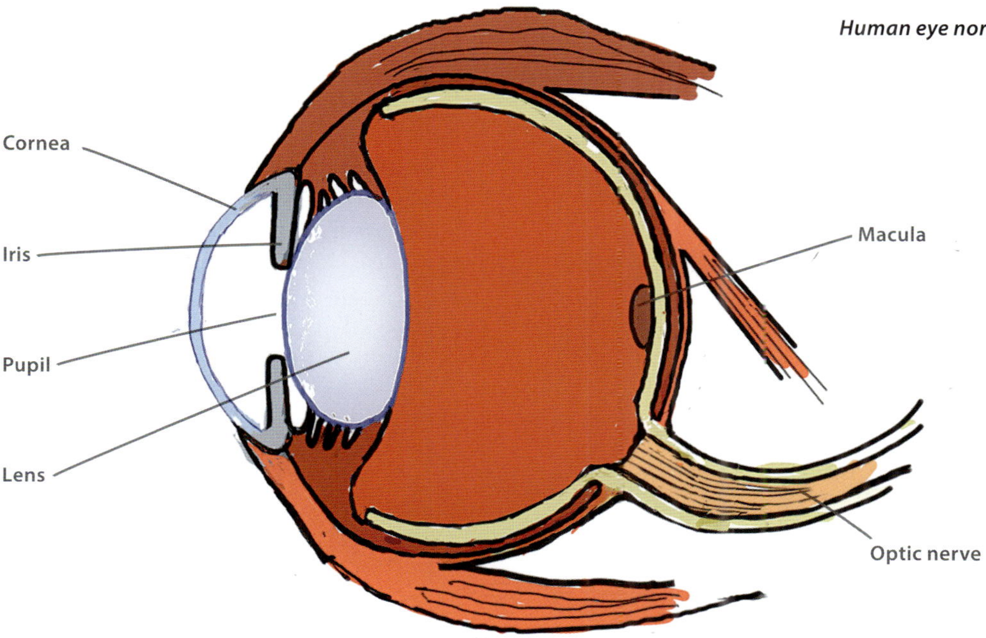

CONJUNCTIVITIS

VIRUS

Signs and symptoms

The most common cause, especially in children, is a viral infection accompanied by symptoms such as a runny nose, cough and sore throat. In addition to red eyes, inflammation may cause increased tear flow, a gritty sensation and itching.

Treatment

- Do not rub the eyes.
- Use a suitable lubricating eye ointment.
- Antibiotics are usually not needed unless complicated by a bacterial infection (see below).

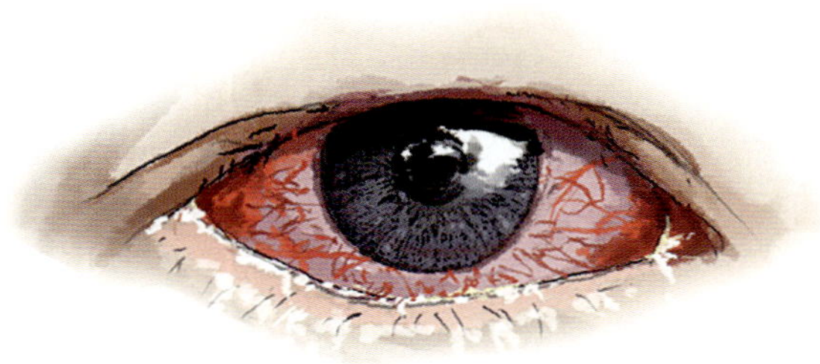

Red eye. Conjunctivitis.

BACTERIA

Signs and symptoms

A purulent discharge indicates a bacterial infection, which often spreads to both eyes within a day or two. A yellow-green secretion may dry overnight, causing the eyes to stick shut. This may require careful moistening with water. Symptoms are otherwise similar to viral conjunctivitis.

Treatment

- Do not rub the eyes.
- Clean the eyes several times daily with lukewarm water or saline solution.
- Antibiotic ointments may be used, particularly when far from help.
- Avoid spreading the infection by using separate towels and maintaining strict hand hygiene.

The condition usually heals within a week with no other treatment than cleaning.

Bacterial conjunctivitis with purulent secretion.

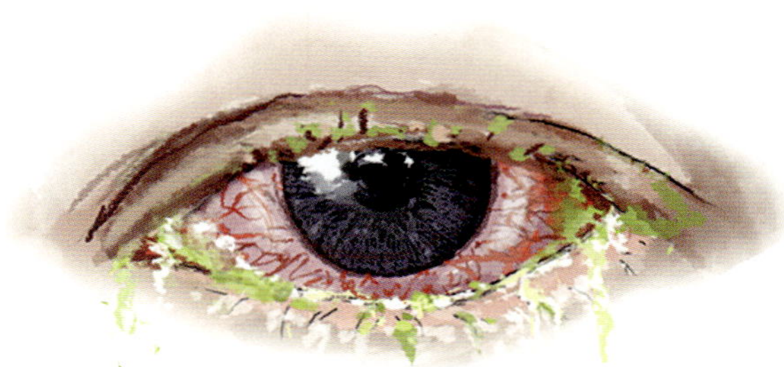

SAILOR'S EYE (DIVER'S EYE)

'Sailor's eye' is similar to 'snow blindness' and occurs after exposure to strong sunlight reflected off water, sand or snow, affecting both eyes.

Signs and symptoms

Severe inflammation of the cornea (keratitis) and conjunctiva with intense redness, swollen eyelids, excessive tearing and painful eye movements. While it doesn't cause true blindness, vision impairment is common. The severe discomfort makes it impossible to keep the eyes open and see normally.

Treatment

- Protect the eyes from light using an eye patch.
- Apply eye drops or ointments containing hydrocortisone 1%.

Prevention

Be cautious with your eyes and vision. Avoid exposure to too strong sunlight.

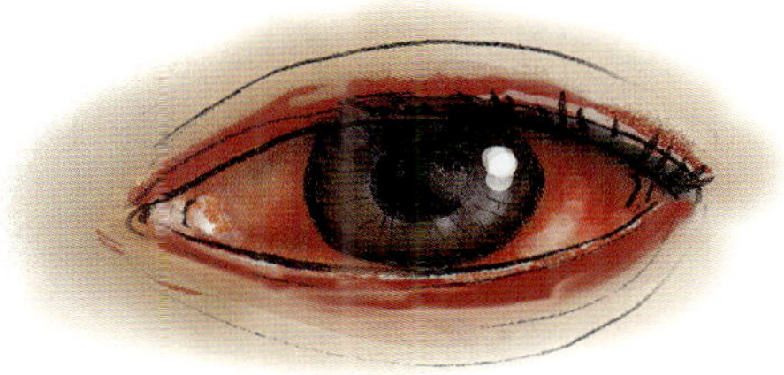

Sailor's eye with painful and extreme redness.

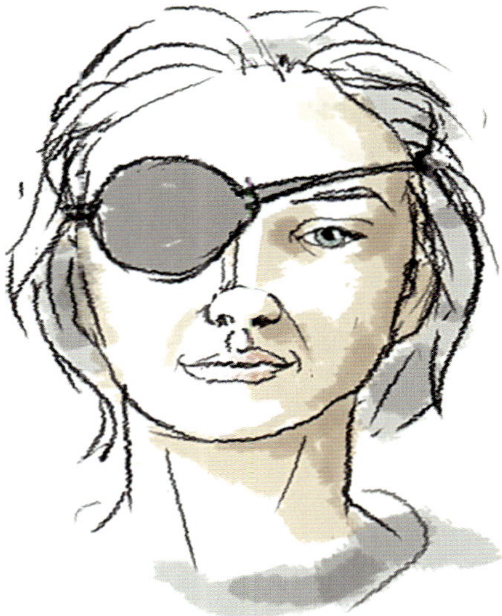

Eye patch.

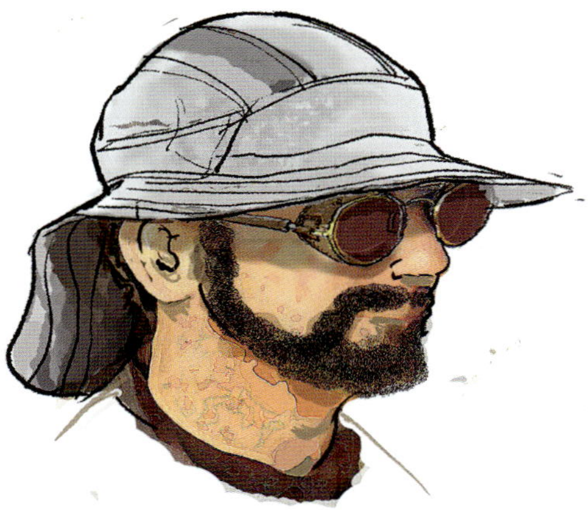

Use high-quality sunglasses with polarised lenses and side protection. Combine with a broad-brimmed hat for shade.

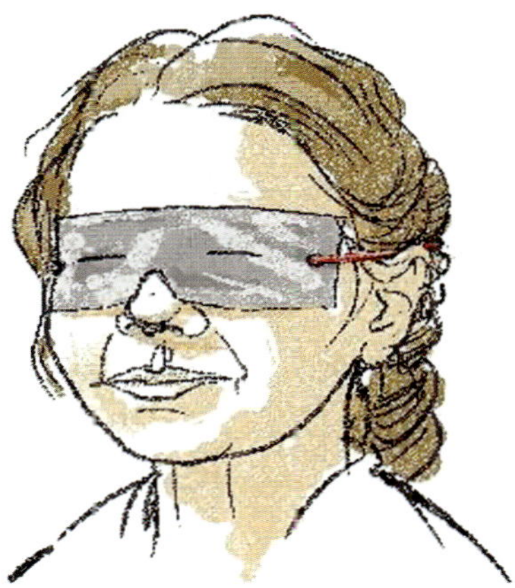

A makeshift solution is a double layer of duct tape with incisions for vision and a band to hold it – a primitive but very effective way to protect the eyes from UV radiation as well as for therapeutic use, allowing the eye to heal a keratitis.

SUBCONJUNCTIVAL HAEMORRHAGE (HYPOSPHAGMA)

This condition involves sudden, noticeable red bleeding on the conjunctiva. It is often harmless but may be associated with minor trauma, high blood pressure or blood-thinning medications.

Signs and symptoms

- Visible red bleeding on the white part of the eye
- Usually minor or no discomfort

Treatment

No specific treatment is necessary, it resolves spontaneously within a week.

Prevention

- Avoid rubbing the eyes.
- Monitor blood pressure and medications.

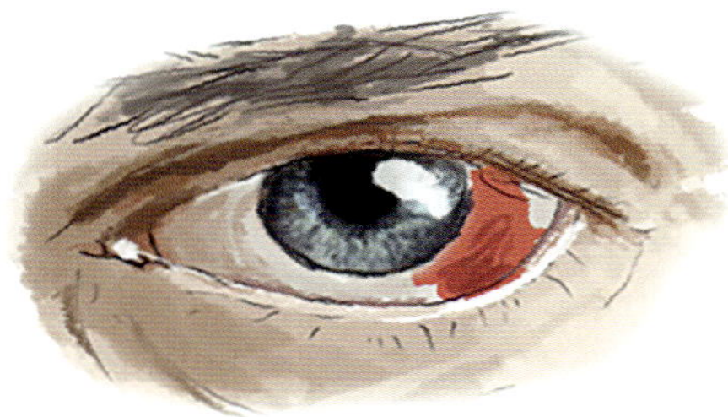

Typical appearance of a subconjunctival bleed (hyposphagma).

FOREIGN BODY

A foreign particle in the eye causes discomfort, increased tearing, blinking and light sensitivity. The severity depends on the particle type. Metal shards can embed in the outer layer of the eye. An object with higher speed may get stuck in the cornea. Light-coloured sand particles may be difficult to locate.

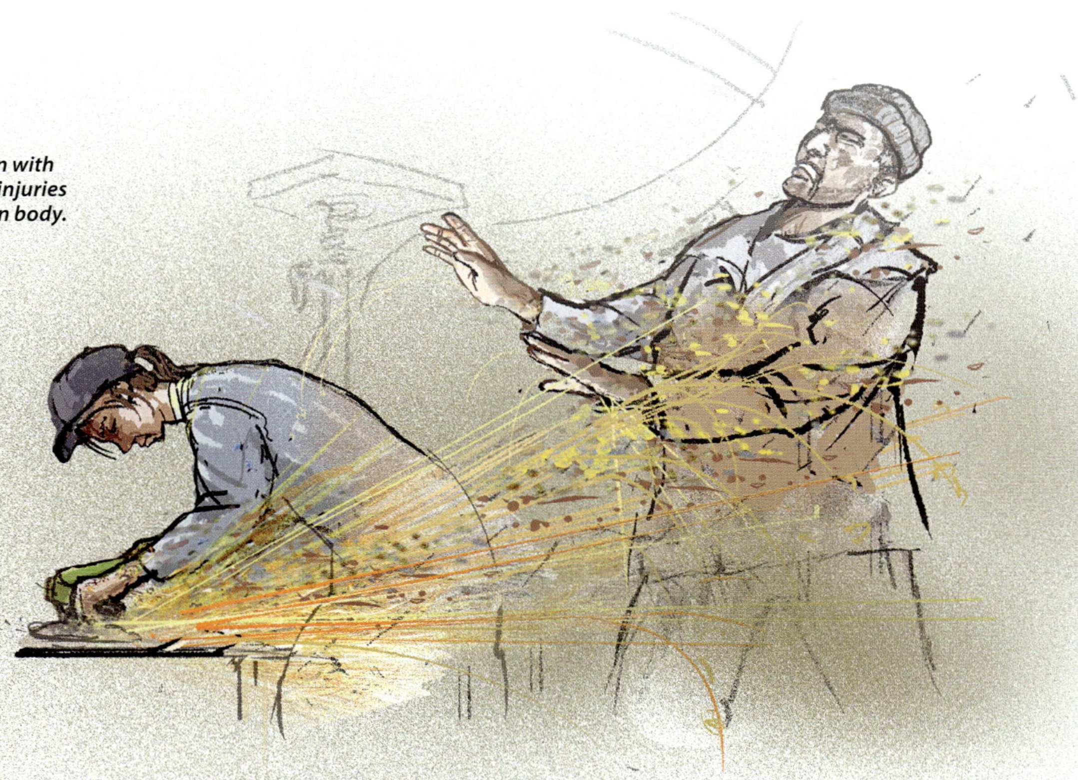

Typical situation with high risk of eye injuries such as a foreign body.

Immediate action

- Remove any visible particle.
- Rinse the eye thoroughly with lukewarm water under a tap or use an eye bath.
- If rinsing fails, locate the particle by having the person look in different directions.

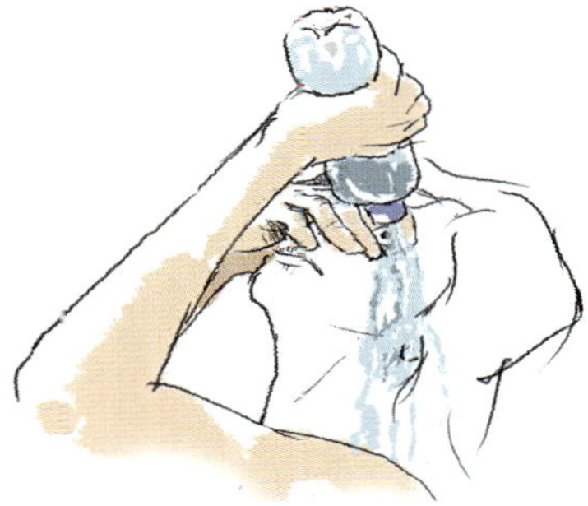

Rinse the eye with water. Use drinking water if it is the best available source.

Treatment

If the particle is behind the lower lid:

- Wash your hands or use gloves.
- Pull the lower eyelid downwards and inspect.
- Remove the particle using a damp cotton swab or clean stick.
- If the particle is not found, ask the person to look vigorously in all directions (up, down, right, left) to locate it.

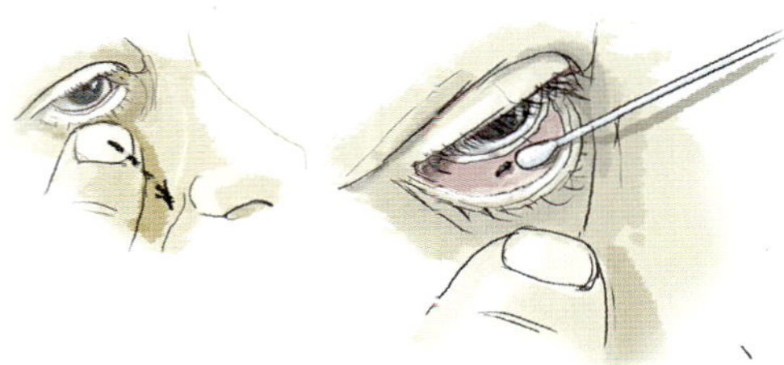

Removal of a foreign body behind the lower lid.

If the particle is behind the upper eyelid:

1. Dry around the eye.
2. Ask the person to look downwards with open eyes.
3. Grab the eyelashes and pull the eyelid downwards/outwards to release it from the eye.
4. At the same time, press downwards on the soft upper part of the eyelid with a cotton swab.
5. Gently and slowly pull the eyelid upwards to turn it inside out.
6. Remove the particle using a cotton swab.

Apply lubricating eye ointment afterwards. If unsuccessful, seek medical attention.

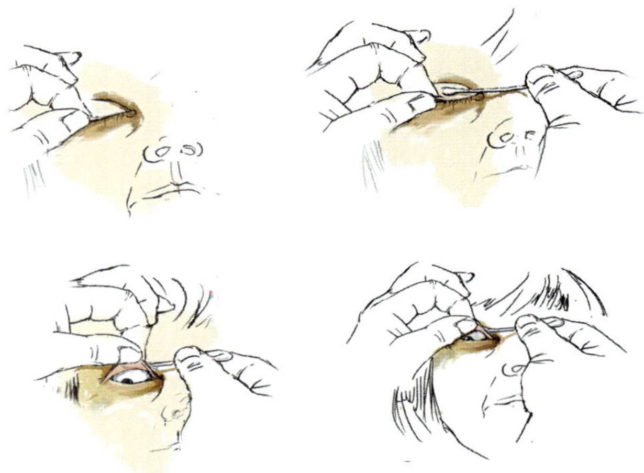

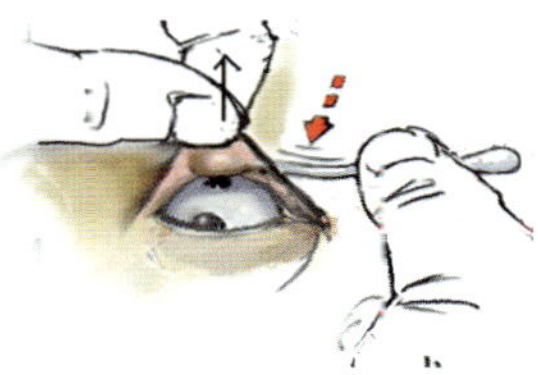

Technique for turning the upper eyelid.

Far from help

Use your communication equipment to seek advice from an eye specialist. If vision is intact, the advice is likely to use eye ointment until you reach the port and can consult a doctor.

Prevention

Always use protective glasses when performing activities that risk eye injuries.

EYE INJURY

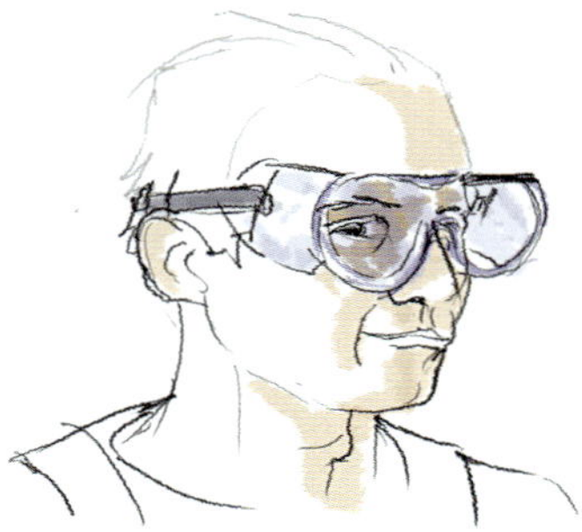

Protective glasses: simple and effective prevention.

TRAUMATIC NON-CHEMICAL INJURIES

An eye can be injured by sharp objects such as a knife or a tree branch, or through blunt trauma caused by a snapping line, a ball, or other blunt objects. Injuries may range from superficial scratches on the conjunctiva to severe penetrating or blunt injuries requiring urgent surgery.

Immediate action

- Cover the injured eye and apply antibiotic ointment or drops until examination by an eye specialist.
- Seek medical advice immediately, as vision may be at risk.

Far from help

- Options may be limited. Advice from a specialist will be needed.
- Evacuation might be necessary, especially if vision is affected.

CHEMICALS

Accidents involving corrosive or unknown liquids in the eye require immediate attention.

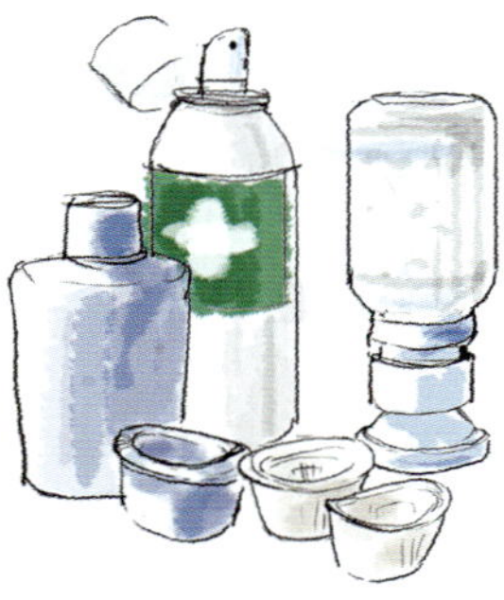

Thorough rinsing after chemical exposure using running tap water or an eye bath.

Immediate action

- Rinse the eye immediately and continuously with a large volume (2–3 litres) of lukewarm water for at least 20 to 30 minutes.
- For the best effect, let the water flow gently while blinking repeatedly.
- Alternatively, use an eye bath.

Treatment

- Apply lubricating ointment or drops.
- Seek medical attention on the same day.

Far from help

Seek advice from a specialist.

Prevention

Always use protective glasses when working with fluids containing irritants.

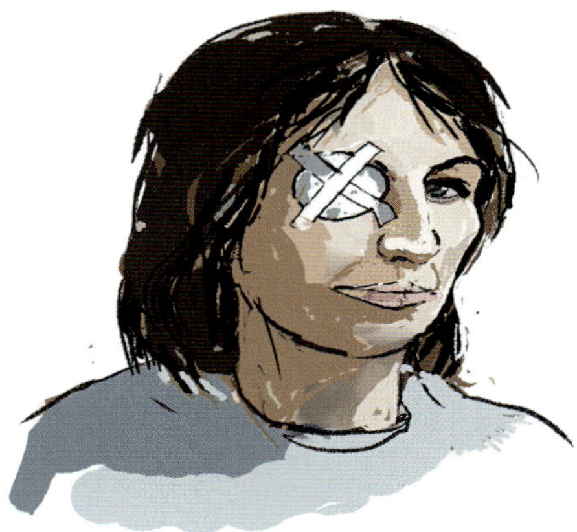

An injured eye is covered by a patch or a clean compress fixed by surgical tape.

CAUTION: Vision problems requiring immediate specialist examination

- Certain conditions pose a risk of permanent vision loss and require urgent evaluation by a specialist.

ACUTE GLAUCOMA

Glaucoma results from increased pressure inside the eye, which damages the optic nerve.

Signs and symptoms

- Unilateral redness, itching, irritation and watery eyes
- Severe headache, vision disturbances, eye pain and nausea/vomiting
- A dilated pupil that does not react to light.

RETINAL DETACHMENT

A sudden, painless condition that can lead to permanent vision loss.

Signs and symptoms

- A noticeable increase in eye floaters
- Light flashes in the peripheral vision
- A shadow appearing in the field of vision

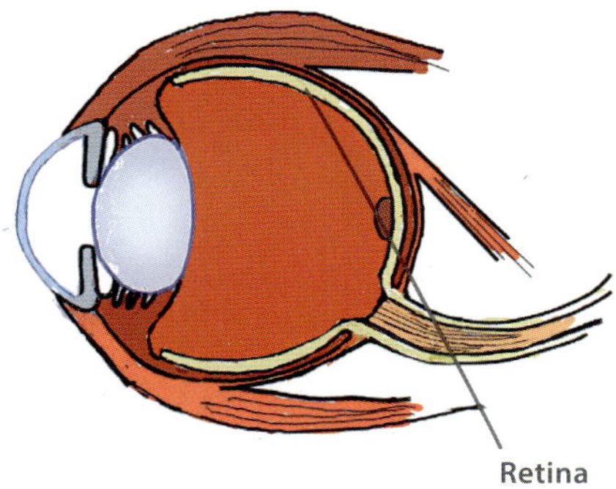

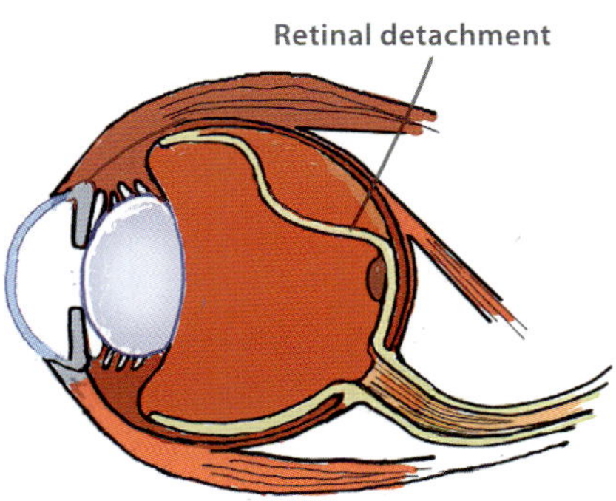

MACULAR DEGENERATION

A sudden, painless change in vision affecting the central field of view.

Signs and symptoms

- Blurred central vision
- Distorted or deformed contours/lines

Far from help

For acute glaucoma, retinal detachment or macular degeneration, immediate intervention is essential to prevent blindness.

- Use communication equipment to seek advice from a specialist.
- Protect the eye with an eye patch until professional care is available.

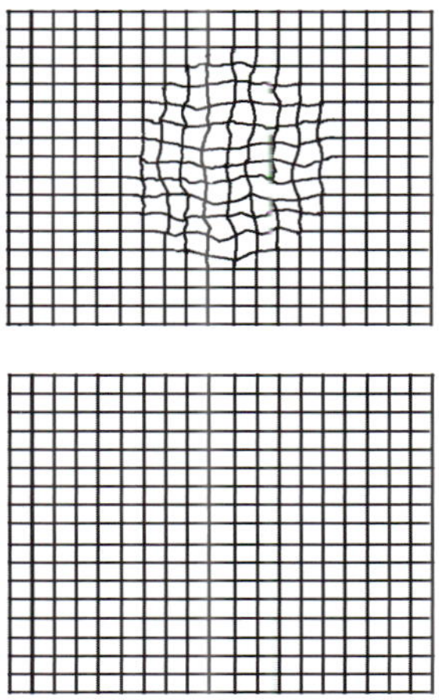

Macular degeneration. Typical early pattern, straight contours become curved.

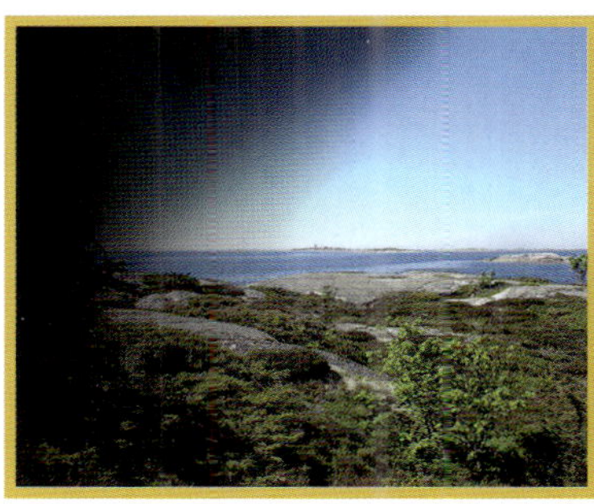

Typical vision field in retinal detachment.

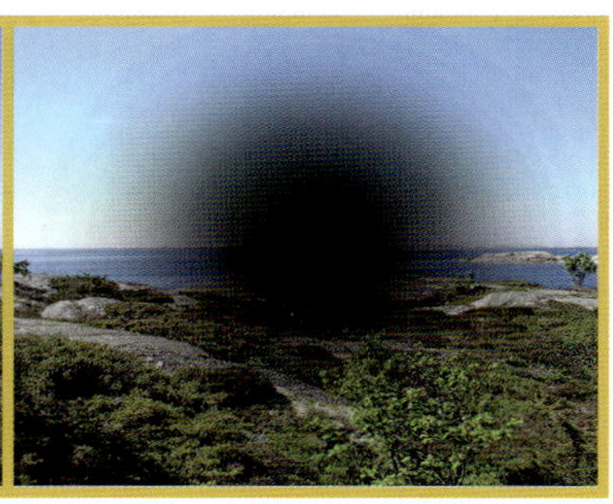

Typical alterations of vision in macular degeneration.

11. CARDIOVASCULAR PROBLEMS

Acute chest pain in myocardial infarction. Call for immediate help!

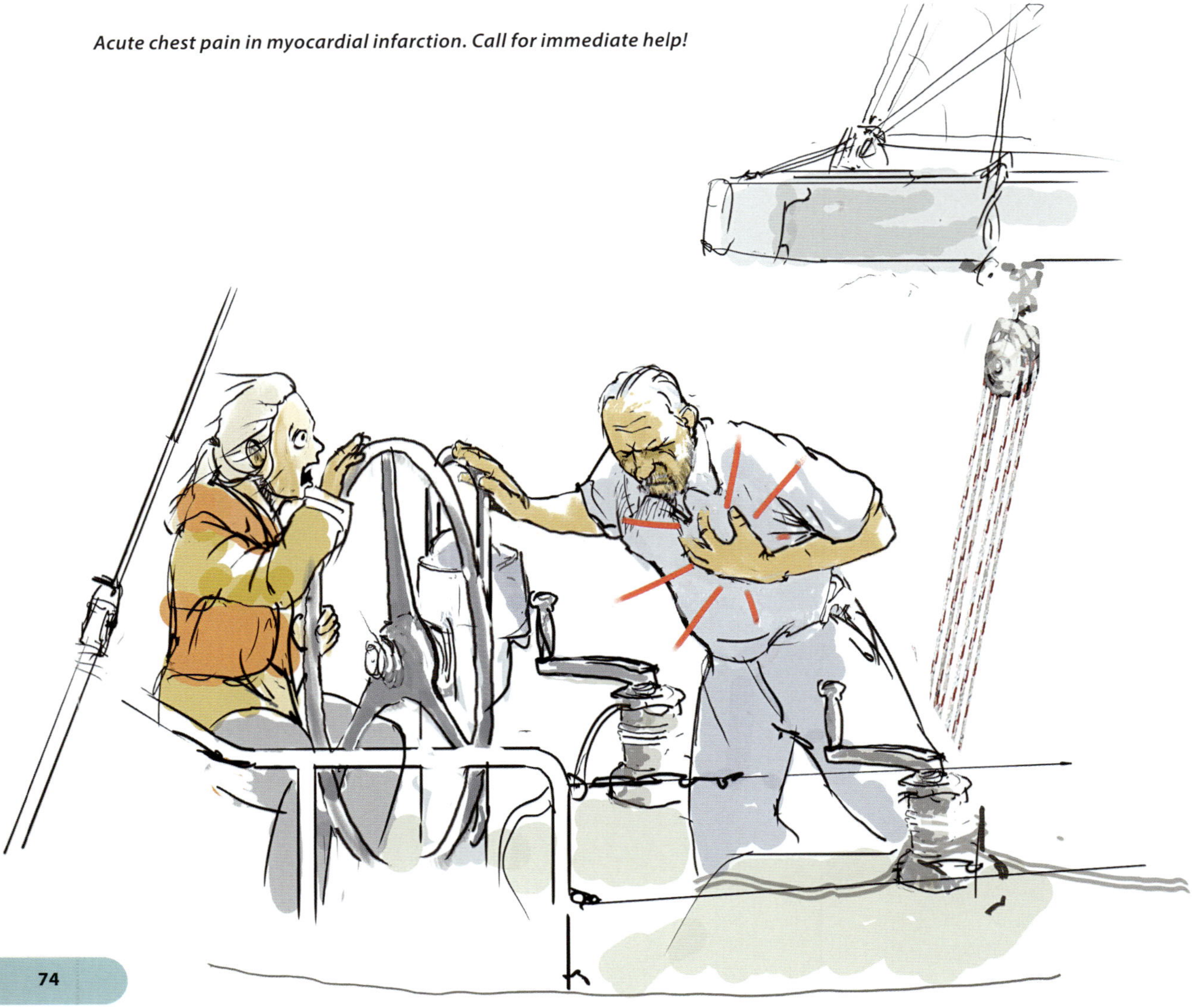

The cardiovascular system comprises the heart, arteries and veins. While they are functionally interconnected, they are structurally distinct and are therefore susceptible to different pathological conditions. In the arteries, arteriosclerosis is the predominant issue, whereas in the venous system, coagulation disorders and other physiological disturbances are more common.

The arteries deliver oxygenated blood to all parts of the body, while the veins return deoxygenated blood to the heart and lungs for filtration and reoxygenation before starting a new cycle.

The human cardiovascular system. Red – arteries. Blue – veins.

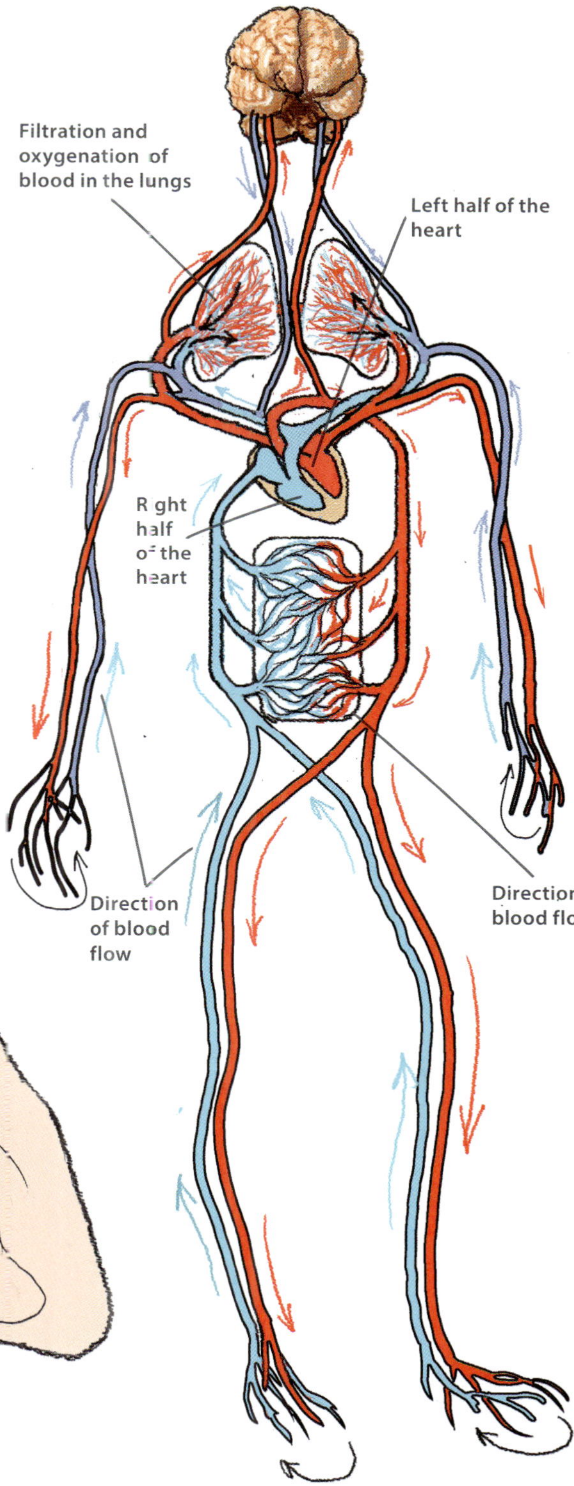

The heart is a complex pump with a smart system of valves, making it possible to run two different but parallel blood circuits. Red – oxygenated blood. Blue – oxygen-depleted blood.

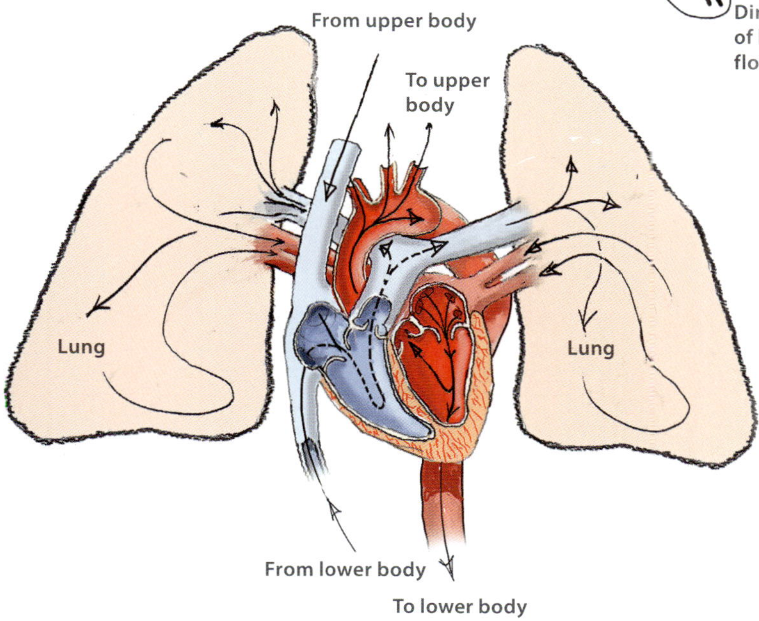

ATHEROSCLEROSIS

The most significant problem affecting arteries and the heart is atherosclerosis, a chronic condition that does not occur in veins. Atherosclerosis involves the gradual build-up of plaques composed of fat and calcium. A plaque may rupture due to high blood pressure and turbulent blood flow, releasing debris and clots that form emboli. These emboli are a common cause of myocardial infarction (MI), stroke, and acute leg ischaemia (see pages 76, 79 and 80).

Another potential source of arterial emboli is the heart, particularly in cases of atrial fibrillation. During fibrillation, small amounts of blood may stagnate in folds of the heart muscle, allowing clots to form. If a clot is dislodged, it can travel through the bloodstream as an embolus.

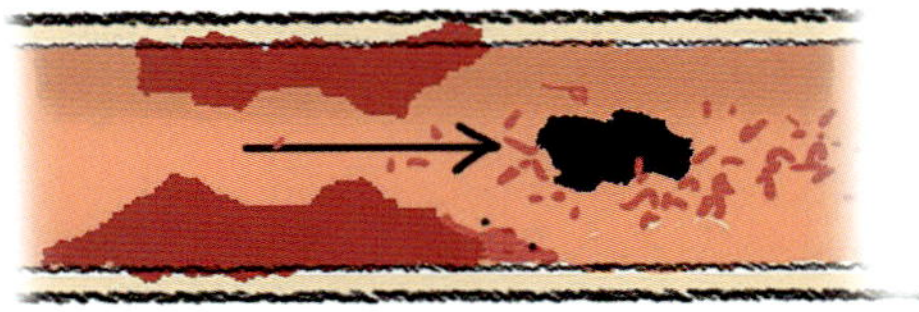

Plaque rupture: debris and clots form emboli, causing acute ischaemia by blocking an artery further downstream.

RISK FACTORS FOR ARTERIOSCLEROSIS

- Age > 60 years
- Smoking
- Diabetes
- Obesity
- Hypertension
- Hyperlipidaemia
- Hereditary predisposition

MYOCARDIAL INFARCTION (MI)

MI remains the leading cause of death in developed countries. The risk increases with age and is further exacerbated by conditions such as diabetes and obesity. MI is typically caused by plaque rupture and subsequent embolisation in a coronary artery branch, depriving a section of the heart muscle of oxygen. This results in impaired pump function and irregular contractions.

MI – acute chest pain (angina), general symptoms, pain, nausea, shortness of breath, anxiety. Always alarming!

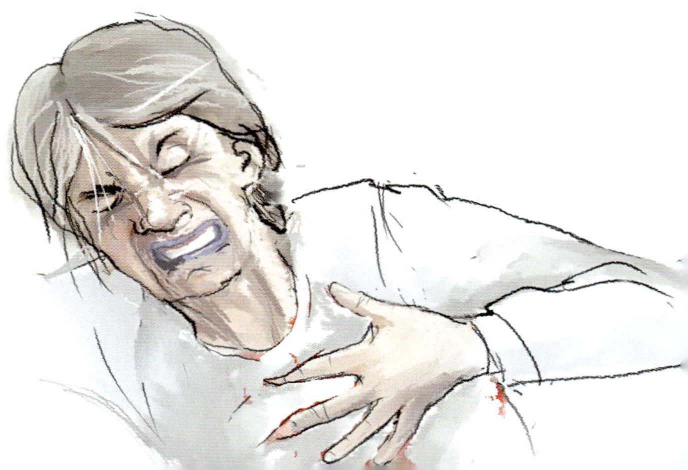

Signs and symptoms

An MI is often preceded by physical or emotional stress.

Typical symptoms of MI include:

- central chest pain, often described as a tightening band around the chest
- pain radiating to the neck, jaw, left shoulder or arm
- general symptoms such as shortness of breath, nausea, vomiting, fatigue and irregular cardiac rhythm

In cases of a large MI, signs of shock may develop. Note: Symptoms in women can be less pronounced or atypical.

Other potential causes of chest pain include oesophagitis and pulmonary embolism (see pages 100 and 86). However, MI must always be ruled out first.

Immediate action

- Place the person in a calm, warm and peaceful location.
- Make an emergency call and request immediate transport to a hospital.

Treatment

- Assess the person's general condition, pulse and breathing. Look for signs of shock.
- If a vasodilator such as nitroglycerine is available, administer it.
- Position the person in the cardiac position: elevate the upper body by 30–45 degrees, with the knees slightly bent and supported by pillows.
- Follow the advice provided by emergency services.

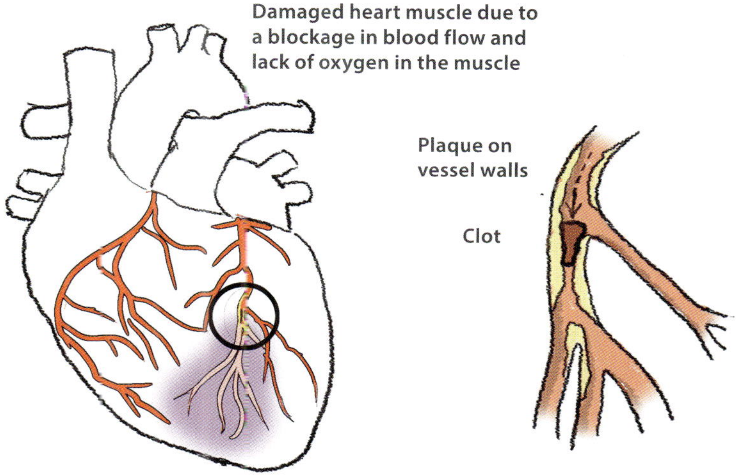

Mechanism behind MI. Blockage of a coronary artery, causing ischaemia in part of the heart muscle with secondary effect on pump function.

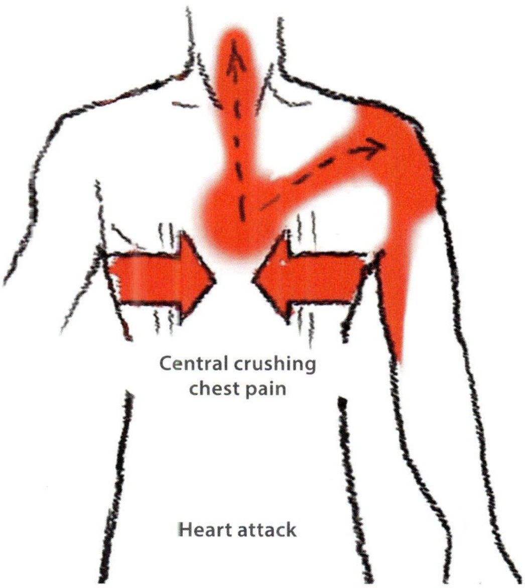

Typical distribution of pain in MI/angina.

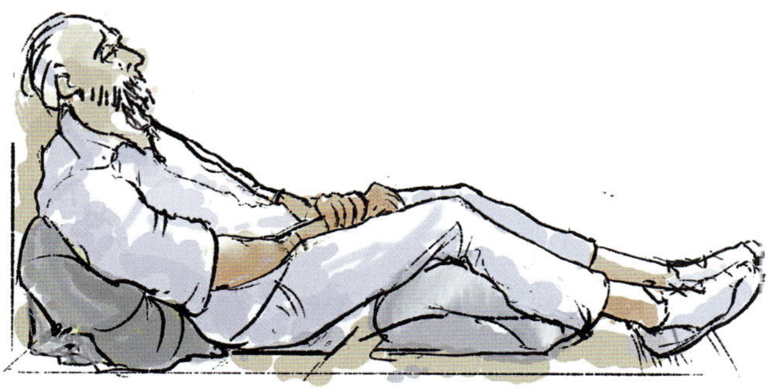

Cardiac position facilitating respiration. Upper body elevated 30–45 degrees, knees slightly bent supported by pillows.

Far from help

If evacuation is not immediately possible:

- Administer aspirin if available, as these can reduce clot formation.
- Provide an analgesic and/or a sedative, such as an opioid if available.
- Monitor for progression to severe shock or cardiac arrest. In such cases, refer to pages 14 and 20 for CPR guidance and protocols for handling life-threatening situations.

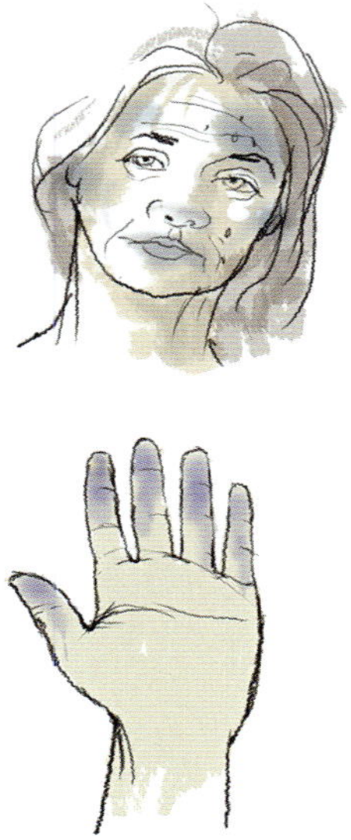

Signs of shock: cold sweat, cyanotic lips, face and fingertips.

Prevention

Individuals with a history of cardiovascular disease should consult their cardiologist to assess the risks of embarking on an adventurous cruise.

As the captain, you are responsible for deciding whether the individual should join the crew and ensuring they have access to necessary medications.

General prevention of arteriosclerosis includes:

- quitting smoking
- maintaining a healthy diet
- regular physical exercise
- using preventive medications for clot formation and high blood pressure when prescribed

Should you bring an AED (defibrillator)?

This decision should be made in consultation with a cardiologist. On longer ocean crossings, the prognosis remains poor for cardiac arrest without immediate intensive care and surgical interventions. The geographic location and available evacuation resources are critical factors in determining the outcome.

The four links in the chain of survival during cardiac arrest:

1. *Recognise early symptoms such as chest pain. Emergency evacuation of the individual at this stage offers the best prognosis.*
2. *In the event of cardiac arrest, begin CPR within three minutes. Each minute of delay reduces survival chances by 10 per cent.*
3. *Use a defibrillator within three minutes if ventricular fibrillation is the cause.*
4. *Arrange immediate transport to a hospital for surgery and intensive care.*

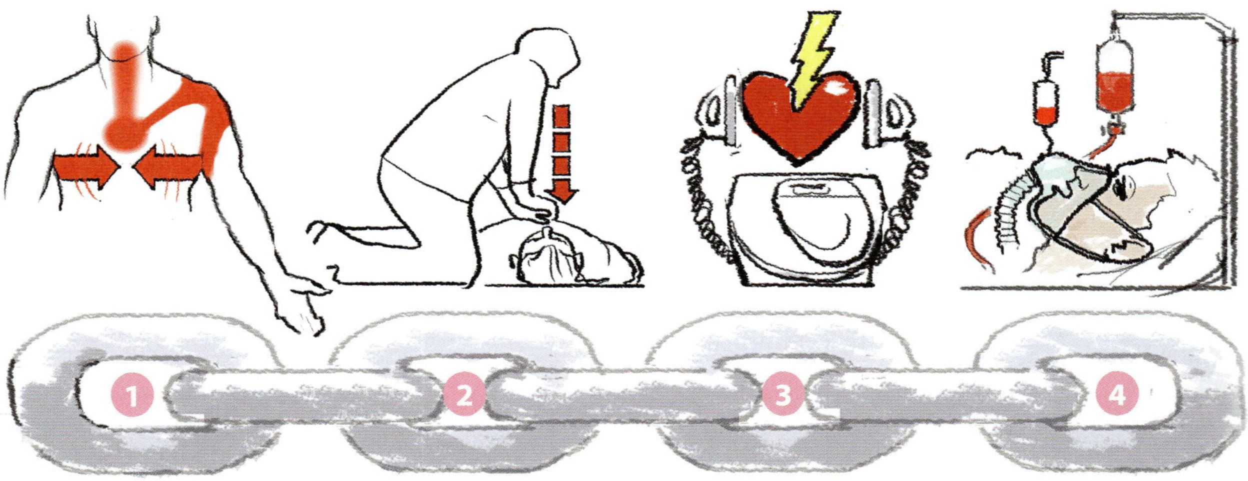

The chain of survival.

STROKE

Most strokes are caused by atherosclerosis and an arterial embolus originating either from the carotid artery, which supplies the brain with oxygenated blood, or from a fibrillating heart. These are referred to as embolic strokes, which are our primary focus. A less common type is a haemorrhagic stroke (see box on page 80).

Arteriosclerotic plaques commonly develop in arterial branches, such as those in the carotid artery. Fragments of a plaque can travel through the bloodstream to the brain, where they occlude an arterial branch, leading to reduced oxygenation in the affected part of the brain.

Signs and symptoms

Stroke symptoms usually have a sudden onset and may include one or more of the following, listed in order of frequency:

- weakness in an arm, a leg, or the entire left or right side of the body
- difficulty speaking or finding words – dysphasia
- facial paralysis, such as a drooping corner of the mouth
- vision problems or temporary blindness, often described as 'like a curtain being raised again after a while'

Note: Headache is not typically associated with embolic strokes.

Immediate action

- Ensure the individual rests in a chair or lies down to avoid falling.
- Remain calm and create a calming environment.
- Perform these diagnostic tests (right).
- If these tests indicate that a stroke is likely, make an emergency call immediately and arrange urgent transportation to hospital.

Modern invasive treatments can significantly improve outcomes for embolic strokes if performed early, within four hours of symptom onset.

Symptoms of stroke or a TIA.

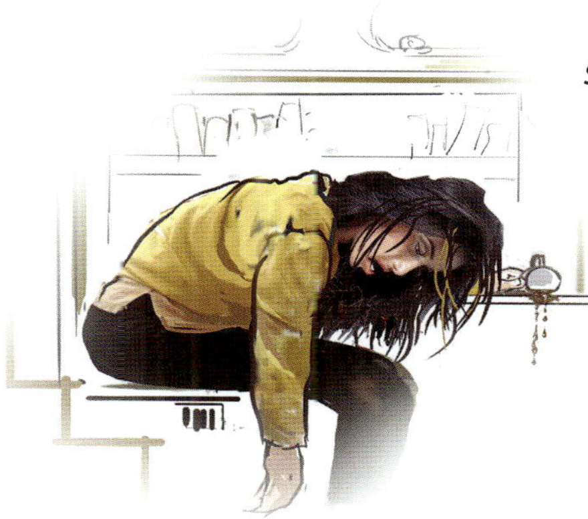

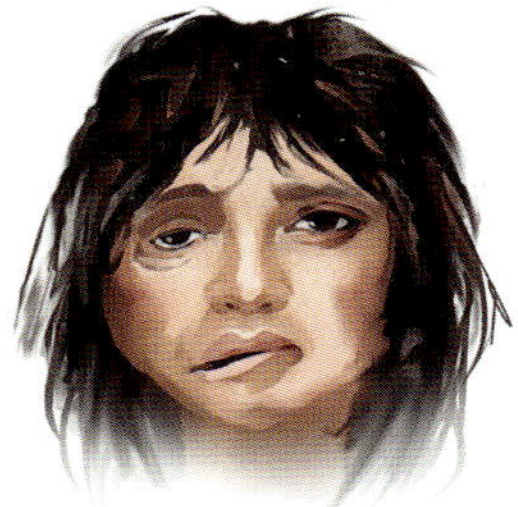

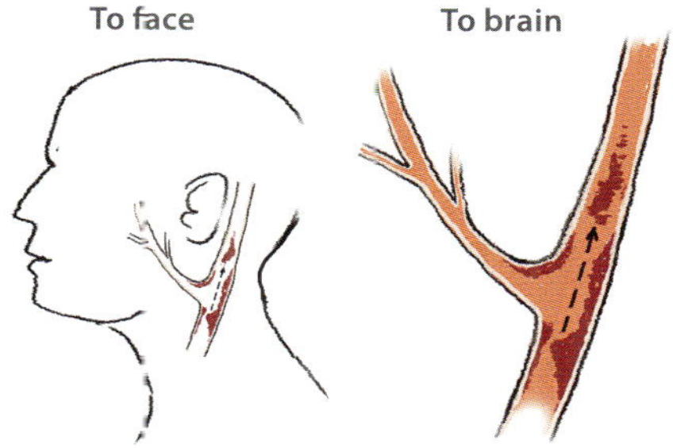

Arteriosclerosis (plaque). Disintegrating small fragments break loose into a clot.

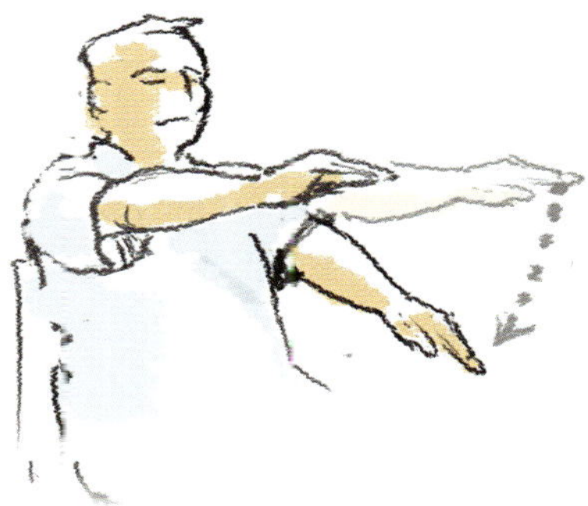

1. Ask the person to hold both arms straight out in front for one minute. If one arm falls earlier, this indicates an acute neurological event – a stroke.

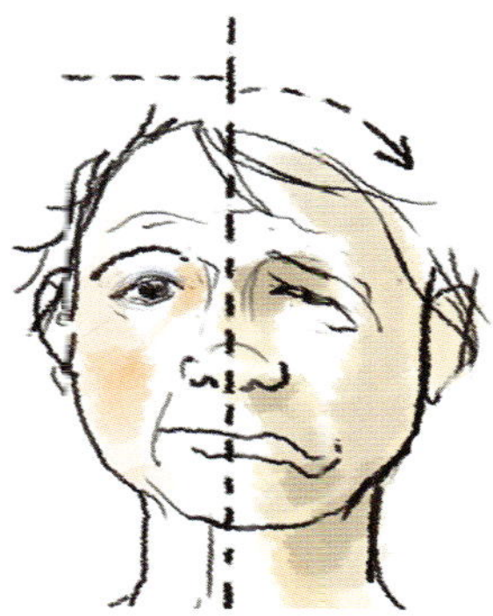

Facial paresis on one side

2. Check for asymmetry of the face. Ask the person to smile or stick out their tongue.

3. Finally, ask the person to say: 'The sun is shining today'. If they fail any of these tests, a stroke is likely. The person requires urgent transportation to hospital. Make an emergency call immediately.

Treatment

- Keep the person warm, calm and reassured.
- Allow them to choose a comfortable position.
- If needed, anxiety can be alleviated with a sedative.
- For pain relief, administer paracetamol. Avoid other analgesics with anticoagulant effects unless professional advice confirms the absence of a haemorrhagic stroke.

Far from help

Managing a fully developed stroke in a remote setting is highly challenging.

- Arrange evacuation as soon as possible.
- Seek medical advice by any available means.
- Provide comfort and care.
- Administer pain relief and sedatives as outlined above.

Prevention

Individuals with atrial fibrillation should be assessed for the need for anticoagulant or antiplatelet medication, which can prevent embolisation in most cases.

For general prevention measures, see page 78 under 'Myocardial infarction'.

TRANSIENT ISCHAEMIC ATTACK

A transient ischaemic attack (TIA) occurs when very small emboli travel to a part of the brain with robust collateral blood supply. Symptoms are similar to those of a stroke but resolve completely within minutes or up to 24 hours.

A TIA is a warning sign of a potential imminent major stroke, and hospital evaluation the same day is essential.

HAEMORRHAGIC STROKES

Haemorrhagic strokes are less common and are often related to uncontrolled hypertension or vascular malformations. They occur due to bleeding from a ruptured blood vessel.

Neurological symptoms are similar to those of an embolic stroke, but a headache, often severe, is more typical.

Important: Avoid analgesics with anticoagulant effects, such as aspirin or ibuprofen, without professional advice. A sedative may be given if necessary.

ACUTE ISCHAEMIA (ARTERIAL EMBOLUS IN A LEG)

It is important to recognise acute ischaemia caused by an arterial embolus, as it is potentially a very serious condition requiring urgent hospital treatment.

The most common cause is an embolus originating from a fibrillating heart.

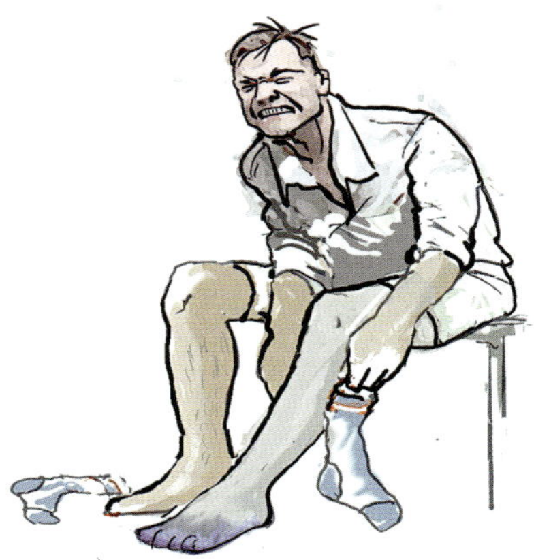

Acute severe ischaemia in one leg.

Signs and symptoms

The most characteristic symptom is acute, often sudden, severe pain in the foot and calf. However, the severity and presentation may vary depending on the size and location of the embolus.

Always compare the affected side with the unaffected side.

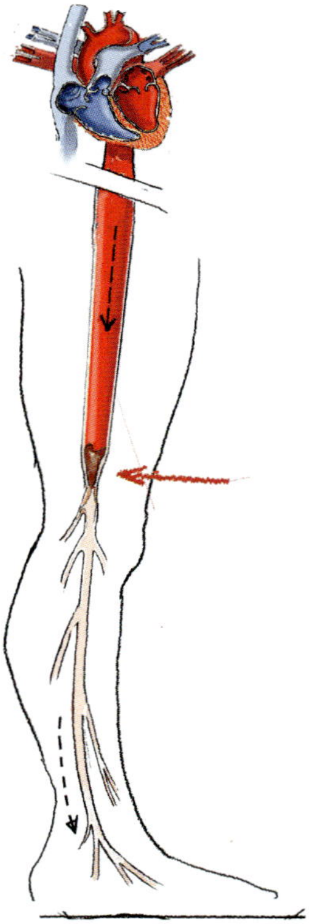

An embolus lodged in the knee artery causes acute ischaemia, leading to a lack of blood supply and oxygen, with sudden severe pain in the foot and calf.

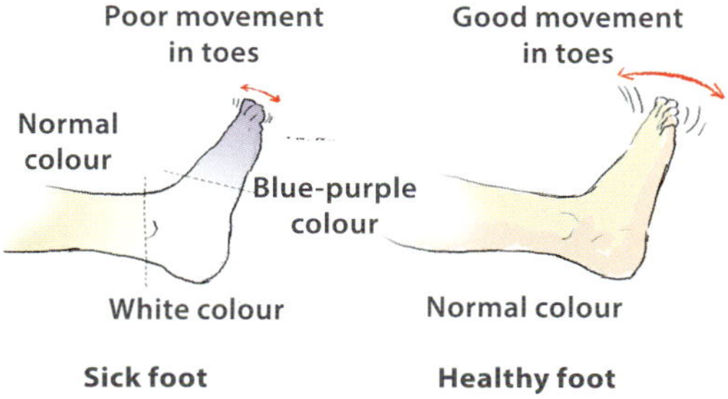

In a typical case, the ischaemic foot appears pale, white, or even cyanotic (blue). Movement of the toes is normal on the unaffected side but absent on the ischaemic side.

Check sensation and temperature.

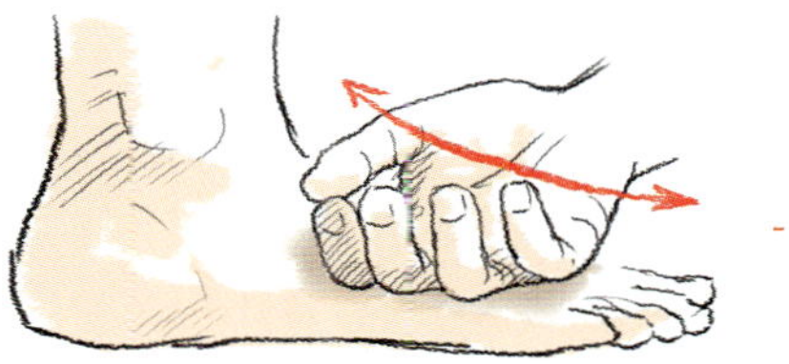

Use the back of your hand to compare temperature and sensitivity. An ischaemic foot is cold, and the sense of touch is diminished.

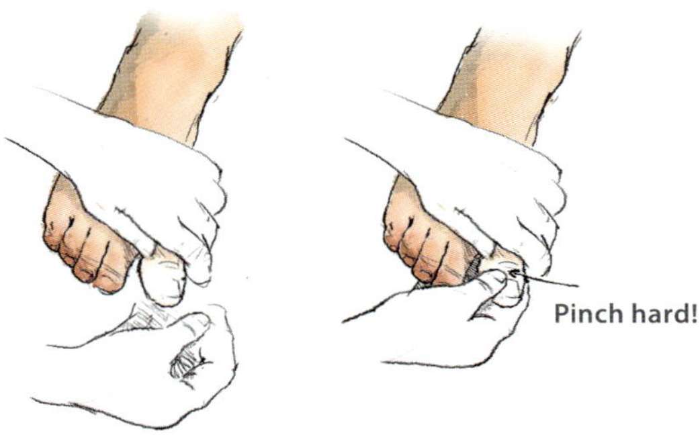

Capillary refill test: Press the big toe firmly between your thumb and index finger. On release, the nail bed will initially appear white but should normally return to pink within seconds if circulation is adequate. Compare with the unaffected side. Delayed return of colour indicates ischaemia.

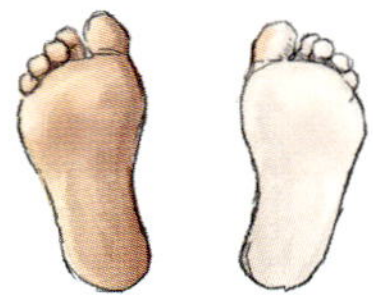

After a few minutes, a colour change begins to occur.

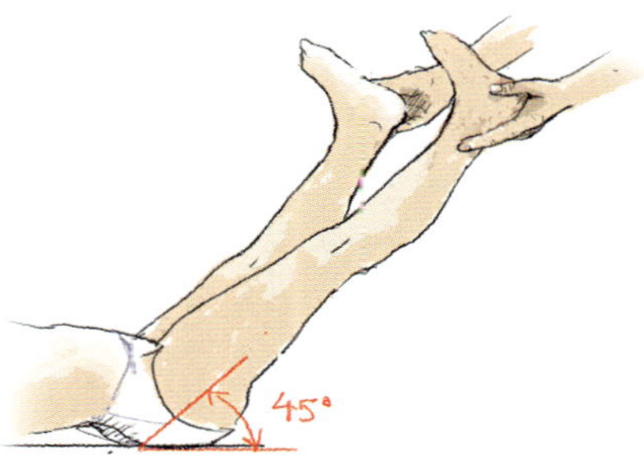

An elevation test is useful in less obvious cases. Elevate both legs to 45 degrees for two minutes while observing the colour of the soles. The ischaemic foot will turn white, while the unaffected foot retains its normal colour.

Immediate action

- Ensure the person rests to prevent falls due to impaired leg function.
- Examine the individual as described above.
- Seek professional medical support and guidance.
- Limb-threatening acute ischaemia usually requires emergency intervention within four to six hours.
- Prepare for evacuation.

Treatment

- Administer analgesics, as opioids will likely be needed.
- Aspirin may have a beneficial effect by inhibiting platelets and reducing further clot formation.

Far from help

This presents an extremely challenging situation if medical assistance is delayed for days. You may need to manage:

- Severe pain.
- The onset of gangrene.
- Progressive failure of vital functions.
- Provide care, warmth (blankets), fluids, and analgesics. Sedatives, if available, can also help. sedatives as outlined above.

Immediate evacuation is essential.

Prevention

See page 78 under 'Myocardial infarction'. If you have atrial fibrillation, consult your GP regarding preventive medication.

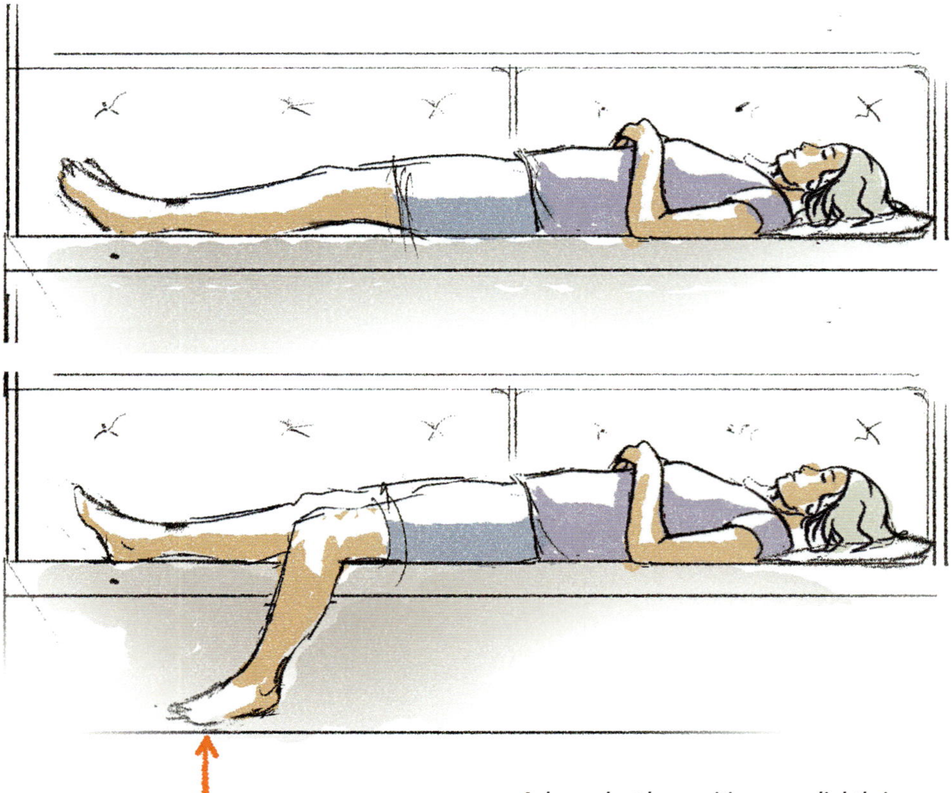

A dependent leg position may slightly improve blood supply and is often preferred by patients with acute or chronic ischaemia.

RUPTURED AORTIC ANEURYSM

An aneurysm is defined as a localised dilation of a blood vessel, most commonly in the aorta between the renal arteries and the pelvic branches. The primary cause is a pathological process, most commonly atherosclerosis, often linked to smoking, high blood pressure, or genetic factors that weaken the vessel wall.

The associated risk is that the aneurysm may increase in size and eventually rupture, causing life-threatening bleeding.

Signs and symptoms

An aortic aneurysm is usually asymptomatic until it ruptures. Symptoms of rupture typically include:

- sudden onset of severe abdominal and back pain
- signs of shock, such as cold sweat and fainting

Rupture is often triggered by severe coughing, heavy lifting or straining, which increases intra-abdominal pressure.

Immediate action

- Lay the person flat and keep them warm.
- Call for immediate transport to a hospital.
- If shock progresses and the person becomes unconscious, try lowering their head and elevating their legs.
- For the recovery position, see page 16.

Far from help

If left untreated, the mortality rate is close to 100 per cent within 24 to 48 hours. If evacuation or professional help is unavailable within this time frame, you will have to provide end-of-life care for a dying crew-mate.

Prevention

Men over 65, with a family history of ruptured aortic aneurysms, who smoke or have high blood pressure, should consider an ultrasound screening of the aorta, especially if planning long voyages.

If a large aneurysm (diameter > 5cm) is detected, discuss the benefits of surgical repair. Although less common, the condition can also occur in women.

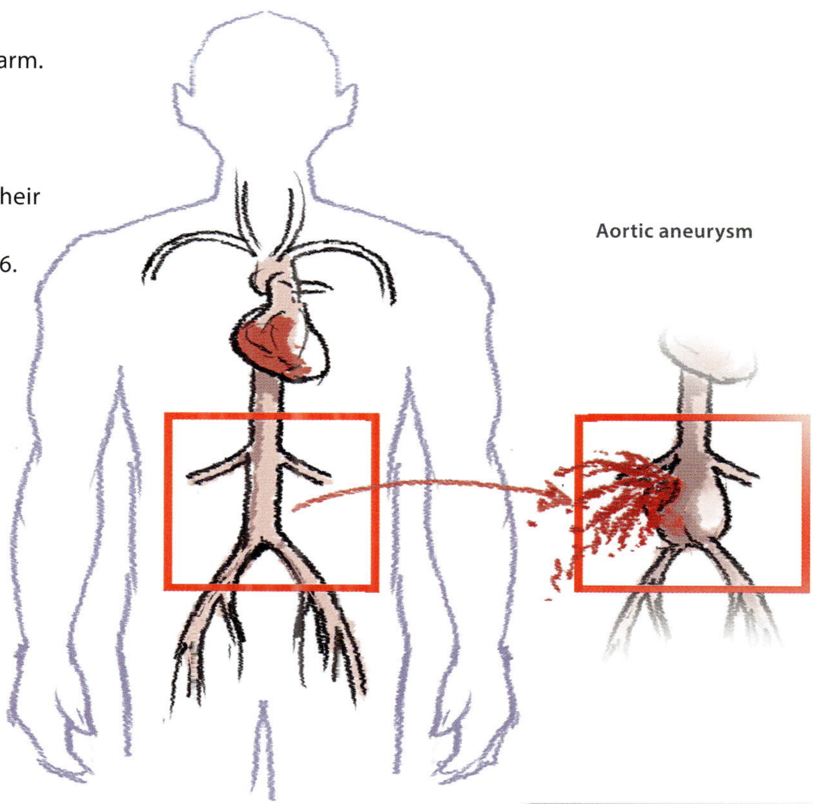

The most common location of an aortic aneurysm. Left: Normal aorta. Right: Aorta with a ruptured large aneurysm.

VENOUS DISORDERS

The body contains numerous superficial subcutaneous veins, but they rarely cause significant problems. When discussing venous issues, the primary concern is with the larger veins located deeper in the body. Blood flow and pressure in veins is much lower than in arteries. Hyperactive coagulation and reduced blood flow are the main concerns in venous problems.

DEEP VEIN THROMBOSIS (DVT)

When blood flow is impaired – for example, by obesity, pregnancy, or a condition compressing a vein – and/or when the coagulation system is overactivated, as seen in smokers or with oral contraceptive use, conditions arise that can allow the formation of a clot, or venous thrombosis.

Immobility, such as during long flights or prolonged sitting in a boat cockpit, can also increase the risk of venous thrombosis. DVT most often occurs in the legs or pelvic veins.

Signs and symptoms

The onset of DVT is typically slow, developing over hours or even days. Symptoms include:

- leg swelling that varies depending on the location and size of the thrombus
- a feeling of heaviness and dull pain
- tenderness around the area of the thrombus

Diagnosing DVT is challenging and requires blood tests, ultrasound or venogram for confirmation.

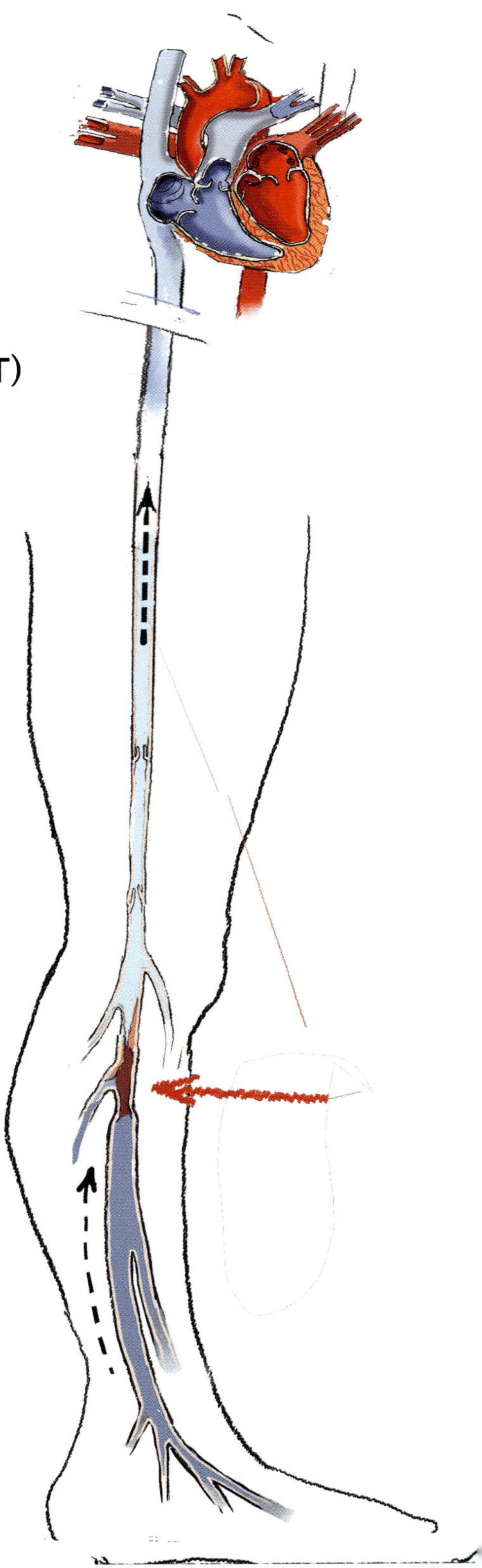

A thrombus in a deep calf vein obstructs the return blood flow from the foot, leading to swelling and increased foot temperature.

MYTH BUSTER

Swelling in one leg is very common and is not always indicative of venous thrombosis. Common causes include immobilisation, prolonged sitting or standing, or minor issues with venous valves causing increased backflow.

Immediate action

Immediate action is usually unnecessary unless directed under treatment recommendations (see below).

Treatment

The best course of action is to have the diagnosis confirmed by a doctor within a day. While awaiting medical confirmation:

- Apply a compression bandage (see image). It is best to do this in the morning before leaving bed, when the swelling is minimal.
- If antithrombotic medications such as NSAIDs are available on board, they may be used.
- Pain relief can be provided with aspirin or paracetamol.

Final treatment often involves anticoagulants, sometimes clot-dissolving agents, and the use of compression stockings.

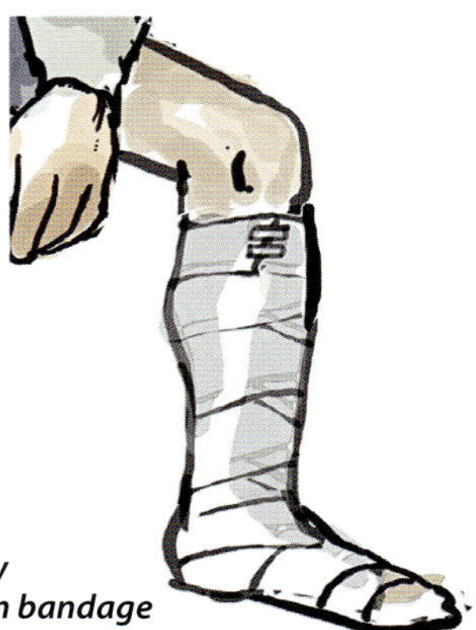

A temporary compression bandage applied for suspected deep vein thrombosis.

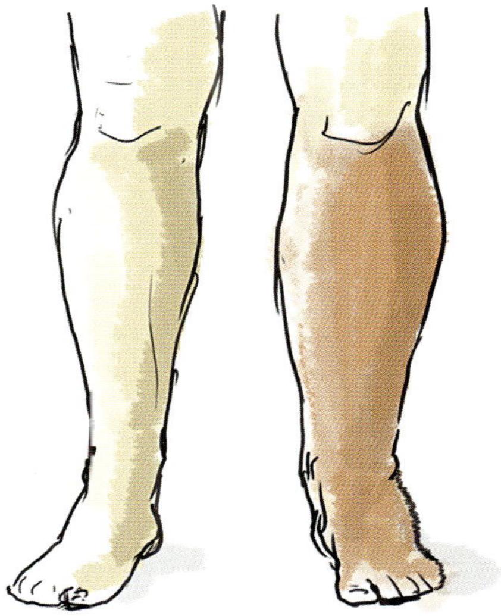

Swelling in the left leg caused by a venous thrombosis at knee level. The leg is warm and red, and superficial veins are prominent.

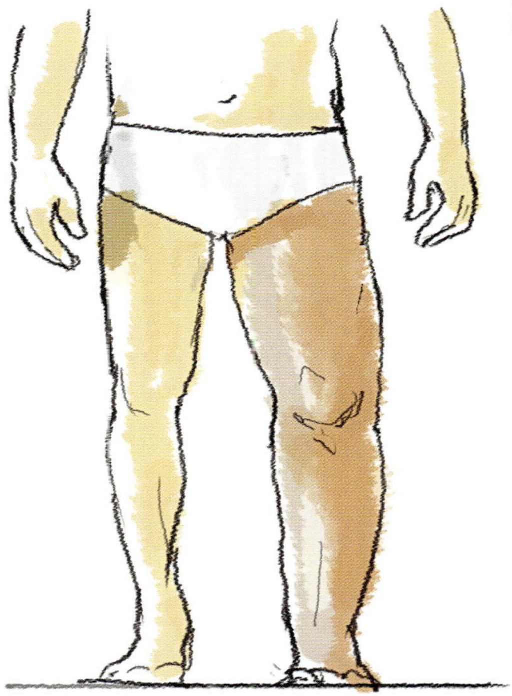

A thrombus in a pelvic vein causes swelling of the entire leg.

Far from help

- Seek medical guidance as soon as possible.
- Follow the advice on compression, pain relief and medications to reduce clot formation.
- Be vigilant for symptoms of pulmonary embolism, such as sudden shortness of breath or chest pain (see below).

Prevention

- During long passages, avoid sitting still – MOVE around regularly!
- Consider wearing compression stockings.
- If you are pregnant, on oral contraceptives, undergoing hormone therapy, or have a chronic illness, consult your doctor about preventive measures if planning extended time at sea.

PULMONARY EMBOLISM

As in the arterial system, a venous thrombus can dislodge and move with the bloodstream, becoming a venous embolus. This typically involves a deep vein thrombosis in a leg or pelvic vein. The embolus travels with the venous blood through the heart and into the lungs, where it becomes lodged, causing a pulmonary embolism. This usually results in severe damage to the lung tissue and its vital function.

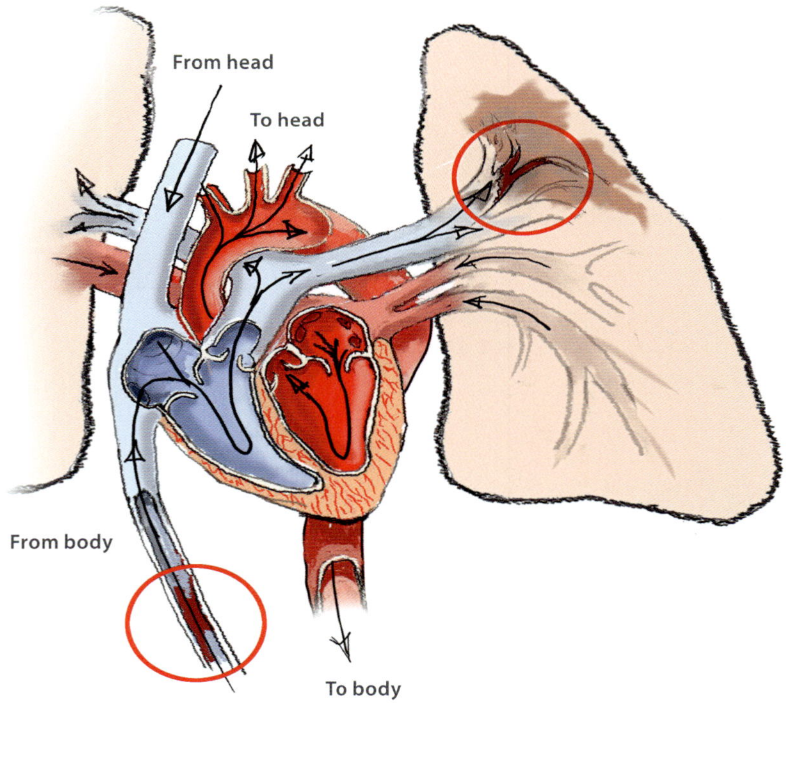

A venous thrombus has dislodged and travels with the venous blood through the right side of the heart and into the lungs. The affected part of the lung will suffer serious functional disturbances.

Signs and symptoms

Typical symptoms include:

- sudden onset of chest pain
- shortness of breath
- coughing
- dyspnoea
- painful breathing

If pulmonary embolism is suspected, it is important to check for signs of venous thrombosis in the legs.

Immediate action

If a pulmonary embolism is suspected, immediate contact with a hospital is essential. Diagnostic tests and emergency treatment are mandatory. Attempt to differentiate from other causes of chest pain, such as angina or myocardial infarction. Begin planning for evacuation.

Treatment

- Put the person at rest in a comfortable position.
- Provide warmth and reassurance.
- Administer an analgesic and a sedative.
- Use aspirin or an NSAID if available, due to their platelet-inhibiting effects.

Far from help

- Establish contact for medical guidance.
- Administer medication as described above under 'Treatment'.
- Position the person comfortably, often sitting and leaning backwards at approximately 30 degrees.
- A large embolus can be life-threatening – keep the person warm and provide comforting care.

Suggested positions for managing acute pulmonary problems.

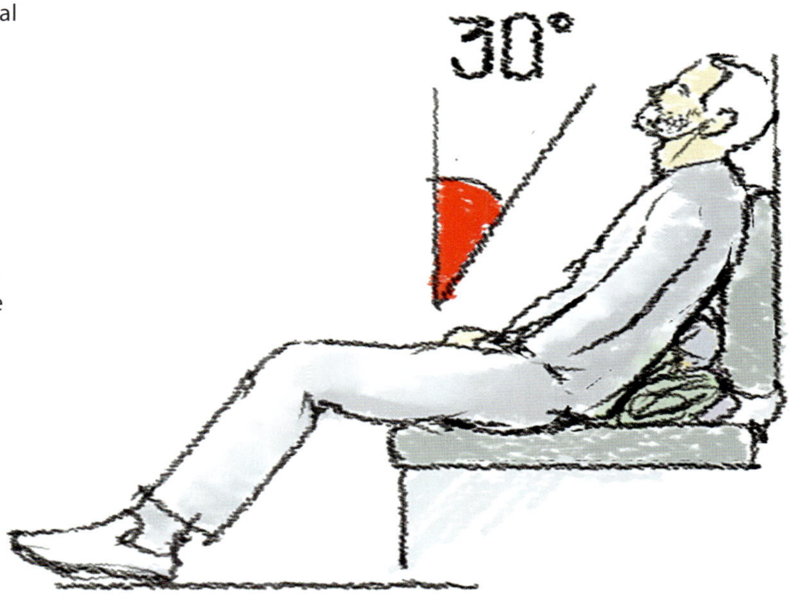

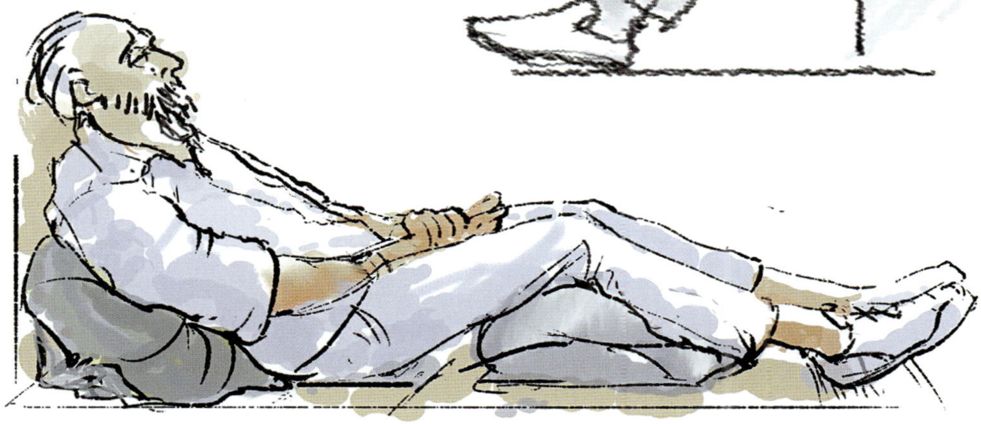

THROMBUS IN VARICOSE VEIN (THROMBOPHLEBITIS)

Varicose veins – dilated, winding superficial veins with defective valve function – are very common in the calves and thighs of adults. Low blood flow increases the risk of thrombus formation, resulting in painful inflammation around the occluded vein (thrombophlebitis). Fortunately, many other veins compensate for the function of the affected vein. A superficial thrombus in a varicose vein will not dislodge to become a pulmonary embolus.

Signs and symptoms

Typical location of varicose veins on the inside of the calf and thigh.

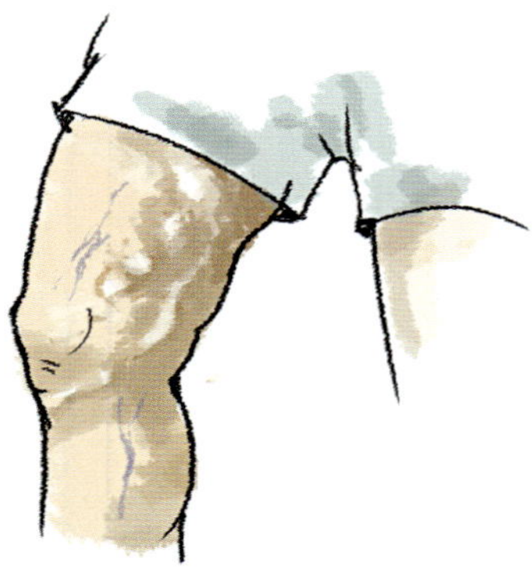

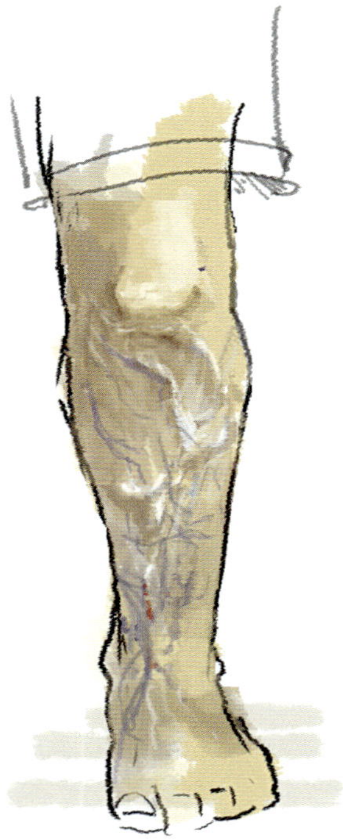

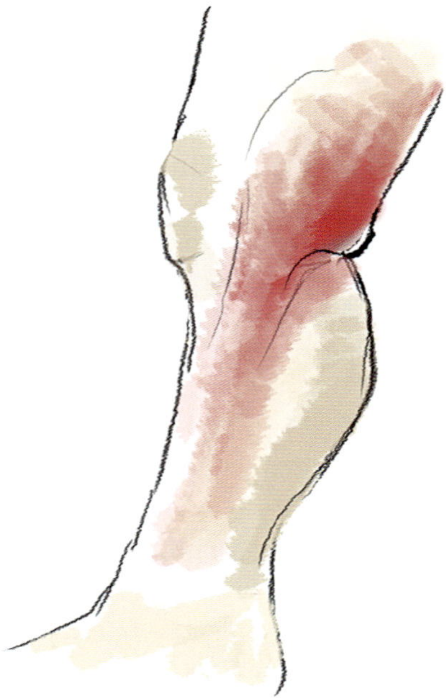

Thrombus in a varicose vein (thrombophlebitis) with prominent hard swelling, redness, tenderness and heat. The thrombosed vein can easily be felt under skin.

Immediate action

No immediate action is required beyond the treatment steps detailed opposite.

Far from help

See section under 'Treatment'.

Treatment

- Apply an anti-inflammatory cream or use anti-inflammatory tablets.
- Consult a doctor at the earliest convenience; this is rarely an emergency.
- Use a compression bandage or stocking.
- For pain relief, administer ibuprofen or paracetamol.

BLEEDING FROM A VARICOSE VEIN

The skin over a varicose vein is often thin, and minor skin trauma can result in bleeding, which may appear alarming.

Signs and symptoms

- Skin is perforated right over a bleeding varicose vein.

Immediate action

- The following steps are often highly effective:
- Lay the person down.
- Elevate the affected limb.
- Apply a pressure bandage for 15–20 minutes.

Treatment

Even if the bleeding stops, it is advisable to keep the pressure bandage on for at least a day. Occasionally, a minor surgical procedure may be necessary if the bleeding recurs.

Prevention

- Treat dry, brittle skin with ointments.
- Use protective and compression bandages if necessary.
- Consult a surgeon to discuss surgical or invasive treatment options for varicose veins.

Far from help

Follow the steps outlined under 'Immediate Action' and 'Treatment'.

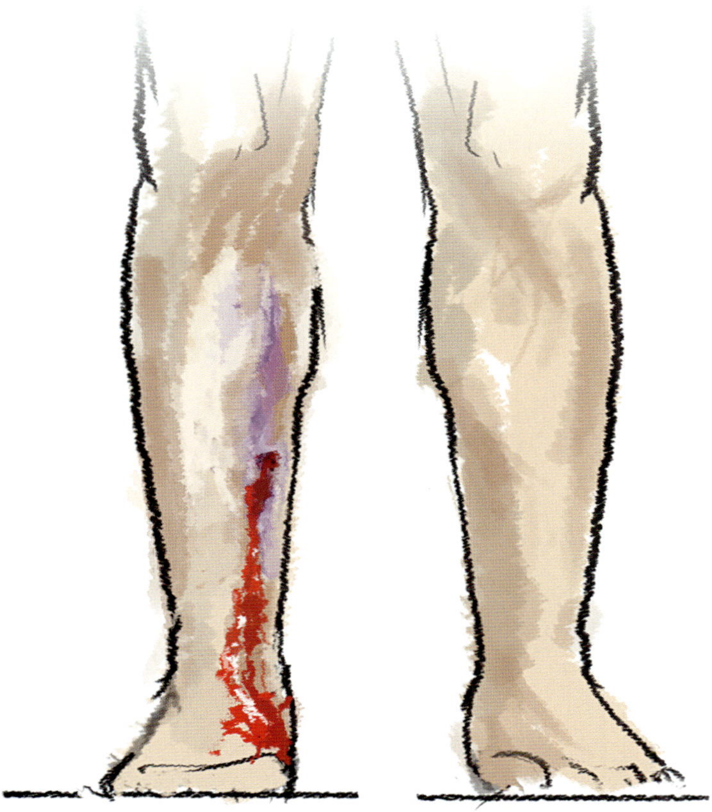

Bleeding from a varicose vein.

12. ACUTE ABDOMEN

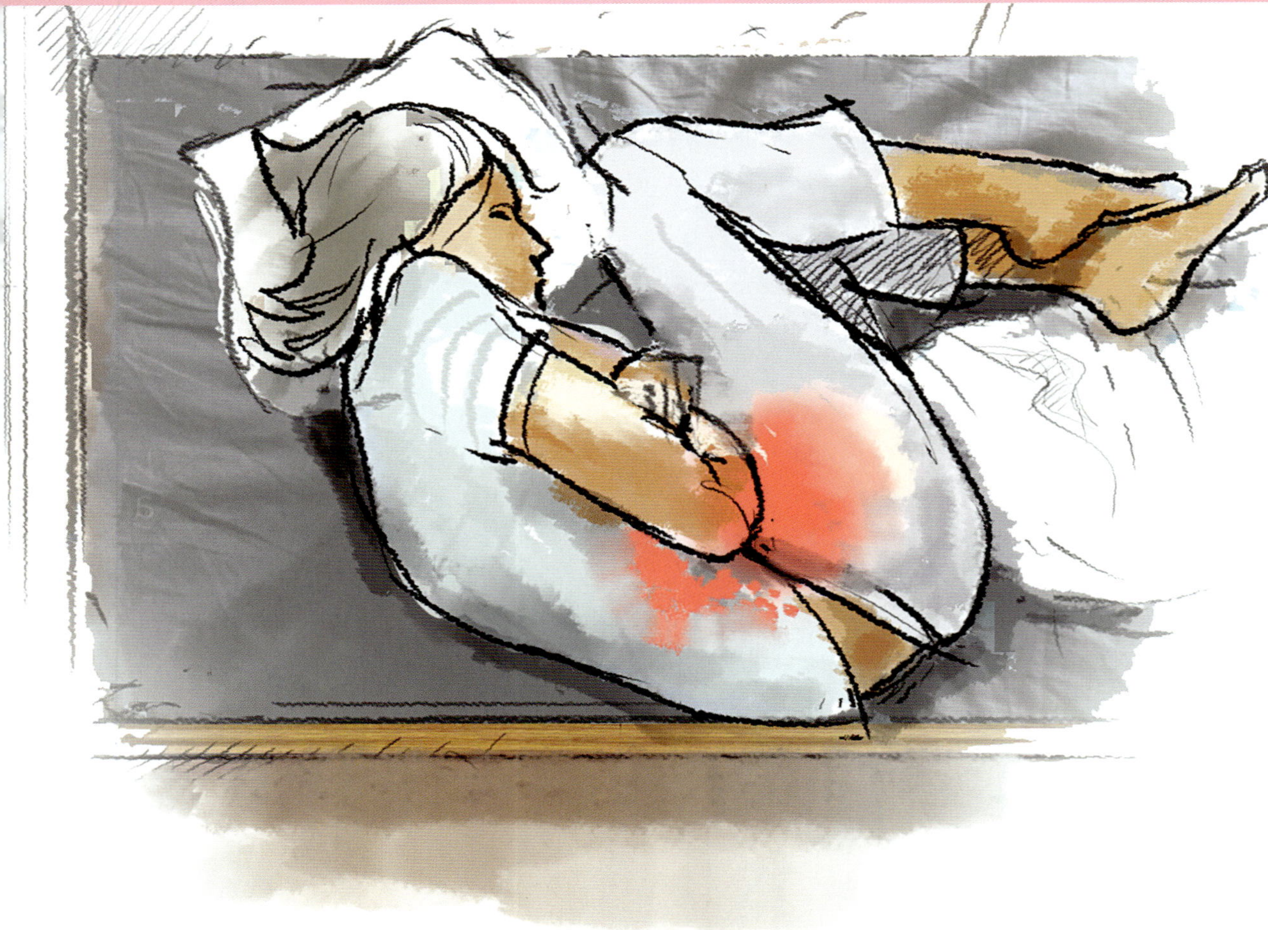

Typical foetal position often preferred in an acute inflammatory abdominal process.

Abdominal pain is a common symptom that can be caused by a variety of conditions, some of which may require urgent medical attention. It can result from harmless, recurrent conditions that resolve spontaneously, such as menstrual pain or constipation. Evaluating an 'acute abdomen' can be challenging and should ideally be performed by a doctor in a hospital setting. However, when far from professional help, an attempt must be made to conduct an initial assessment and seek advice using available communication equipment.

REASONS TO CONTACT A DOCTOR

Reasons to contact a doctor for acute abdominal pain that you do not recognise:

- severe pain lasting more than one to two hours
- unbearable pain
- increasing pain
- combination with other symptoms like nausea, vomiting, fever, general malaise

ASSESSMENT

The immediate goal is to obtain a preliminary diagnosis by focusing on the person's general appearance and the characteristics of the pain, using the following four steps. A preliminary diagnosis will guide subsequent actions, detailed for each specific illness.

Step 1: How did the pain start? Type of pain?

The table below describes causes of abdominal pain based on character and onset.

Consider:

- The intensity of the pain – is it improving or worsening?
- Any history of previous abdominal surgery.
- Changes over time – does the pain worsen or improve, and is it affected by movement or eating/drinking?

Abrupt onset	Escalating pain	Interval pain	Burning pain
Intestinal obstruction with circulatory impairment	Appendicitis	Mild pancreatitis	Oesophgitis (heartburn)
Emboli acute ischaemia	Inflamed intestinal pocket (diverticulitis)	Intestinal obstruction	Gastritis
Rupture (aorta, cyst)	Cholecystitis	Kidney stone	Gastric ulcer
Perforation (gastric ulcer, intestine)		Gallstone	
Severe pancreatitis		Gastroenteritis	
Ovarian torsion			
Kidney stone			

Step 2: Where is the pain located?

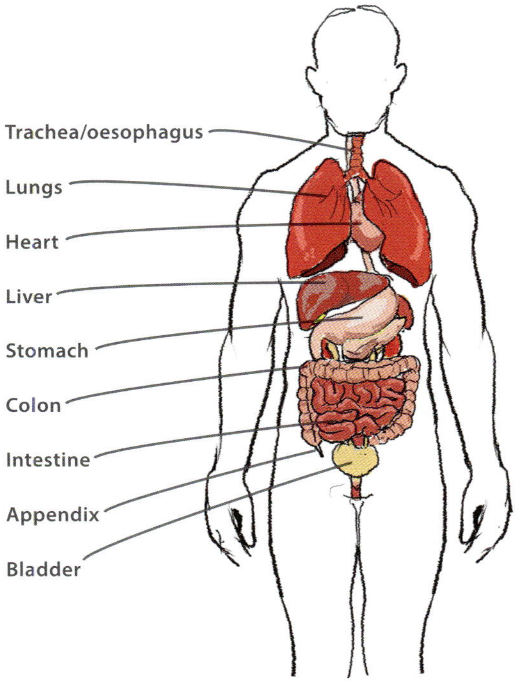

Normal anatomy of internal organs.

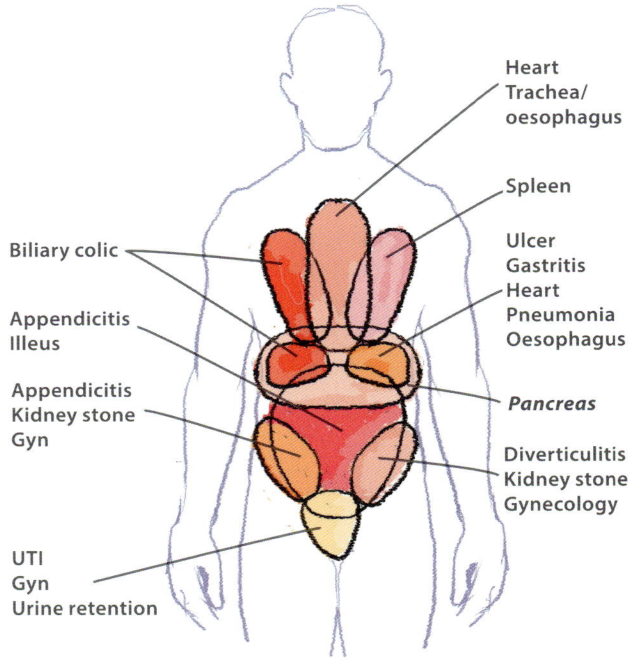

The complexity of the anatomy of the internal organs and their pain distribution.

Consider the location of the pain and whether it radiates to other areas, such as the chest. Some chest conditions, such as a heart attack or pneumonia, can cause abdominal pain, and vice versa.

Step 3: Physical examination

Conducting a physical examination of an acute abdomen as a non-medical professional can be challenging but may provide valuable clues for diagnosis. Ensure the person is comfortable and relaxed.

- Inspection: Look for signs of abdominal distension. In a normal abdomen, the contours of the rib arches are visible when lying flat. In cases of abdominal distension, these contours are hidden by the distended abdomen.

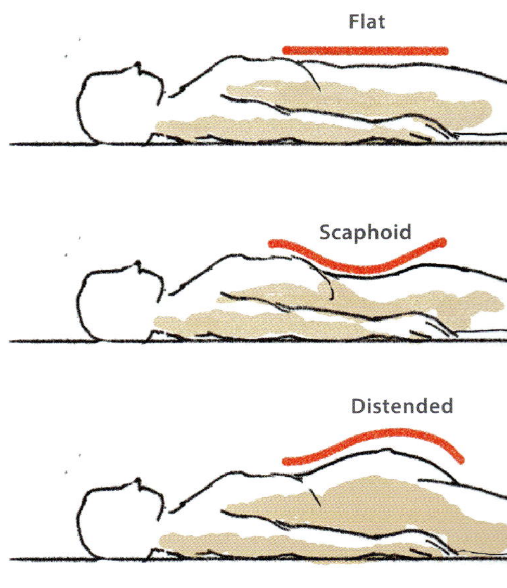

Normal configurations of abdomen, flat or scaphoid. Distended abdomen may indicate some acute pathological process.

- Palpation: Check for local or general tenderness. Divide the abdomen into four quadrants. Begin palpating away from the area of pain, examining the less tender quadrants first.

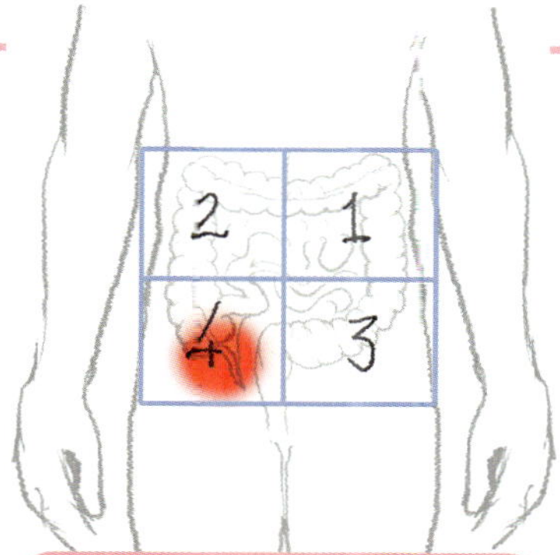

Palpation: divide the abdomen into four quadrants.

Ensure your fingers are warm! Gently press into the abdomen, starting with a depth of 1–2cm, then gradually increase pressure. Identify areas of tenderness, rigidity or 'muscle guarding'.

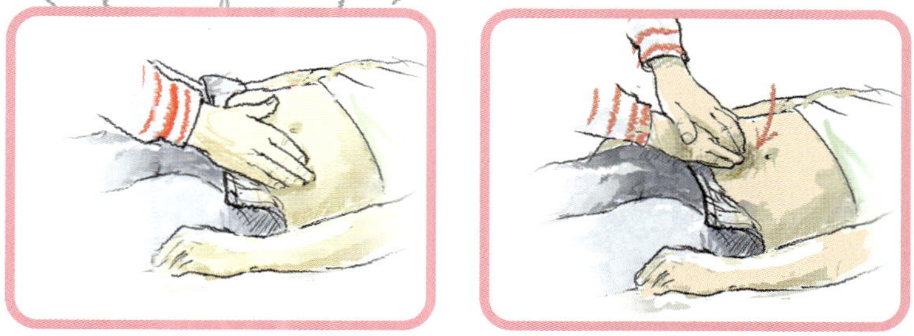

Palpation of abdomen. Is it soft or rigid? Any deeper tenderness? Any masses?

- Rebound tenderness: Place one hand flat on the abdominal flank and gently thump it with the other hand. This may provoke pain in inflamed organs such as the kidneys, gallbladder or appendix.

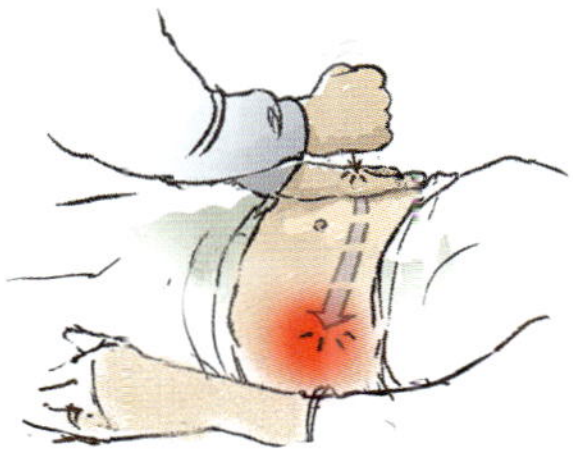

Technique for checking rebound tenderness.

- Listening for bowel sounds:
  - » Lay your ear on the abdomen (or use a stethoscope, if available) and listen for at least 30 seconds. Note whether bowel sounds are overactive or absent.
  - » No sounds: suggests bowel paralysis or loss of circulation.
  - » Excessive sounds: indicates irritation or obstruction.
  - » Metallic sounds: indicate obstruction.

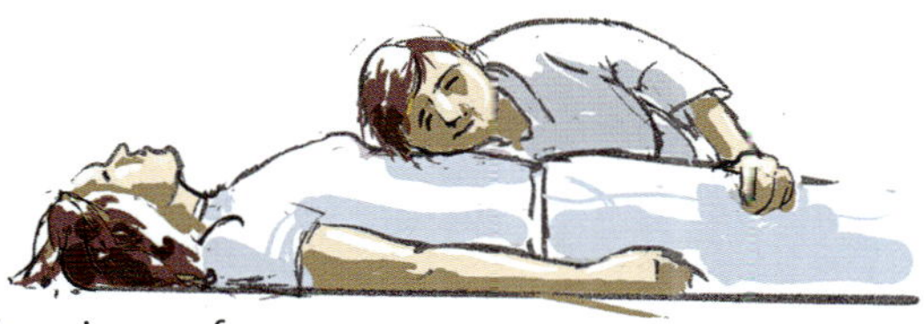

Listen for bowel sounds directly with your ear if a stethoscope is unavailable. Practise to learn normal bowel sound!

Step 4: General appearance

Most important is to check for signs of dehydration (see next page).

- Check for fever.
- Check pulse rate and breathing patterns.
- Monitor urine colour and volume.
- Vomiting: Note volume and colour (for example, digested food, bile, blood or 'coffee grounds', which indicates upper gastrointestinal bleeding).
- Stools: Assess for constipation, passage of faeces and gas. Black and tarry indicates upper gastrointestinal bleeding. Blood in or on the faeces indicates lower gastrointestinal bleeding.
- Position: Observe whether the person is curled in the foetal position or restless.

Stomach problems complicated with tropical climate is a risk for dehydration.

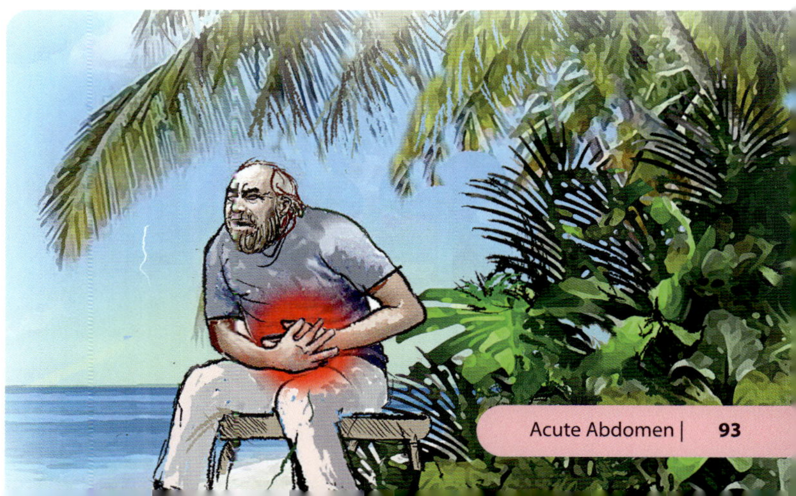

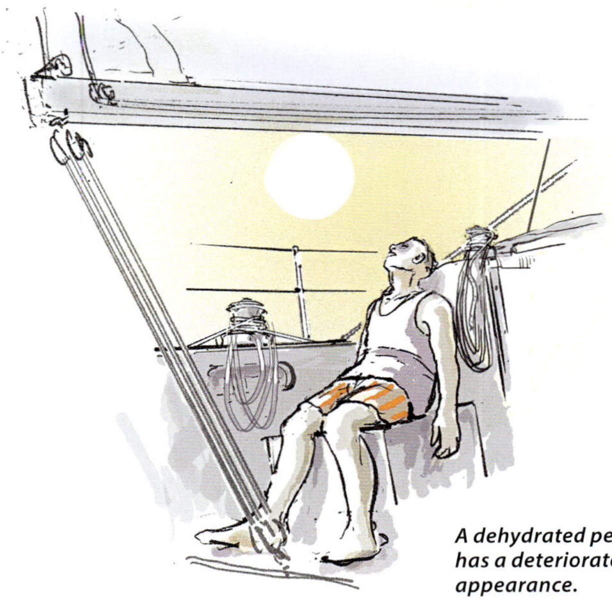

A dehydrated person often has a deteriorated general appearance.

DEHYDRATION

Dehydration is a common complication in cases of acute abdominal illness. Fever, diarrhoea and vomiting can rapidly cause dehydration, especially in tropical climates. However, other conditions – such as seasickness, hyperthermia, septicaemia and burns – may also lead to dehydration. It is important to recognise the signs and symptoms of dehydration and assess its severity.

Normal fluid intake for a healthy 70-kilogram person is 2–3 litres per day. Perspiration alone accounts for approximately 1 litre per day.

Signs and symptoms

Moderate dehydration **5% of bodyweight**	**Severe dehydration** **10% of bodyweight**
Tiredness Headache Thirst Dry mucous membranes in the mouth Reduced urine volume	Confusion Drowsiness Pale appearance Very dry mucous membranes in the mouth Elevated pulse Very small urine volume Pre-shock symptoms

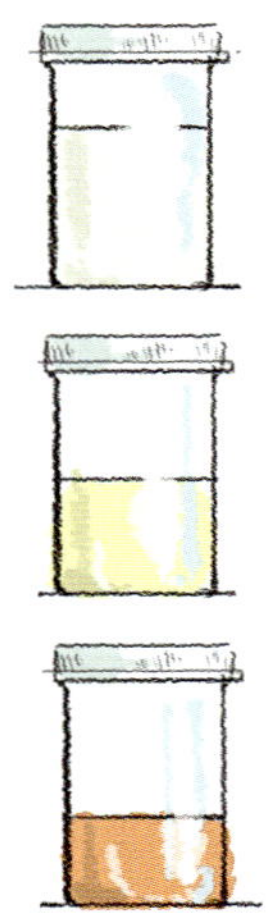

Urine colour and volume are key indicators. Adequate hydration results in bright yellow urine and a high output. In dehydration, urine output decreases significantly, and the colour darkens. Strong yellow or brown urine indicates dehydration. Normal urine production is 1–2 litres per day.

Urinate in a glass container. Check the colour and volume.

Treatment

Rehydrate with plenty of fluids. A guideline is 500ml in the first hour. Dehydration leads to salt loss, so fluid replacement must include salt. Never give plain water, particularly from a water-maker. Use cola, water with added salt and sugar, or a commercial oral rehydration solution (ORS).

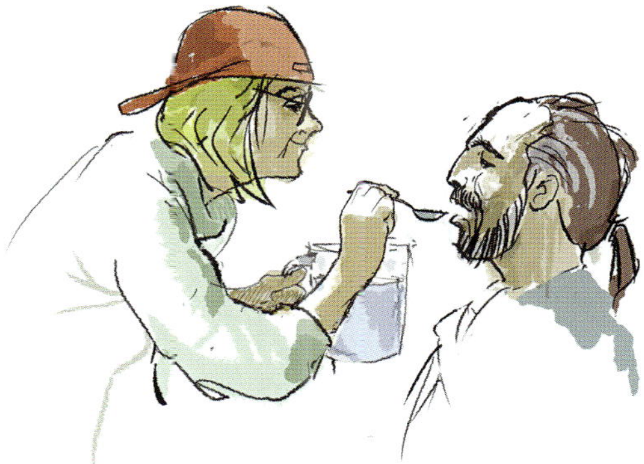

Spoon-by-spoon technique for treating dehydration.

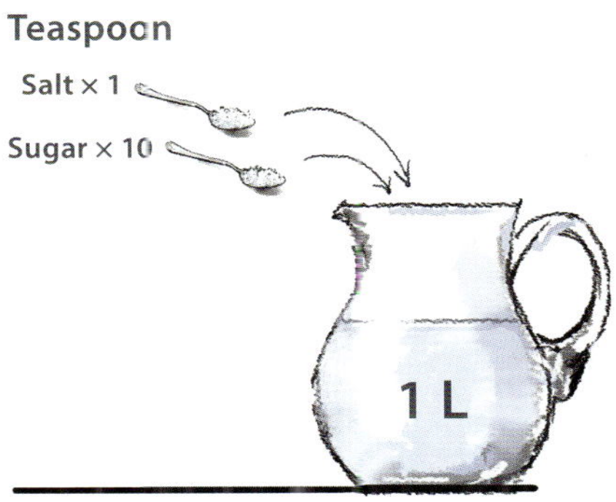

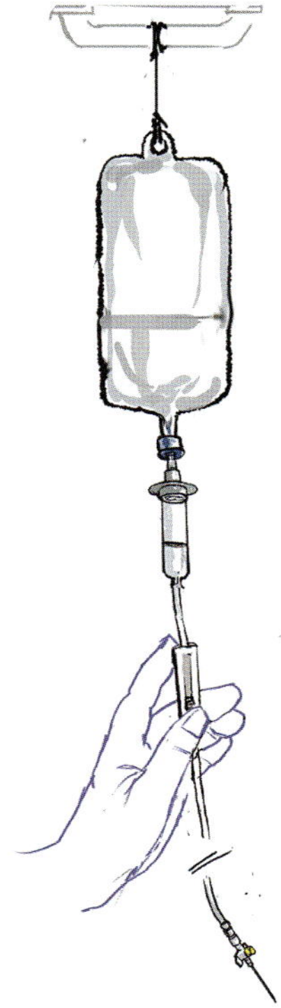

Equipment needed for intravenous fluid therapy.

Oral route

This is the easiest way to rehydrate a person who can drink and swallow. If the person is vomiting, administer small, repeated amounts, spoon by spoon, until their general appearance and urine output improve. Larger volumes may worsen the situation by inducing vomiting. Never attempt oral hydration if the person is not fully conscious.

Intravenous route

If the necessary skills (a nurse or doctor) and equipment are available on board, the intravenous route is the most effective method of rehydration in severe dehydration due to acute gastrointestinal disease. Only sterile intravenous (IV) fluid should be used.

Rectal route

If neither the oral nor intravenous route is possible, rectal hydration may be an option. This procedure can be messy due to the casualty's reflex to defecate when fluid is infused into the rectum/colon. Infuse fluid slowly at 50–100ml per hour via a soft tube inserted 10–15cm.

DEHYDRATION IN CHILDREN

It is difficult to assess dehydration in children, who are far more sensitive to its effects. An early sign is faster-than-usual breathing. In severe dehydration, the child's skin may feel dry, and they may become quiet and floppy. If dehydration is suspected in a child, seek healthcare advice immediately.

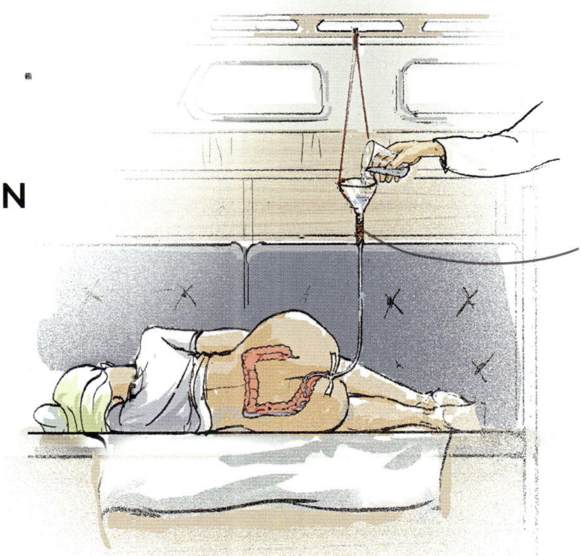

Fluid substitution via rectal infusion. It is important to lie on the left side, allowing the fluid to reach the colon.

GASTROENTERITIS

Gastroenteritis, commonly referred to as 'stomach flu', is a collective term for infections caused by viruses, bacteria or other microorganisms. Poor food and hand hygiene, contaminated food and water, and person-to-person transmission in a shared household are common routes of infection.

BACTERIAL FOOD POISONING

Hygienic issues in the storage and handling of food can lead to bacterial contamination, with organisms such as staphylococci and Escherichia coli (E. coli) being common culprits. Some bacteria release toxins that can cause illness.

Signs and symptoms

Symptoms typically appear within a few hours after consuming contaminated food. Onset is usually acute and sudden, with:

- nausea
- intense vomiting (often described as 'cascade vomiting')
- severe painful stomach cramps due to intense bowel movements
- a pronounced feeling of illness, accompanied by paleness and cold sweats
- a rapid spike of fever, which usually subsides within a few hours
- watery diarrhoea may occur simultaneously

Symptoms last one to two days, until the body eliminates the toxin.

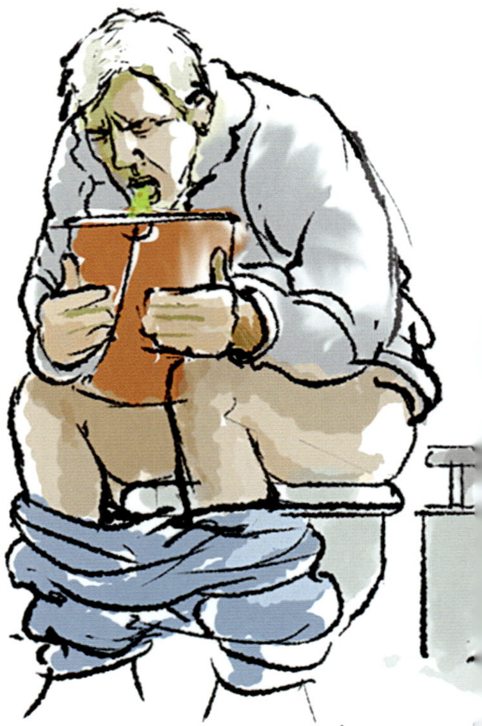

Simultaneous intense vomiting and watery diarrhoea are common in acute food poisoning. Risk of dehydration!

Treatment

For suspected food poisoning, activated charcoal can be administered to absorb toxins and expedite recovery. Anti-nausea medications (for example, ondansetron) and anti-diarrhoeal drugs (for example, loperamide) may be used, but their administration is complicated if the person is vomiting or experiencing diarrhoea. Acute food poisoning is generally manageable on board.

TRAVELLER'S DIARRHOEA

Traveller's diarrhoea can result from various bacteria – including Salmonella, Campylobacter, Yersinia, Escherichia coli – and the disease typhoid fever. The latter often causes diarrhoea, which may be bloody, accompanied by fever and cramping abdominal pain (colic).

Salmonella is transmitted through undercooked meat, eggs or dairy products, while Campylobacter is primarily spread via poultry and unpasteurised milk. E. coli, abundant in human intestines, can produce toxins that cause traveller's diarrhoea.

These bacterial infections often spread through food, faeces, direct contact or contaminated water. They tend to have a longer course and more general symptoms, such as fever, compared to viral infections. Typhoid fever can lead to sepsis and may require hospitalisation. However, most cases resolve spontaneously within a few days. In some instances, antibiotics may be necessary.

Immediate action

It is crucial to consider the risk of dehydration and take appropriate measures. Refer to the previous section for guidance on managing dehydration.

Treatment

Seeking advice from healthcare professionals is valuable, especially in cases of suspected dehydration or bacterial causes. Antibiotics for acute gastroenteritis are often of limited value but may be considered for a severe or prolonged course with fever and bloody diarrhoea, particularly when far from medical assistance. Ciprofloxacin 500mg every 8 hours for 5 days is an option in such cases.

Far from help

Refer to the treatment section above. Early consultation with healthcare professionals is essential to optimise management.

Prevention

- Ensure thorough food hygiene.
- Avoid consuming old leftovers.
- Store food in small packages to minimise leftovers.
- Practise rigorous hand hygiene using soap and water or hand sanitiser, and avoid wearing rings.
- Use disposable gloves if you have infected wounds.
- Be cautious when dining at 'hole-in-the-wall' type restaurants, especially before embarking on a long overseas voyage.
- Exercise caution when consuming fresh salads, vegetables, or ice, as they may have been exposed to contaminated water.
- Consider vaccination, such as for typhoid.

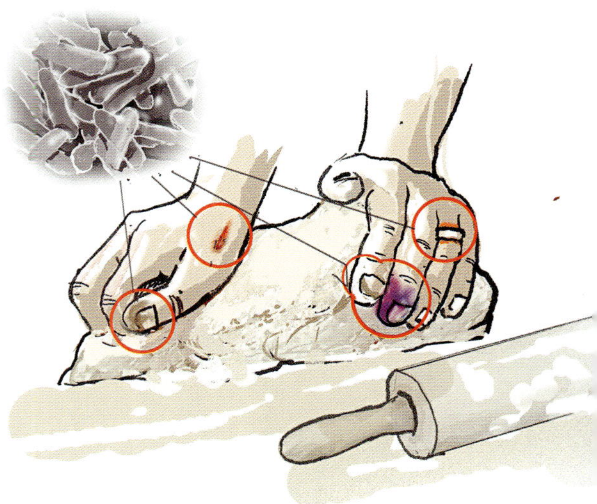

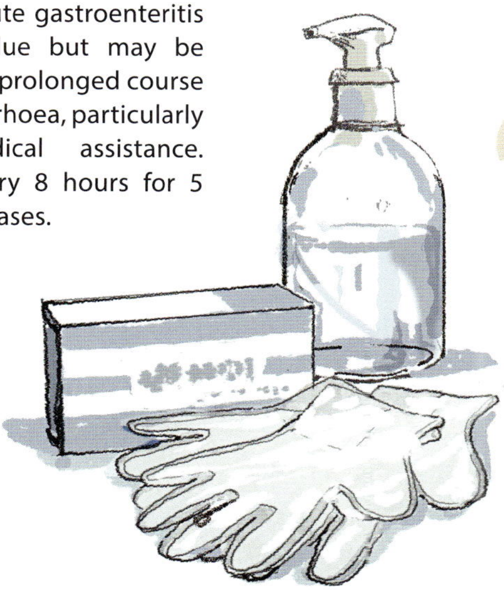

Hand sanitiser and disposable gloves should be included in on-board equipment. Avoid handling food if you have infected wounds, or use gloves, and do not wear rings. Infected wounds can contaminate food.

APPENDICITIS

Historically, appendicitis was a sailor's dread. Today, it is usually manageable even when far from help. Appendicitis is most common between the ages of 5 and 20, and the lifetime risk is approximately 5 per cent. The cause is unclear, but it is speculated that inflammation results from the accumulation of bowel content in the narrow appendix.

Signs and symptoms

- Discomfort, pain in the upper abdomen
- Loss of appetite and a general feeling of illness
- Nausea and vomiting
- Fever
- Pain migrating to the right groin area in about 50 per cent of cases
- Pain worsening with movement
- Tenderness in the lower right abdomen

Symptoms may not always follow the classic pattern, especially in pregnant women, children and the elderly.

Immediate action

- Place the person in bed.
- Allow the stomach to rest by avoiding solid food and providing only fluids (see 'Treatment' under 'Dehydration' on page 95).
- Seek professional advice and arrange transport to hospital

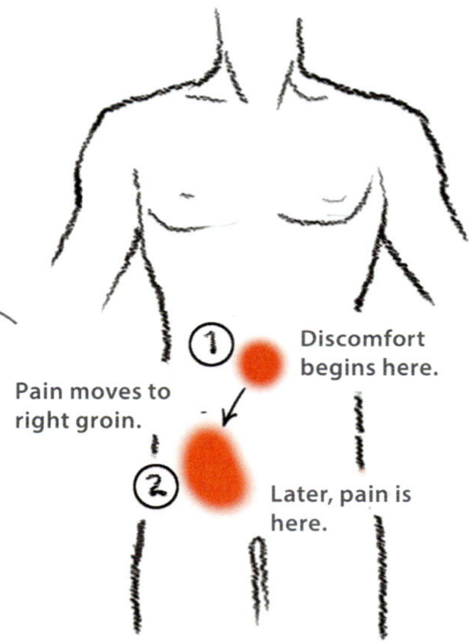

Pain distribution in appendicitis.

Location of a healthy appendix and its appearance when inflamed or perforated, with intestinal content leaking out into the abdomen.

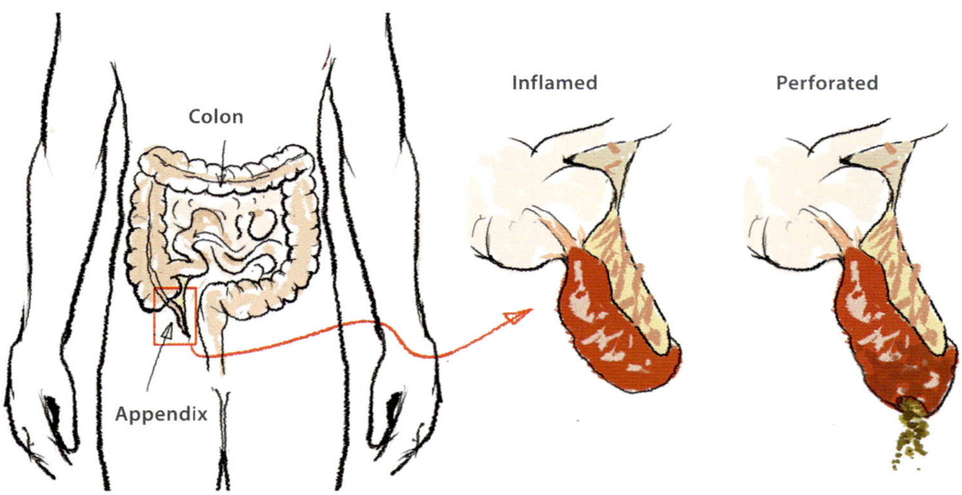

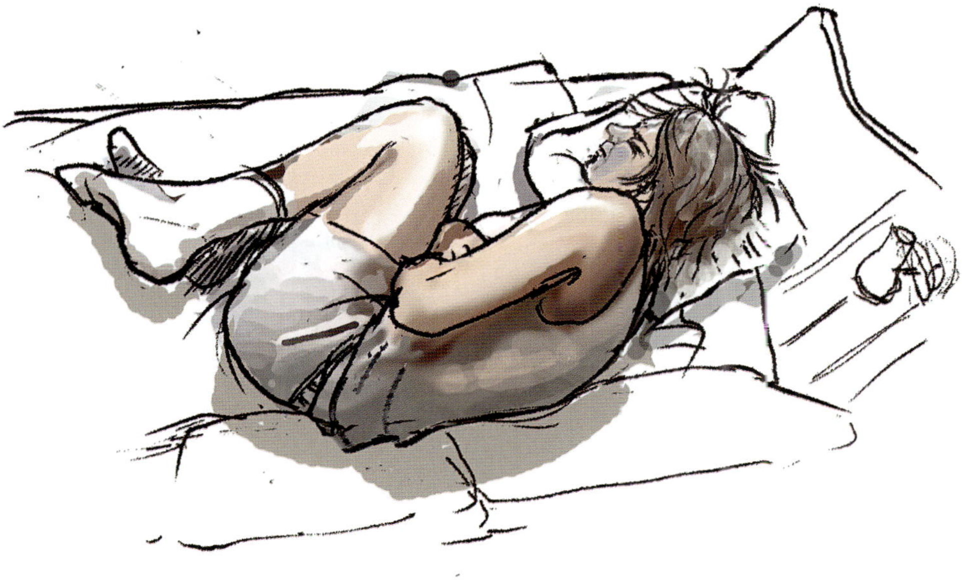

A person with appendicitis often lies still in the foetal position to reduce the pain, which worsens with movement. General appearance sick and pale.

Treatment

Contact healthcare professionals for advice on management and transportation planning. Most cases require surgery within a day, but some may be managed with antibiotics and delayed surgery. If the appendix perforates, it can cause peritonitis, characterised by a rapid worsening of symptoms such as sharp abdominal pain, a 'rigid' abdomen, septic fever and general malaise. Suspected perforation requires immediate evacuation.

Pain relief with medications like paracetamol 1000mg (two 500mg tablets), codeine, or even morphine may be necessary if transport is delayed.

Far from help

Evacuation remains the best option. Maintain communication with a doctor. It is possible but challenging to manage appendicitis on board. Start antibiotics such as ciprofloxacin 500mg every 12 hours and metronidazole 400mg every 8 hours. Provide fluids only, avoiding solid food (refer to the section on fluid balance/dehydration on page 95). Pain management may require a combination of opioids such as codeine or morphine and paracetamol until reaching medical care.

In some cases, antibiotics during the acute phase followed by surgery months later is an established alternative.

Prevention

There is no known way to prevent appendicitis, and preventive removal of the appendix is not recommended as it carries risks of adhesions and bowel obstruction.

MYTH BUSTER

Is it 'over' if you get appendicitis out at sea? No! Today, there is strong scientific evidence that appendicitis can be treated with antibiotics. A significant proportion of cases can heal without surgery, and surgery can be delayed in some instances. Mild appendicitis may even resolve on its own. Increased pain is a sign to contact healthcare services.

GASTRITIS/GASTRIC ULCER/OESOPHAGITIS

Dyspepsia and discomfort often attributed to gastritis or gastric ulcers are common complaints. Elevated acid production and bacterial infection with Helicobacter pylori are significant contributors, as are stress, lifestyle factors, smoking and alcohol consumption. Modern medical treatments, including acid-reducing medications and antibiotics (for example, amoxicillin), have reduced the incidence of ulcers in recent decades. Gastritis or gastric ulcers can also lead to reflux of stomach acids into the oesophagus, causing oesophagitis.

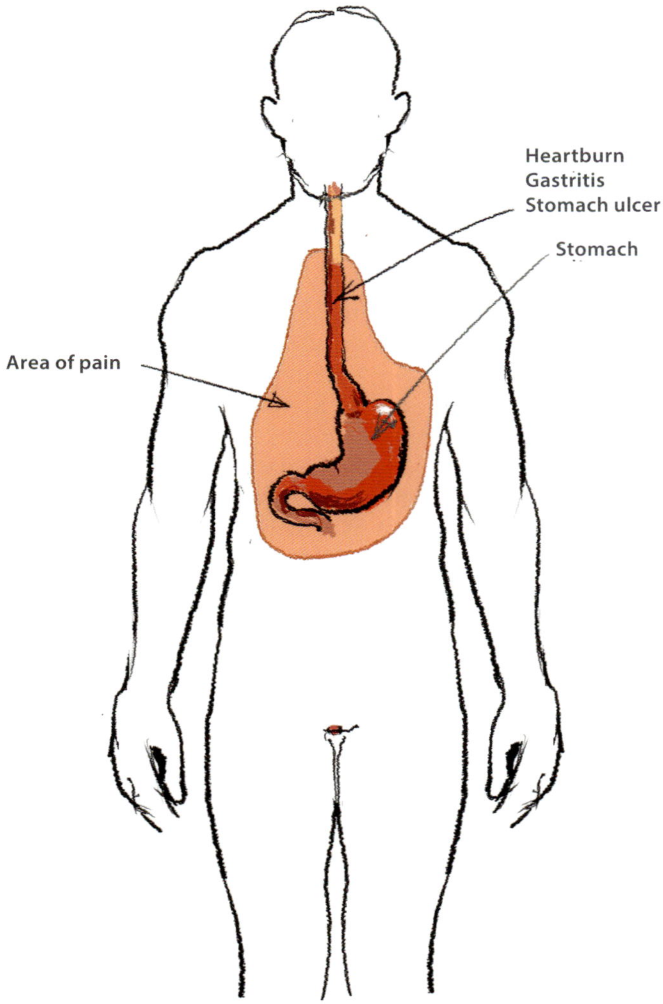

Anatomy of the oesophagus, stomach and duodenum. Pain distribution in gastritis, gastric ulcer and oesophagitis. Note difficulties to distinguish from heart-related pain.

Signs and symptoms

Common symptoms include heartburn, pain, nausea and dyspepsia, which usually improve after eating. Reflux is often worse at night when lying down, making it sometimes difficult to distinguish from heart-related pain.

Immediate action

It is essential to differentiate these symptoms from other potential causes and obtain a proper diagnosis.

Treatment

Uncomplicated gastritis or ulcers can often be successfully treated with acid-neutralising medications or esomeprazole. Elevating the upper part of the bed or body can improve nightly reflux.

Far from help

Refer to the previous section for guidance on treatment. Establish contact with healthcare professionals for advice and support.

Prevention

- Avoid stress, alcohol and smoking.
- Discuss with your doctor the need for eradication of bacteria and other preventive measures, particularly for longer voyages.
- Note that the risk of a gastric ulcer leading to perforation or bleeding still exists and can occur without preceding gastritis (see opposite).

PERFORATED GASTRIC ULCER

The risk of a perforated ulcer is increased among smokers, those under high stress, and people taking anti-inflammatory medicines (NSAIDs, such as ibuprofen) or steroids.

Signs and symptoms

Perforated ulcers are often preceded by symptoms of gastritis or ulcers, followed by sudden, severe, acute pain in the upper abdomen, which then spreads across the belly. The pain typically starts abruptly, as though a switch has been flipped. Stomach acid erodes a hole through the entire stomach or duodenal wall. Although the hole is usually no larger than 5mm, it allows stomach acid to leak into the abdominal cavity, causing peritonitis. This is associated with a rigid, tender abdomen, nausea, vomiting and fever.

Immediate action

When a perforated ulcer is suspected on board:

- Contact healthcare professionals immediately.
- Arrange transport to a hospital.

Treatment

Treatment typically involves surgery, but in some less severe cases, medical management may suffice.

Far from help

- Establish contact with healthcare professionals for advice.
- Rest in bed; avoid solid food and provide only fluids (refer to the section on fluid balance/dehydration on page 95).
- Administer acid-neutralising medications and esomeprazole.
- Monitor the condition closely. Managing a perforated ulcer on board is highly challenging, and dehydration poses a significant risk. Antibiotics may be required in some cases.
- In the best-case scenario, the body's defence mechanisms may partially or fully seal a small perforation.

Prevention

If a person with a history of ulcers is on board, they should have modern ulcer medications, such as esomeprazole or antacids, readily available. For longer voyages, discuss preventive measures, including Helicobacter pylori eradication, with a healthcare professional.

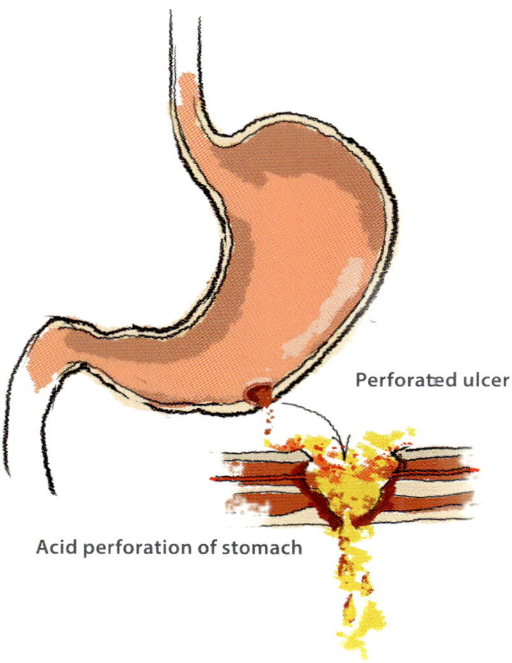

Ulcer in the stomach causing erosion through the entire stomach wall, leading to leakage of stomach acid and peritonitis.

BLEEDING GASTRIC ULCER

An ulcer located near a blood vessel in the stomach can erode the blood vessel due to stomach acid. Bleeding of varying severity can occur even without a previous history of gastric ulcers. The risk is increased in those taking NSAIDs (for example, diclofenac or ibuprofen), anticoagulants, steroids, or consuming excessive alcohol.

Signs and symptoms

Pain is a rare symptom in this group. In cases of slower bleeding, the initial sign is usually black, tarry-looking, foul-smelling stools. After a few days, symptoms of anaemia may develop, including paleness, fatigue and lack of energy. In more significant bleeding, the person may vomit blood clots, which often resemble 'black coffee grounds'. Substantial bleeding can cause rapid signs of circulatory distress/shock: paleness, cold sweat, rapid pulse exceeding 100bpm (see page 20).

Immediate action

- Determine whether the bleeding is slow or significant.
- For ongoing bleeding, immediate evacuation is required.
- While awaiting evacuation, follow the DRABC protocol (page 12).
- If circulatory distress is present, have the person rest with elevated legs.
- If consciousness is affected, place the person in the recovery position (see page 16).
- Monitor the condition closely; deterioration can occur rapidly.
- For slower bleeding (for example, tarry stools), hospital admission the same day is advised.

Treatment

Refer to the instructions under 'Immediate action'. Seek professional assistance immediately.

Far from help

- Establish contact with healthcare professionals.
- Rest in bed; avoid solid food and provide only fluids.
- Administer acid-neutralising medications and esomeprazole.
- Monitor the individual closely, paying particular attention to general appearance, breathing and pulse.
- Managing a bleeding gastric ulcer on board is extremely challenging; evacuation is essential.
- A bleeding ulcer typically requires intensive care, and life may be at risk if evacuation is not possible.

Prevention

Refer to the prevention recommendations under 'Perforated gastric ulcer'.

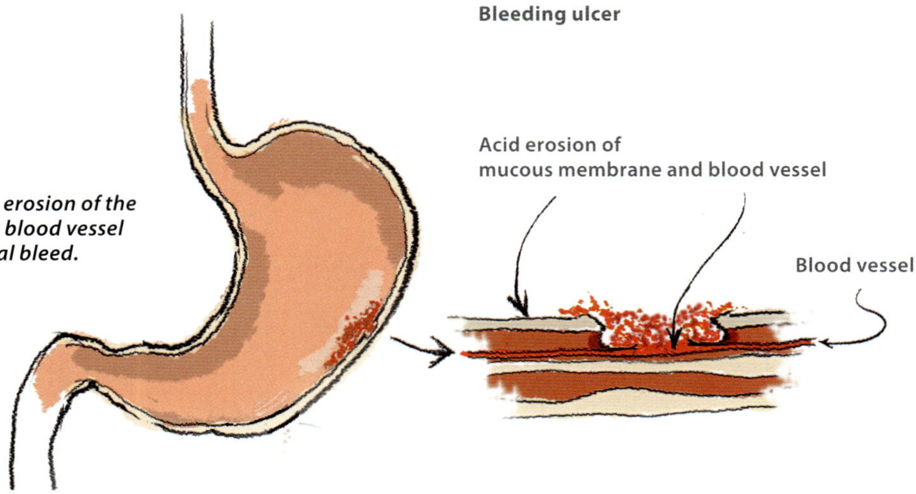

Ulcer in the stomach with erosion of the mucous membrane and a blood vessel causing a gastro-intestinal bleed.

GALLSTONES, CHOLECYSTITIS

Approximately 30 per cent of people over 40 years of age have gallstones, formed in the gallbladder primarily from cholesterol. However, only about a third experience symptoms requiring surgery. Many individuals have gallstones without any symptoms. Consumption of fatty foods, seafood, hard-to-digest fruits and vegetables, and eggs can trigger gallstone spasms and biliary colic. Persons with known gallstones usually know which foods to avoid.

The mechanism of biliary colic involves certain foods triggering the need for extra bile to aid digestion. The gallbladder contracts to release bile into the intestine, potentially lodging a stone within the biliary system. This can cause painful cramps or lead to gallbladder inflammation, known as cholecystitis.

Anatomy of the bile system. The gallbladder contracts, forcing stones into the narrow duct, causing cramping pain.

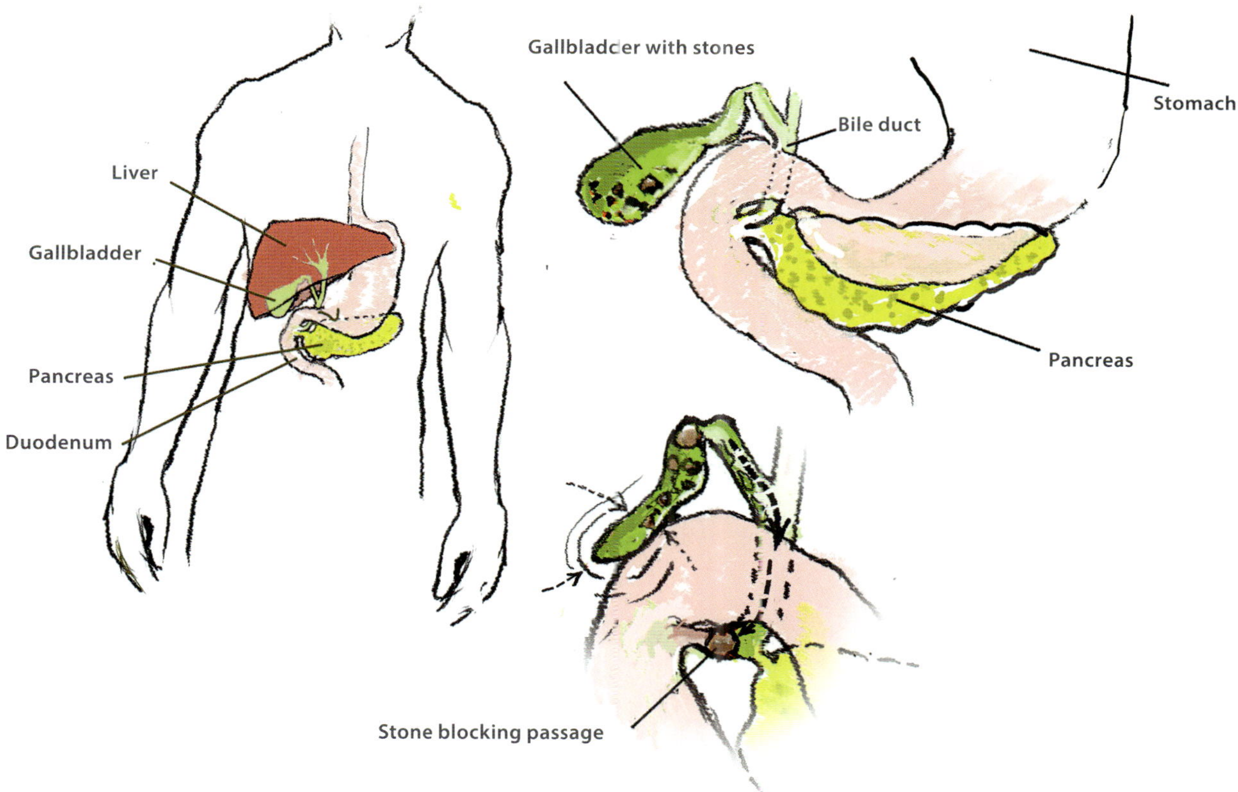

Typical pain distribution during biliary colic.

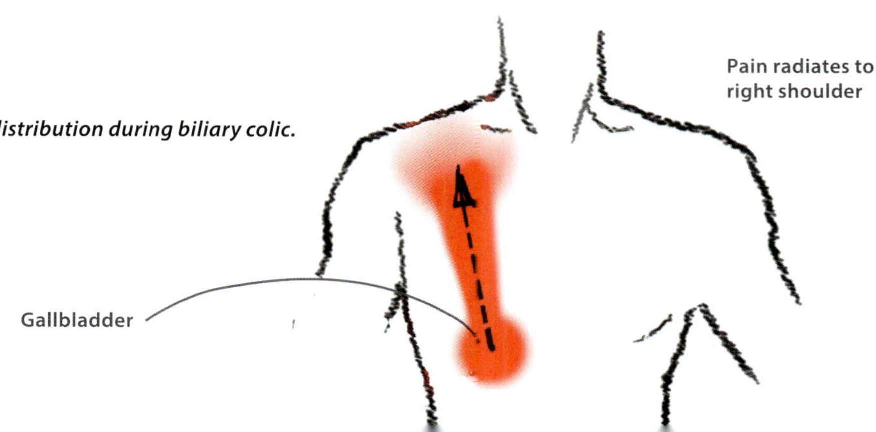

Signs and symptoms

The onset of biliary colic is gradual and includes:

- episodes of dull pain beneath the right ribcage
- pain radiating to the right shoulder and back
- nausea and vomiting

The pain caused by gallbladder spasms is due to irritation from stones and typically lasts from a few hours to a full day.

If gallbladder inflammation (cholecystitis) develops, it is accompanied by:

- continuous pain beneath the right ribcage, radiating to the right side of the back
- tenderness beneath the right ribcage
- pain that worsens with movement and deep breathing
- fever
- general malaise

If a gallstone blocks the deep bile duct, bile cannot enter the intestine. Instead, it is absorbed into the bloodstream, resulting in:

- dark (port-wine-coloured) urine
- yellowing of the whites of the eyes, later followed by jaundice of the skin

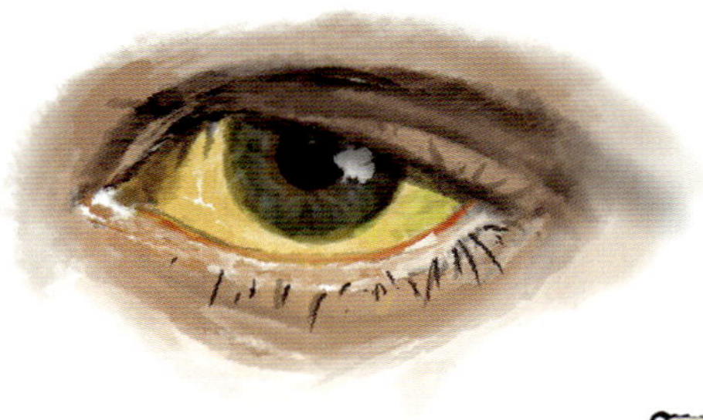

Jaundice is first noticed as yellow discoloration of the eyes.

Immediate action

Administer an anti-inflammatory NSAID, such as ibuprofen or diclofenac (tablet or suppository), to relieve spasms in the bile duct muscles. Avoid solid food during this time but ensure proper hydration by providing fluids.

Treatment

- Ensure adequate fluid intake, and avoid solid food until symptoms subside.
- Administer anti-inflammatory medication, such as diclofenac (50mg) as a tablet 2–3 times per day or as a suppository (100mg) once a day, to reduce spasms in the bile ducts.
- Combine with paracetamol (500mg, 2 tablets) 3 to 4 times daily for additional pain relief.

Far from help

- Follow the above advice and carefully monitor the patient's condition.
- Pay extra attention to more pronounced general symptoms, increasing abdominal pain, or fever. Consultation with a doctor is strongly recommended.
- Antibiotics, such as ciprofloxacin and metronidazole (see table on page 249), may be necessary.
- Evacuation might be required as the condition can worsen rapidly.

Prevention

- Avoid foods that trigger biliary colic.
- If you have known gallstones that have caused symptoms, discuss surgery with a surgeon before embarking on a longer voyage.

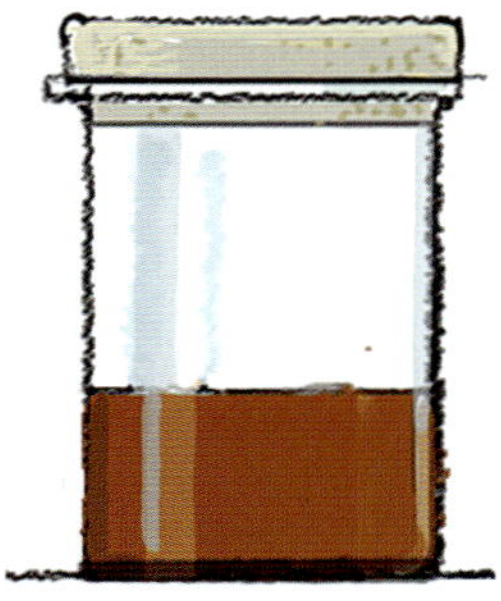

Biliary obstruction causes port-wine-coloured urine.

INFLAMMATION OF THE PANCREAS (PANCREATITIS)

Together with the bile system, the pancreas and its enzymes are vital for digestion. Inflammation of the pancreas can cause acute abdominal pain and may progress to a severe, potentially life-threatening condition. The pancreas and gallbladder share a common duct near the point where it empties into the duodenum. If a gallstone becomes lodged in this duct, it can prevent the pancreas from draining enzymes normally.

The most common cause of pancreatitis in women is gallstones, while in men it is excessive alcohol consumption.

Signs and symptoms

- Severe pain in the upper abdomen
- Pain radiating to the back
- Nausea and vomiting
- Fever
- General malaise

Immediate action

Fasting is essential – no solid food or fluids should be given. A person with suspected acute pancreatitis must be transported to hospital as soon as possible.

Treatment

Hospital care is required. Most patients recover within a few days with fasting, hydration and pain relief. Intravenous fluids and strong painkillers, such as morphine, are usually necessary. However, 20 per cent of patients may experience a life-threatening severe and complicated course of the disease.

Far from help

- Pancreatitis is a challenging and potentially dangerous condition. Professional medical advice and support are crucial.
- Where advanced hospital care is unavailable, 'fasting' should be limited to drinking fluids, with no solid food intake.
- Opioid painkillers are likely to be required to manage pain effectively.

Prevention

- Avoid excessive alcohol consumption. If you have a history of pancreatitis, it is advisable to abstain completely during a voyage.
- If you have gallstones, avoid foods that trigger symptoms and discuss potential surgery with your doctor before a long voyage.

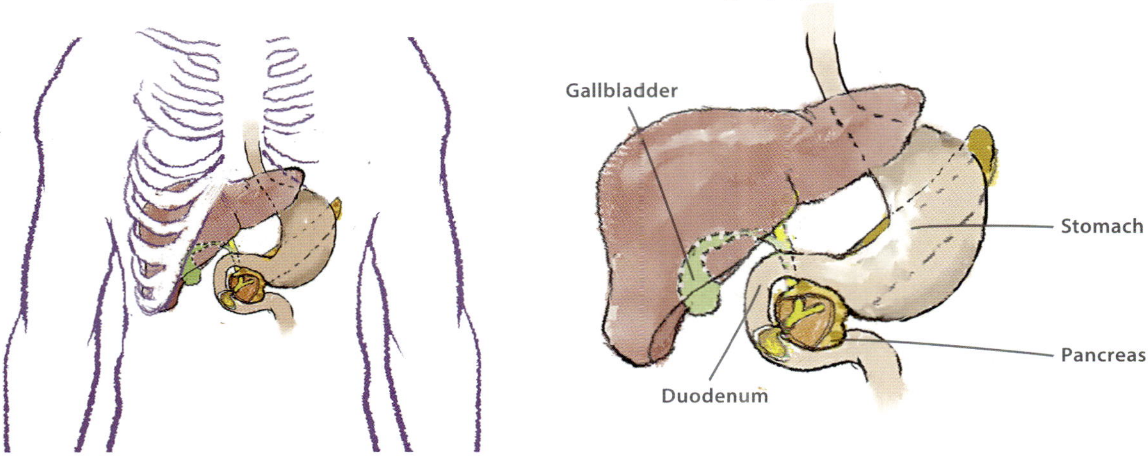

Anatomy of the pancreas. The pancreas is located behind the stomach, close to the gallbladder, with which it shares a common duct leading into the intestine.

BOWEL OBSTRUCTION – ILEUS

Bowel obstruction refers to a blockage in the flow of intestinal contents. The most common cause is mechanical, where the intestine becomes tangled around adhesions or twists upon itself. Adhesions often form after previous abdominal surgeries, but the condition can also occur without prior procedures. Ordinary hernias carry a risk of strangulation and bowel obstruction.

When an obstruction occurs, the intestine tries to push its contents past the blockage, causing it to dilate and resulting in severe colicky pain. Acute circulatory issues, such as an embolism causing paralysis, can also lead to obstruction by depriving the intestine of circulation and mobility.

Signs and symptoms

- Colicky pain in intervals
- Reduced or absent passing of gas and stool
- Increasing abdominal distension
- Nausea and vomiting
- Tenderness over the abdomen
- General malaise

Colicky pain is characterised by bouts of pain lasting a few minutes, which then subside completely before returning. Symptoms may vary depending on the location of the obstruction in the 5-metre-long intestine. A hallmark of circulatory issues causing obstruction is the very sudden onset of intense symptoms.

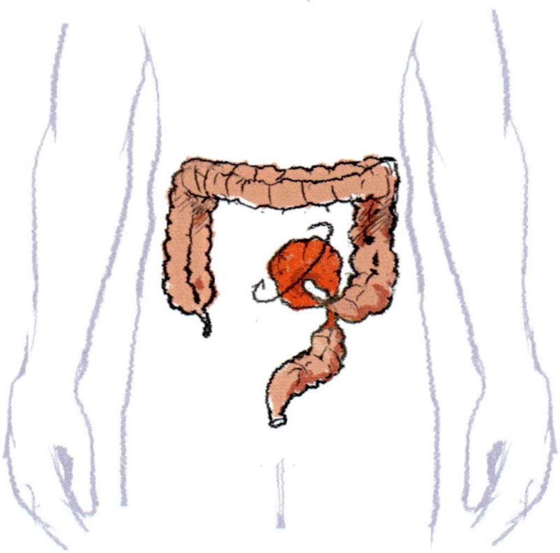

Twisted bowel, colon, causing blockage of intestinal flow.

Immediate action

If obstruction is suspected, urgent transport to a hospital is crucial. Seek professional advice and support without delay.

Treatment

Treatment is typically surgical and often requires immediate intervention. This situation will likely necessitate an urgent request for assistance and evacuation. Seek medical attention and arrange transport to a hospital as soon as possible.

Far from help

- Closely monitor the patient.
- Keep them warm and comfortable.
- Avoid solid foods; provide hydration.
- Administer painkillers such as codeine or morphine.

This is a high-risk situation that may be impossible to manage satisfactorily on board.

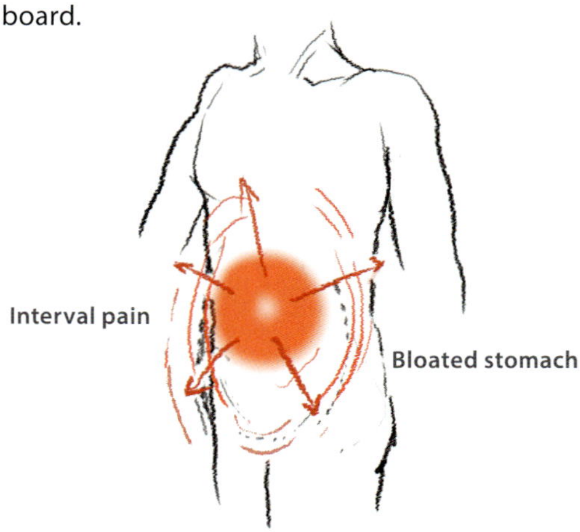

Pain from bowel obstruction typically occurs in intervals and is felt throughout the abdomen.

HERNIA

Another common cause of obstruction is when a loop of intestine becomes trapped in an inguinal hernia, leading to strangulation. If a hernia becomes hard and tender, it may indicate strangulation.

Far from help

If immediate assistance is unavailable, it may be worth attempting to reduce the hernia early.

1. Take a painkiller, possibly combined with a sedative.
2. Lie flat on your back and gently squeeze or press on the hernia.
3. If successful, the hernia may slide back into the abdomen, restoring intestinal flow.

Even if the hernia is reduced, monitor for persistent pain or other symptoms, which may indicate ongoing problems.

Prevention

Preventative measures are essential for those at higher risk, such as individuals with a history of abdominal surgery or previous ileus:

- Review your health status before embarking on long voyages.
- Discuss the repair of known hernias with a surgeon before departure.
- Avoid swallowing large food items (for example, whole orange segments or tough meat).
- If you have had intestinal obstruction before, avoid oranges and mushrooms entirely.
- Drink plenty of fluids with meals.

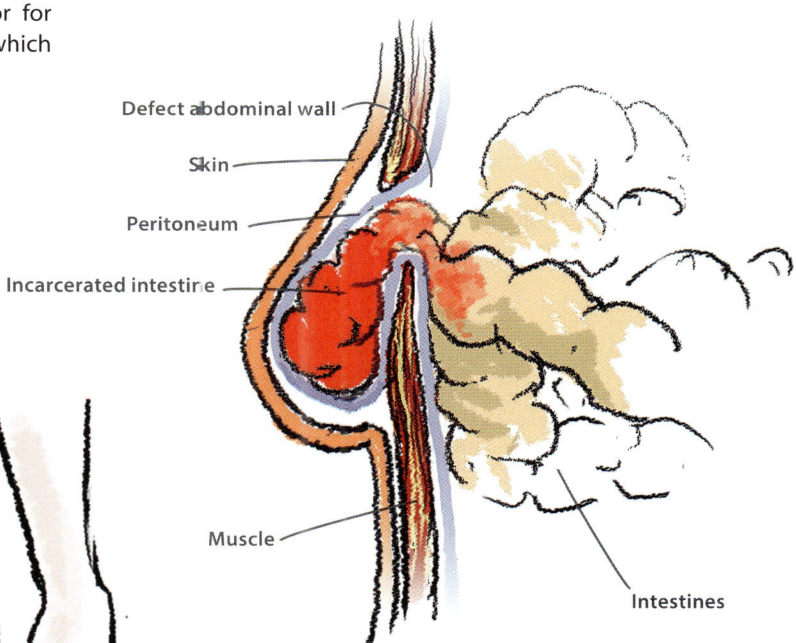

A strangulated hernia where the intestine becomes trapped, leading to obstruction.

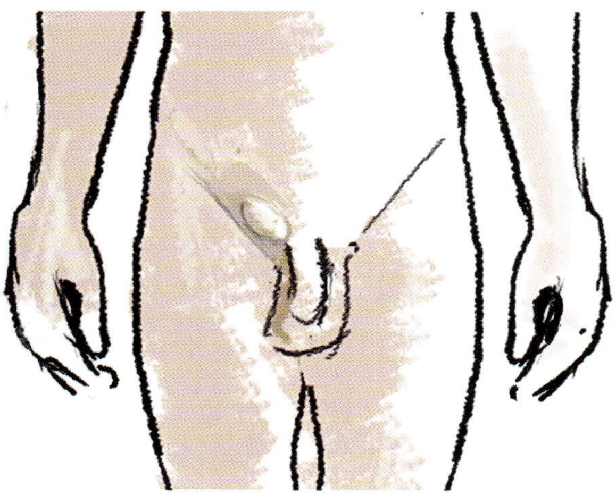

Typical location and appearance of an inguinal hernia.

INFLAMED INTESTINAL POUCH / DIVERTICULITIS

With age, the risk of forming small pouches (diverticula) in the colon wall increases. These are particularly common in the lower left side of the colon. Diverticula form due to increased intestinal pressure, often caused by constipation, combined with weakening of the intestinal wall. The presence of these pouches is called diverticulosis and is usually asymptomatic or mildly symptomatic. Thirty per cent of people over 60 years old have diverticulosis.

When these pouches become inflamed, the condition is called diverticulitis. Unlike appendicitis, diverticulitis progresses less acutely but can still lead to serious complications.

Signs and symptoms

- Initial constipation, sometimes alternating with diarrhoea
- Blood or mucus in the stool
- Pain in the lower abdomen, often on the left side
- Fever and tenderness in the lower abdomen
- If untreated, diverticulitis can perforate, causing peritonitis, sepsis, and severe acute deterioration.

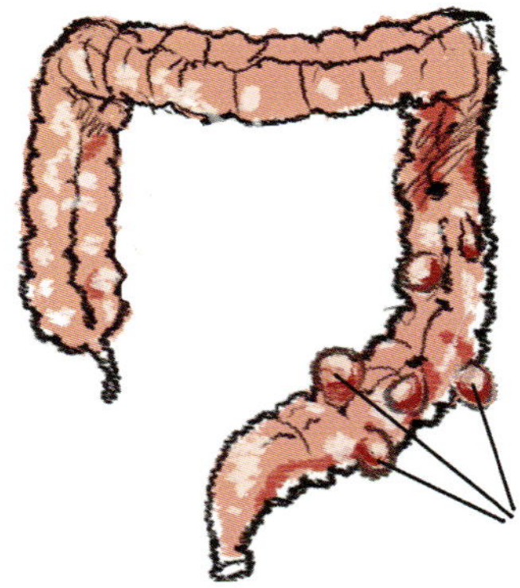

Above: Common location of diverticula. Below: Pain area in diverticulitis.

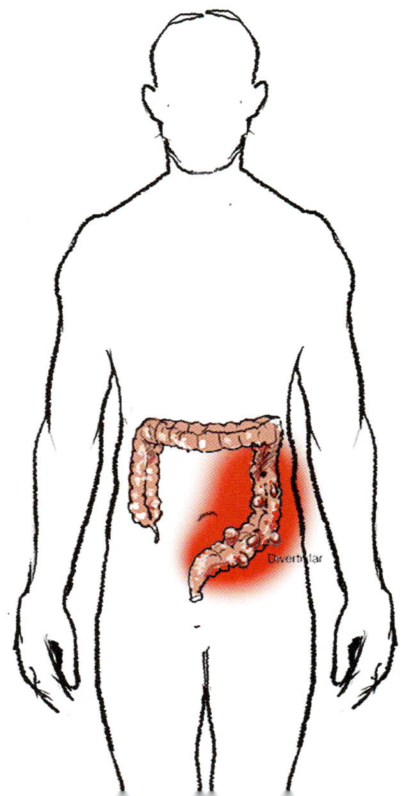

Immediate action

Rest the bowel by avoiding solid food and consuming fluids only.

Treatment

Bowel rest and a liquid diet can reverse the condition in mild cases. If symptoms worsen, including fever and pronounced abdominal pain, consult a doctor for antibiotics and further evaluation.

Far from help

Follow the treatment outlined above but make an early decision about administering antibiotics (for example, ciprofloxacin plus metronidazole). Prevent progression to peritonitis wherever possible. Seek advice from medical professionals and consider evacuation if the condition deteriorates.

Prevention

- Avoid constipation.
- Exercise regularly.
- Follow a fibre-rich diet with softeners such as dried fruit, prunes or figs.
- Drink plenty of fluids.

ANAL FISSURE

An anal fissure is a specific issue related to abdominal health, often secondary to constipation. Hard stools can cause small tears in the anal canal, leading to a painful cycle where fear of defecation worsens constipation.

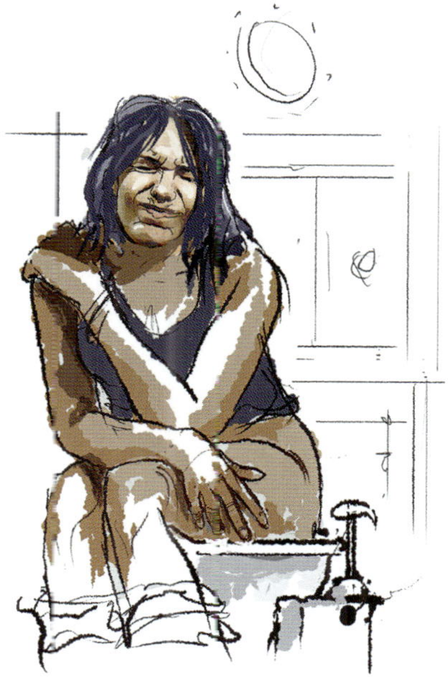

Fear of going to the toilet starts a vicious cycle.

Signs and symptoms

- Tenderness and intense pain during defecation
- Minor bleeding (for example, red spots on wipes)
- Fissure typically located in the posterior aspect of the anal canal

Immediate action

Apply a local anaesthetic gel such as lidocaine before defecation.

Treatment/Far from help

- Address constipation by keeping stools soft.
- Apply anti-inflammatory cream with a steroid and an analgesic to the affected area.
- Use a disposable glove to allow application in the sphincter.
- Relieve secondary anal muscle spasms with warm baths.
- Use a cleaning oil for hygiene to avoid irritation. Excessive washing with soap and water can damage the skin around the anus.

If symptoms persist, consider consulting a surgeon in the next port. Prognosis is usually good with proper treatment.

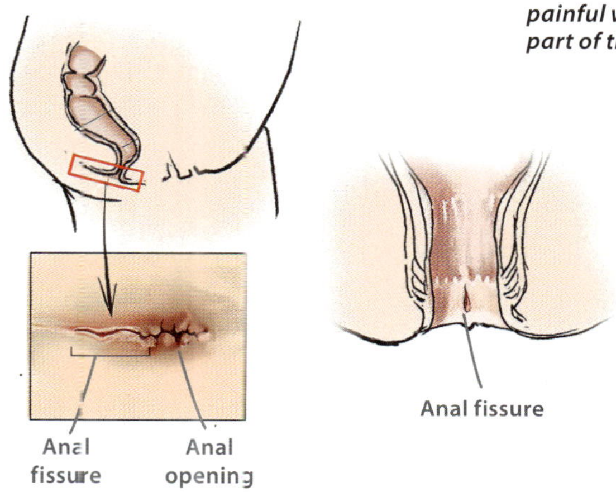

Anal fissure – a very painful wound in the skin part of the anal canal.

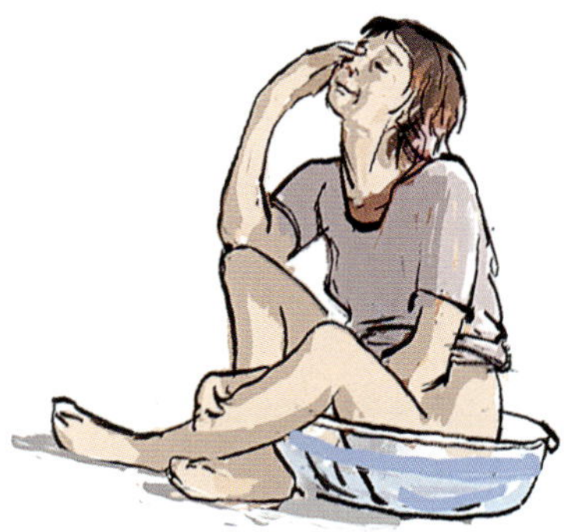

A hot sitting bath will lessen the painful spasm in the anal muscles. Arranging that may be challenging but still worthwhile trying if possible.

OTHER CAUSES OF ACUTE ABDOMINAL PAIN

- Ruptured aortic aneurysm: See page 83 under 'Cardiovascular'.
- Urological causes: Kidney stones, urinary tract infections or urinary retention. See page 120 under 'Urology'.
- Gynaecological causes: Ectopic pregnancy, miscarriage, ovarian cysts or fallopian tube problems. See page 110 under 'Gynaecology' and page 114, 'Pregnancy'.

13. GYNAECOLOGAY

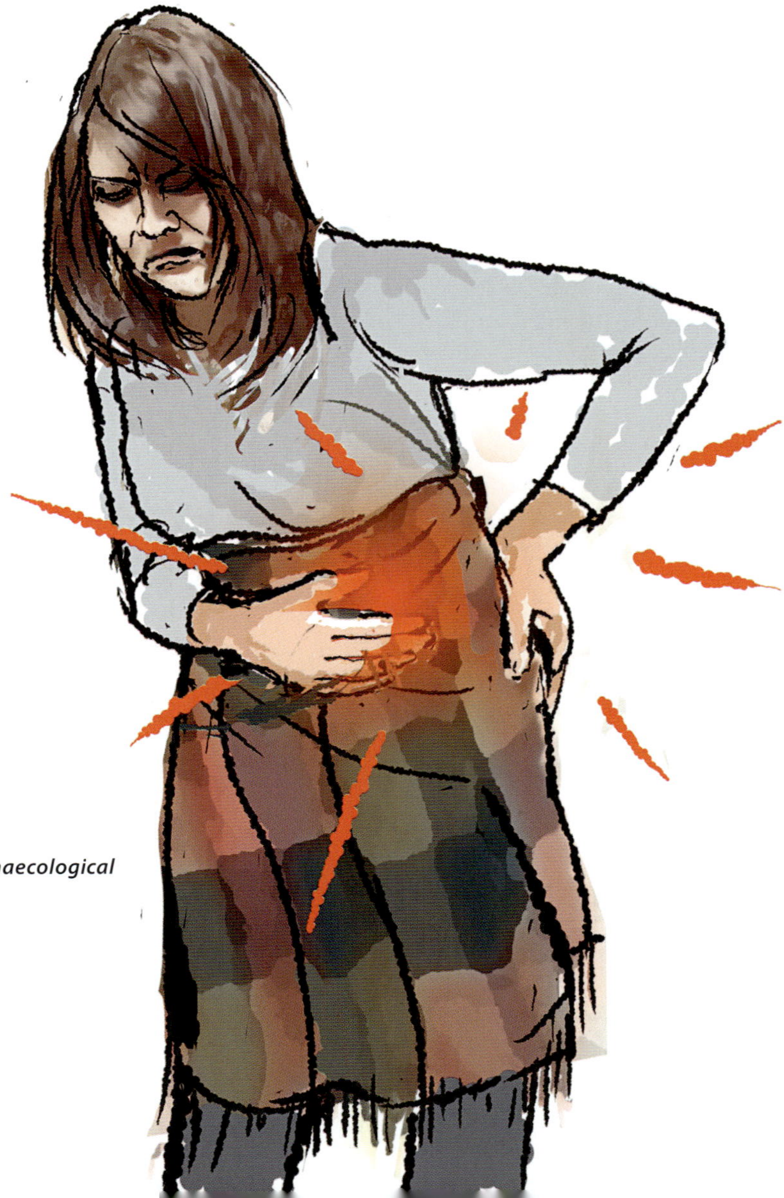

Abdominal or back pain in women – gynaecological disorder must be ruled out.

Acute abdominal pain in women requires special consideration. In addition to causes common to both genders, discomfort originating from the female reproductive organs must be taken into account. Normal conditions that can cause pain, even of high intensity, include menstruation, ovulation and endometriosis. These pains are usually recurrent and recognised, and therefore not unexpected or threatening.

General advice: If a woman does not recognise her symptoms, she should consult a doctor for advice.

Key questions to address:

Pregnant or not? This is a crucial factor in assessing associated risks and should be explored through relevant questions in the medical history:

- How did the pain start? Suddenly or gradually?
- When was the last menstruation? Was it normal?
- Is the woman pregnant?
- Was the pain associated with physical activity?
- Where is the pain located – one side, pelvis, back?
- Is there any bleeding or discharge?
- Has she had previous abdominal surgery?
- What type of contraception is being used?
- Are there general symptoms such as nausea or fever?

Pregnancy and delivery are discussed in a separate chapter (see pages 114–19).

SALPINGITIS

Fallopian tube infection (salpingitis) is relatively common. It may also involve infections in the uterus or urinary bladder and is typically caused by a sexually transmitted bacterial infection.

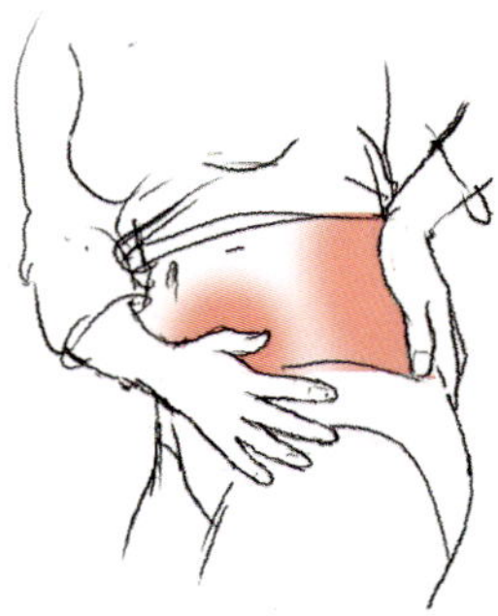

Location of pain in salpingitis.

Signs and symptoms

- Gradually increasing pain in the lower abdomen/pelvic area, radiating to the back
- Foul-smelling discharge and vaginal bleeding
- Fever, general discomfort, fatigue and malaise

Treatment

The woman should consult a doctor. If the pain involves the right side, it may be difficult to distinguish from appendicitis. Treatment typically includes antibiotics and hospitalisation.

Far from help

Contact healthcare professionals for advice. Bed rest and antibiotics (for example, ciprofloxacin; see table on page 249).

Prevention

Practise safe sex and use condoms.

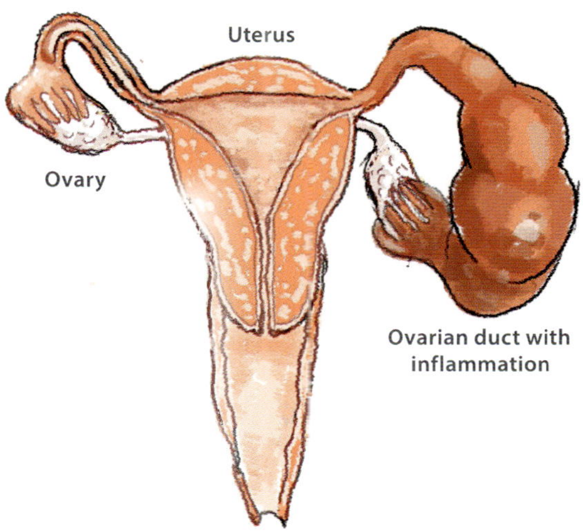

Right tube is swollen, red and inflamed. Left tube is normal.

RUPTURED OVARIAN CYST

Cysts are fluid-filled sacs that can form on the ovaries. Egg release during ovulation may leave behind a small fluid-filled cavity, which can later grow into a cyst. While cysts are generally harmless, they can rupture due to increased force or pressure, such as during physical activity or intercourse.

Signs and symptoms

- Sudden, severe pelvic/lower abdominal pain, often described as pain that starts instantly ('like turning on a light').
- The pain usually subsides within a few hours.

Treatment

Pain often necessitates a hospital visit for diagnosis. With a correct diagnosis, prognosis is good, with recovery within hours. Administer analgesics such as paracetamol or NSAIDs for pain relief.

Far from help

Though initially dramatic and concerning, the pain and anxiety typically subside within hours if the diagnosis is correct. Pain relief as above. Seek medical attention at the next port for follow-up.

Prevention

None known.

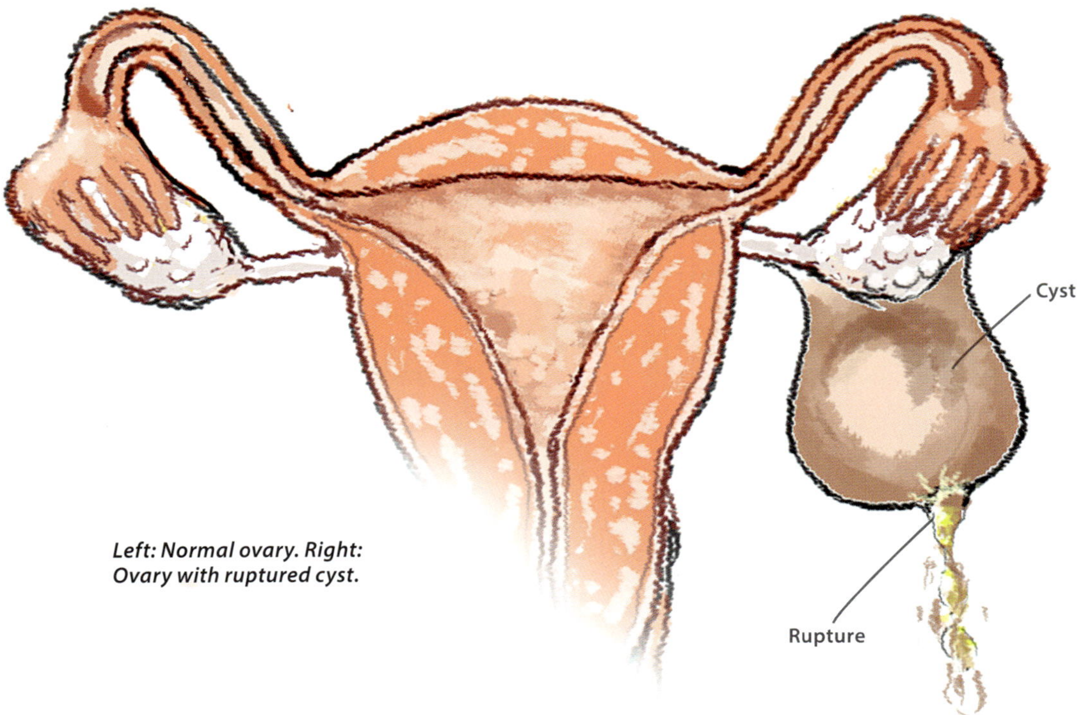

Left: Normal ovary. Right: Ovary with ruptured cyst.

TWISTED OVARY AND TUBE

The ovary's mobility may allow it and the fallopian tube to twist, cutting off circulation to the ovary.

Signs and symptoms

- Sudden, severe, one-sided lower abdominal pain radiating to the back.
- The woman can often pinpoint the exact moment the pain began.

Immediate action

Arrange transport to hospital.

Treatment

Surgery is required to correct the torsion. While not life-threatening, there may be an impact on fertility. Analgesics may be needed.

Far from help

Severe pain may necessitate evacuation. Strong analgesics, including opioids, might be required. As the diagnosis may be uncertain on board, treat as an acute abdomen (see page 90).

Prevention

None known.

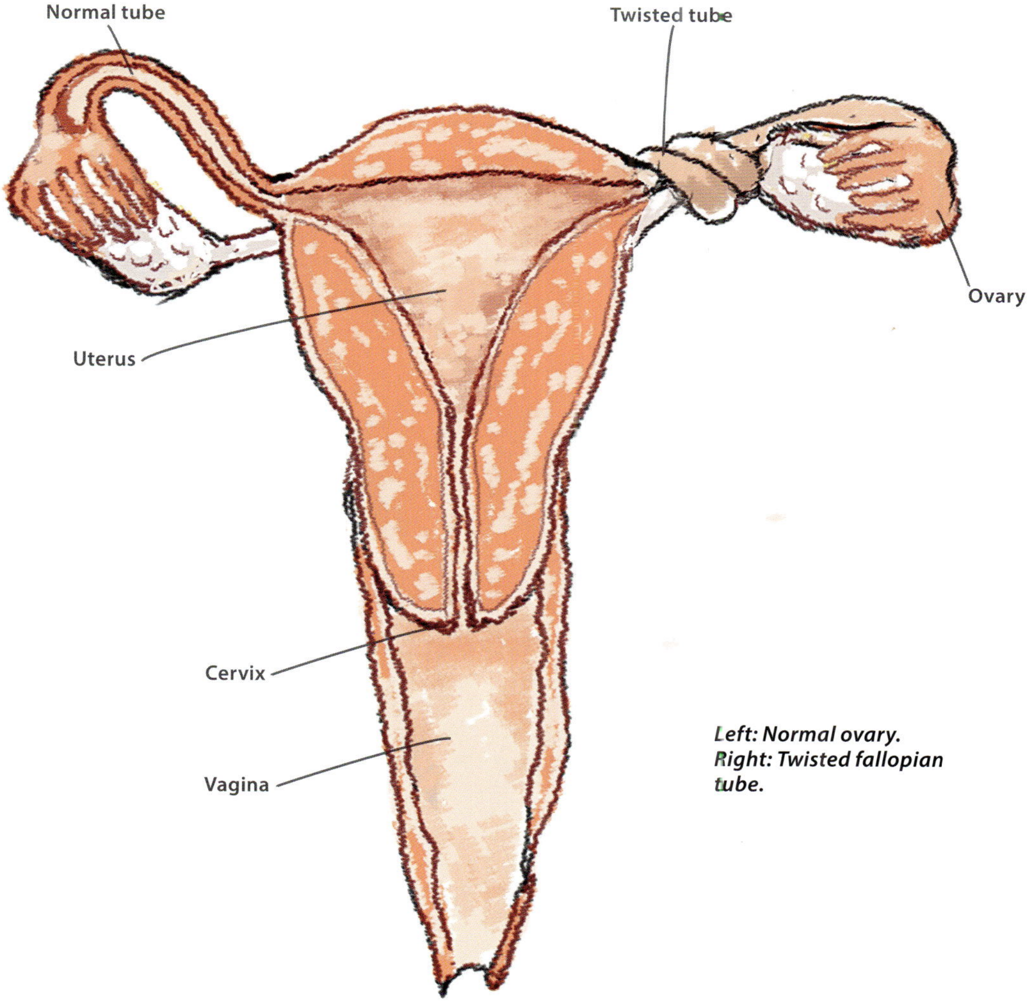

Left: Normal ovary.
Right: Twisted fallopian tube.

14. PREGNANCY – DELIVERY

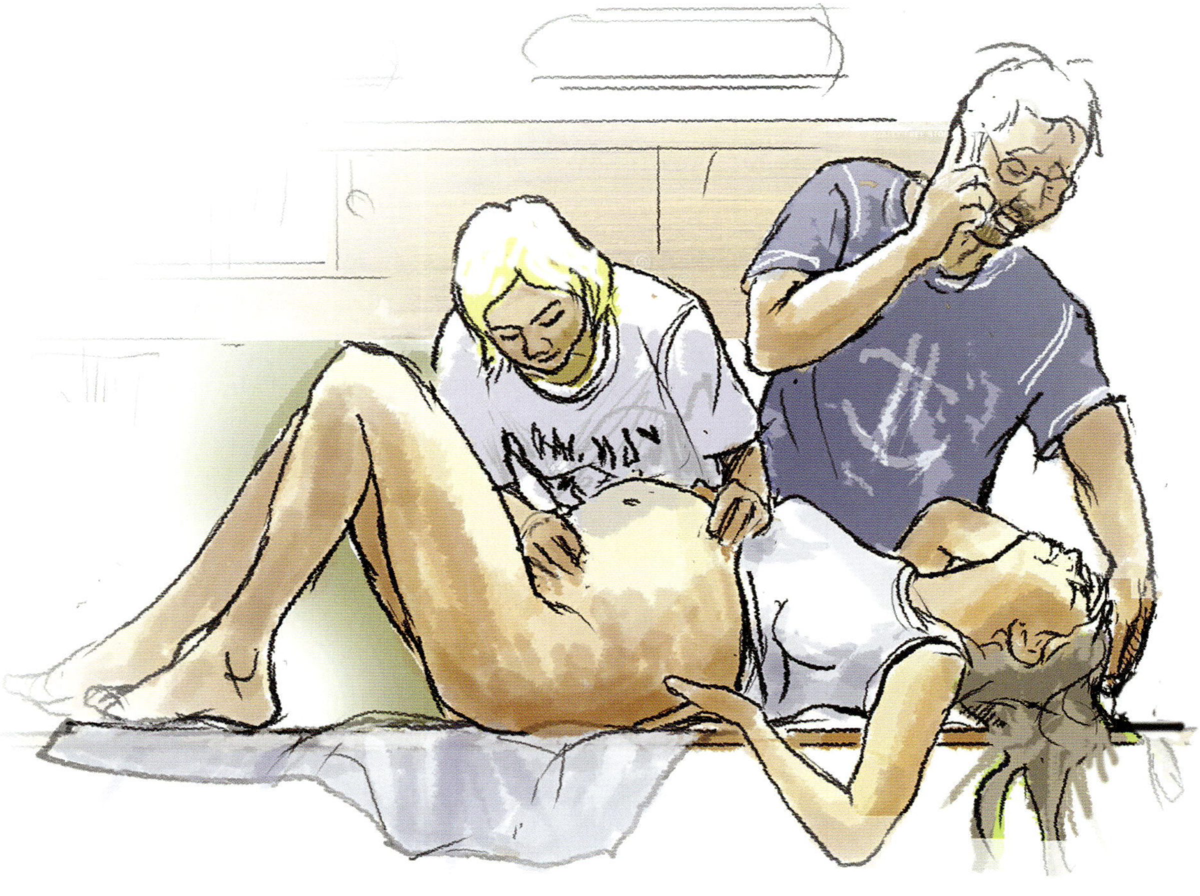

Delivery on board.

It is common for women in early pregnancy to travel, including on longer boat trips. Sometimes, a woman may not even be aware she is pregnant. However, with a pregnant woman on board, there is always a risk of complications, including miscarriage or early, rapid delivery.

From gestational week 22, the foetus is considered viable with proper care. If transport to a hospital is not possible, seek professional assistance via communication equipment. In the absence of professional help, trust in the natural process of childbirth, as humans have been giving birth for millennia without medical intervention.

GENERAL CONSIDERATIONS

- Labour usually begins between 37 and 42 weeks of pregnancy. It is advised to stay near a hospital from week 36 onwards.
- Assess the woman's condition if acute bleeding occurs. Watch for signs of circulatory shock, such as pallor, cold sweats and rapid pulse or breathing.

Signs and symptoms

- Labour begins with contractions, cramp-like pains around the uterus that radiate to the back. Contractions last for about a minute, with a few minutes of rest between each.
- The amniotic membrane ruptures, causing fluid to flow through the vagina.
- Pain intensifies and moves downwards, often experienced as pressure on the rectum.
- Breathing becomes heavy as labour progresses, and the mother begins to push as birth becomes imminent.

Immediate action

If transport to a hospital is impossible, seek professional guidance from an obstetrician, paediatrician or neonatology specialist using available communication equipment.

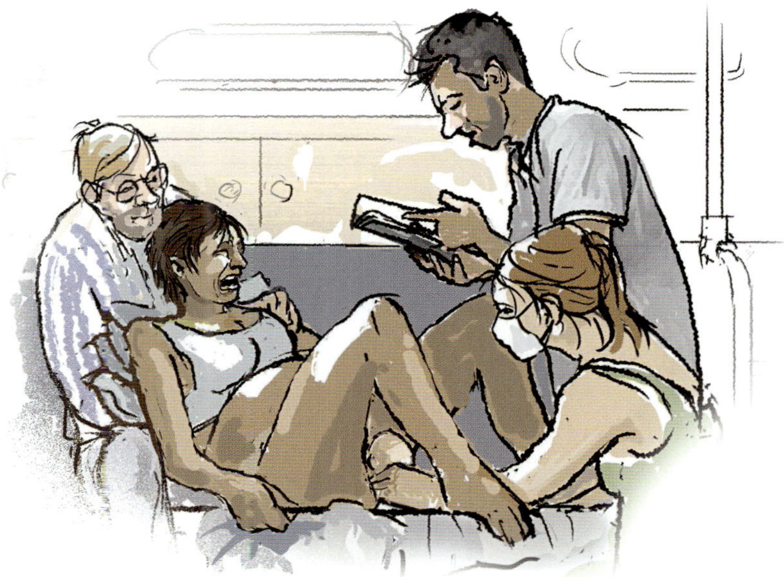

Managing a delivery on board is of course not an ideal situation and should be avoided.

Treatment / Far from help

- Allow the mother to choose a comfortable position for labour and the pace at which she pushes.
- Maintain a calm environment and assist the mother in breathing steadily.
- During the expulsion phase, gently guide the baby's head with one hand to prevent a rapid delivery. Often, the mother is best equipped to guide the baby's head herself.

Gently hold a hand on the head to counteract a too rapid delivery.

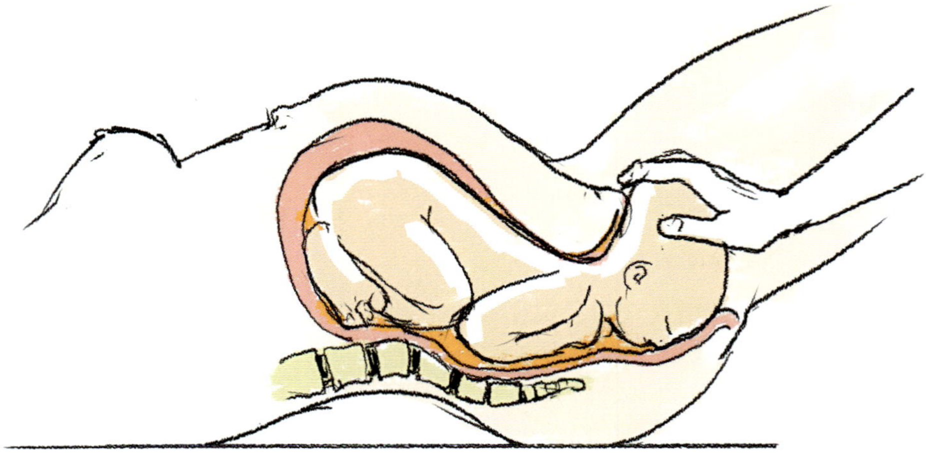

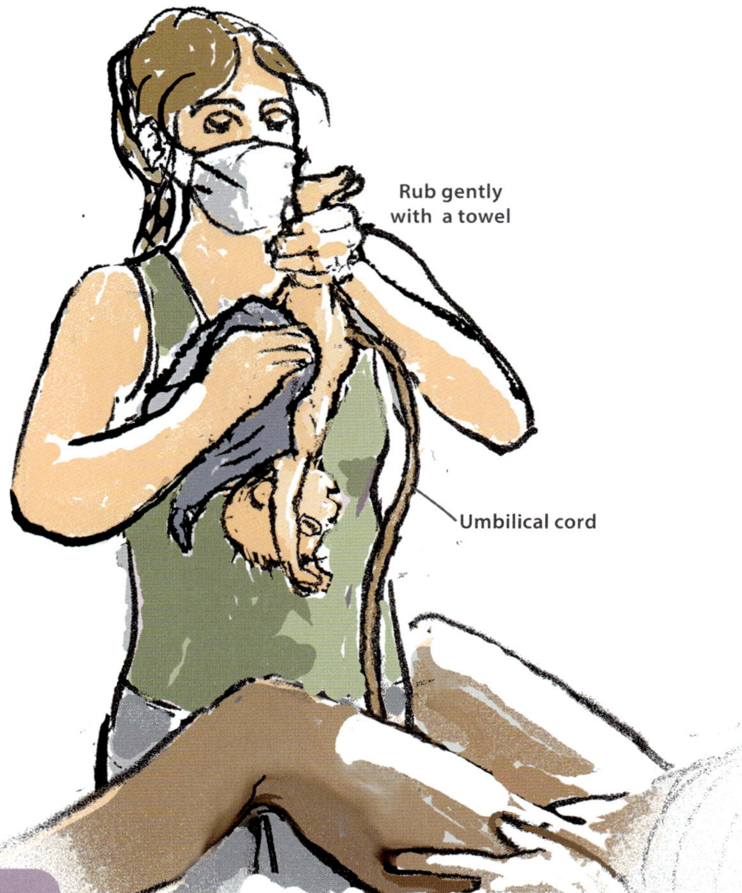

- Be prepared to receive the baby. Use disposable gloves, warm towels and blankets. Newborns are often wet and slippery, so caution is essential to prevent the baby from slipping.
- Dry the baby gently, especially around the mouth and eyes. Hold the baby in a draining position (head down) to encourage breathing and crying within 30 seconds. If the baby does not cry, rub its back gently with a towel.
- Place the baby on the mother's chest, skin-to-skin, to keep it warm.
- The baby remains connected to the placenta via the umbilical cord. Allow blood from the placenta to drain into the baby until the placenta detaches naturally, usually within 30 minutes.

Draining position immediately after delivery.

- When the placenta is expelled:

1. Tie off the cord with two strings or clamps and cut between them.
2. Ensure the knots are secure to prevent bleeding.
3. Encourage the baby to latch on to the mother's nipple for suckling, which helps stimulate uterine contractions and bonding.
4. Continue to keep the baby warm, and both mother and baby must be transported to a hospital at the earliest opportunity.

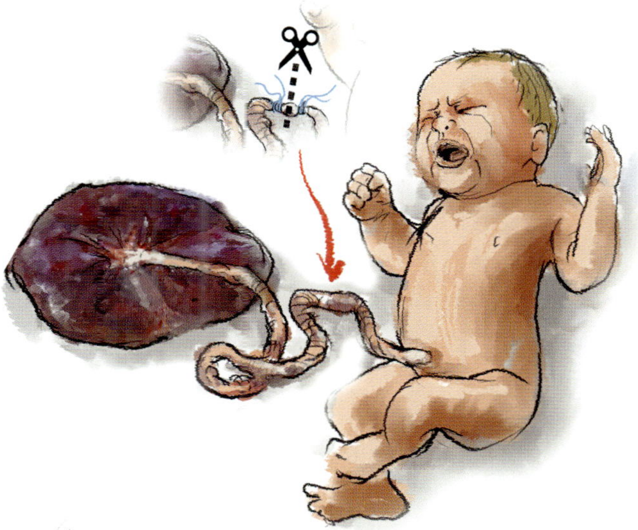

Tie off the umbilical cord with two strings or clamps and cut between them. Check the knots to prevent bleeding.

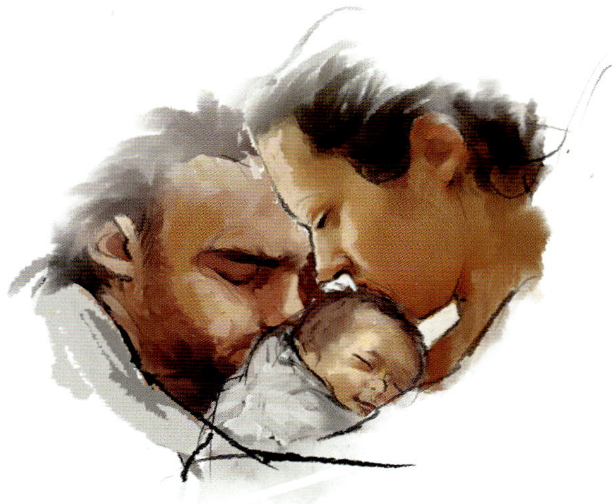

Dry the baby, keep it warm, and place it on the mother's chest – this provides the best comfort.

Premature newborns are facing a tough start in life and need hospital care! If premature and far from help, the prognosis for survival is pessimistic.

Prevention

- Pregnant individuals should prioritise safety by staying ashore and close to medical facilities from week 36 onwards.

INSURANCE

Check that health insurance covers pregnancy-related medical costs after 28 weeks of gestation, especially for international travel. Failure to do so may result in the mother or family bearing significant expenses.

MISCARRIAGES

A woman may be in early, unconfirmed pregnancy, with only a slightly unusual recent menstrual cycle. Miscarriages are most common during the first 12 weeks of pregnancy. After 22 weeks, it is classified as a preterm birth.

Signs and symptoms

- Early miscarriages: Resemble heavier and more painful menstrual bleeding.
- Later miscarriages: Can involve severe labour-like pains and carry a greater risk of heavy bleeding. Discharge often contains blood clots and tissue.

Immediate action

1 Follow DRABC protocols (see page 12) if symptoms are dramatic.

2 Seek emergency care or a maternity ward if the pregnancy has passed 22 weeks of gestation.

3 The woman should rest, stay warm, and urgently see a doctor.

Treatment

A very early miscarriage can possibly be managed on board. Give rest, heat and paracetamol. Seek professional advice. Always seek a gynaecologist for a check-up at the earliest opportunity.

If later in pregnancy, it might present an extreme challenge, including risk to life. Contact healthcare professionals immediately. The woman will likely need medical attention and evacuation as soon as possible, a true challenge during longer passages. Heat, care, fluids and pain relief are what can be offered on board while waiting for help. Antibiotics, such as ciprofloxacin (see table on page 249), may be needed.

Far from help

See above. Early miscarriage is with the best of luck manageable even when far from help. Late miscarriages or the slightest doubt necessitates evacuation and medical support.

Prevention

Captains should evaluate the risks of having a pregnant woman on board and may need to refuse passage. Day cruises in home waters may be considered, but longer voyages are discouraged.

EXTRAUTERINE (ECTOPIC) PREGNANCY

An ectopic pregnancy occurs when a fertilised egg implants outside the uterus, most commonly in the fallopian tube. As the embryo grows, the limited space can cause the tube to rupture, resulting in bleeding that can become life-threatening. This condition is typically detected in time for surgical or medical intervention. Symptoms usually appear 8 to 12 weeks after conception.

Signs and symptoms

Always consider ectopic pregnancy when a woman of childbearing age experiences sudden acute lower abdominal pain radiating to the back. If the bleeding is significant, the woman may become clammy, pale, dizzy, and perhaps faint, showing signs of internal bleeding and shock with a rapid pulse and breathing, see page 20.

Immediate actions

1. Follow DRABC protocols for shock (see page 12).
2. Position the patient appropriately for circulatory shock (see page 20).
3. Make an urgent call for medical assistance.

Treatment

Rest, keep warm and provide fluids. Transport the woman to hospital immediately for surgical or medical intervention.

Far from help

Ectopic pregnancies with significant bleeding are extremely challenging during long voyages. Prioritise rest, warmth and fluids, and administer pain relief. Medical evacuation is critical and must be arranged as soon as possible.

Prevention

Avoid pregnancy or suspend sailing during this period of life. Early pregnancy (5–12 weeks) should be closely monitored for symptoms, with immediate medical consultation for any concerning signs.

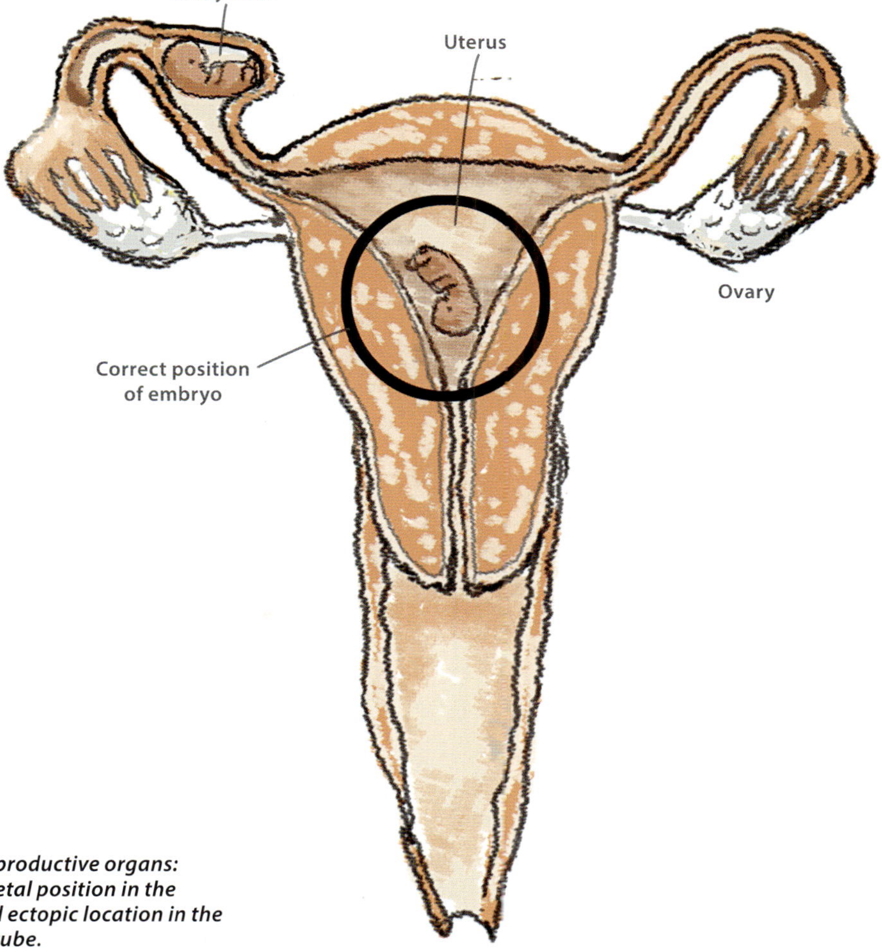

Female reproductive organs: normal foetal position in the uterus and ectopic location in the fallopian tube.

15. UROLOGY

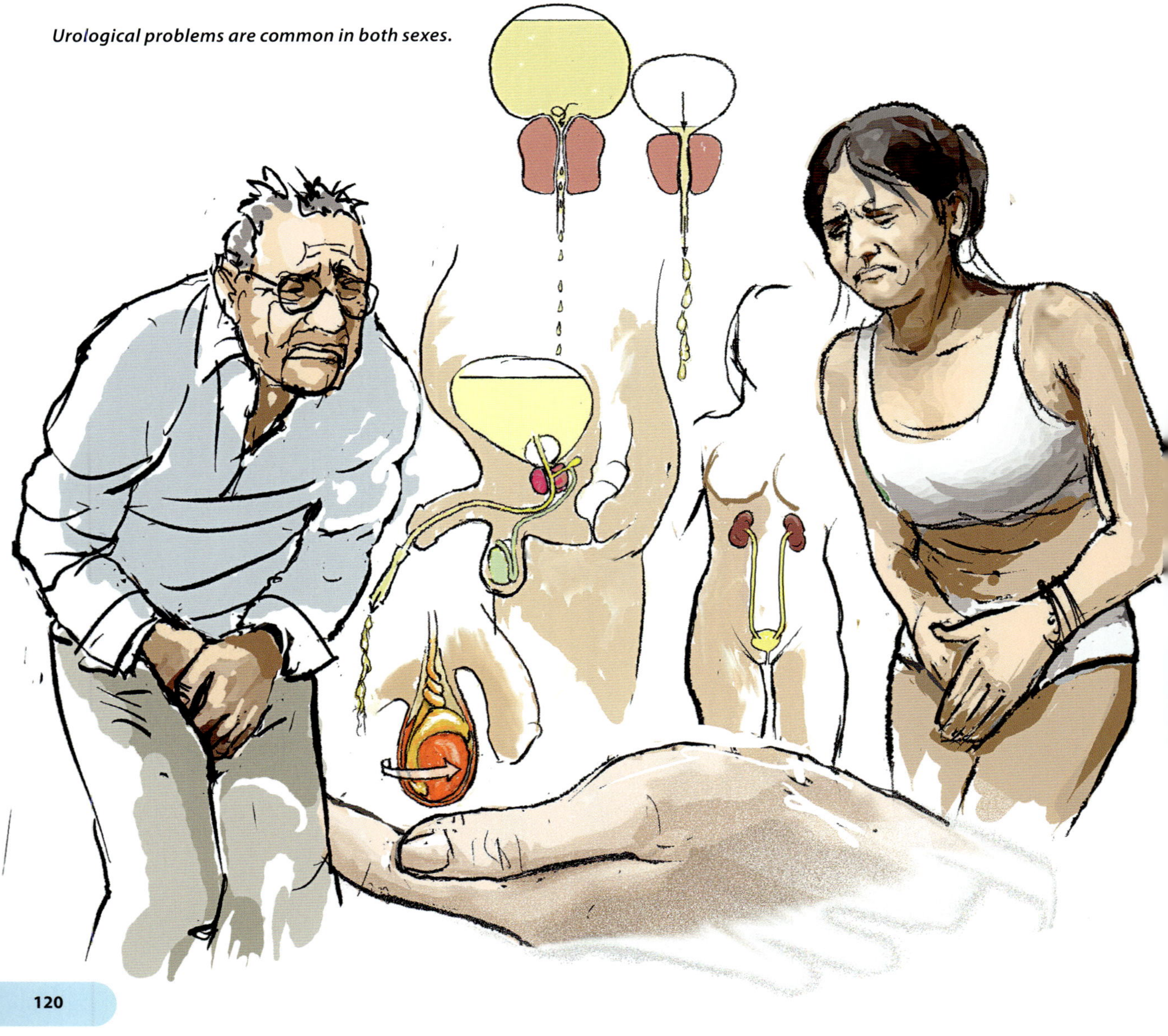

Urological problems are common in both sexes.

Urological problems are indeed common in both sexes but they differ regarding causes, course and complications.

CYSTITIS IN WOMEN

Cystitis (urinary tract infection – UTI) in women is a common reason for outpatient medical visits. It is primarily caused by bacterial contamination from the anal region. Cystitis is common in women but rare in men due to the shorter urethra in women. Half of all women will experience cystitis requiring antibiotic treatment at some point. However, one-third of those with symptoms become symptom-free within one week without antibiotics.

Symptoms of cystitis may also occur in women without detectable bacteria in the urine.

Triggering factors may include:

- high sexual activity
- vulnerable mucous membranes
- excessive hygiene
- local allergy

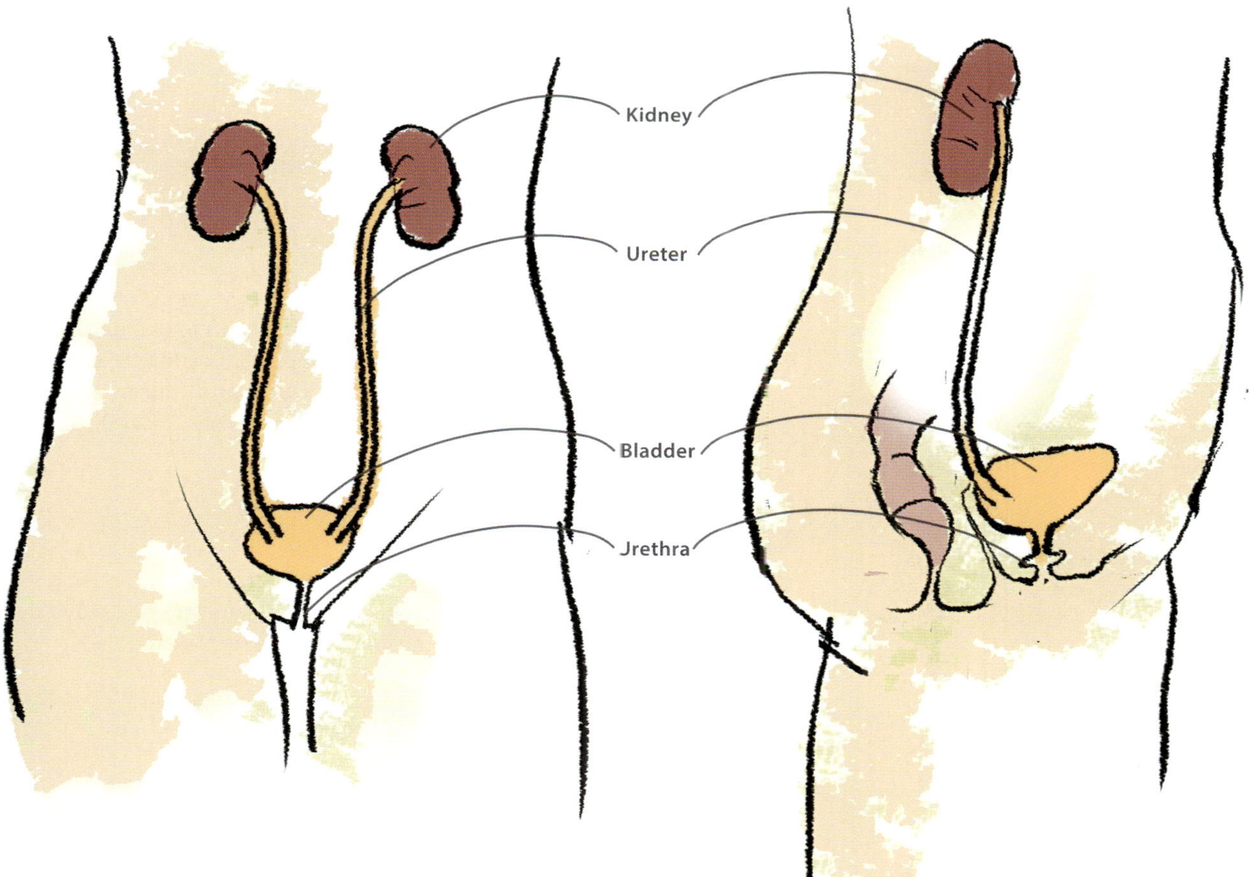

Female urinary tract. Note the short distance between the anal opening and the urethra.

Signs and symptoms

- Urgency to urinate
- Frequent urination
- Foul-smelling urine
- Burning sensation during urination
- Abdominal pain
- Tenderness over the bladder area
- Fever
- Cloudy urine
- Blood in the urine

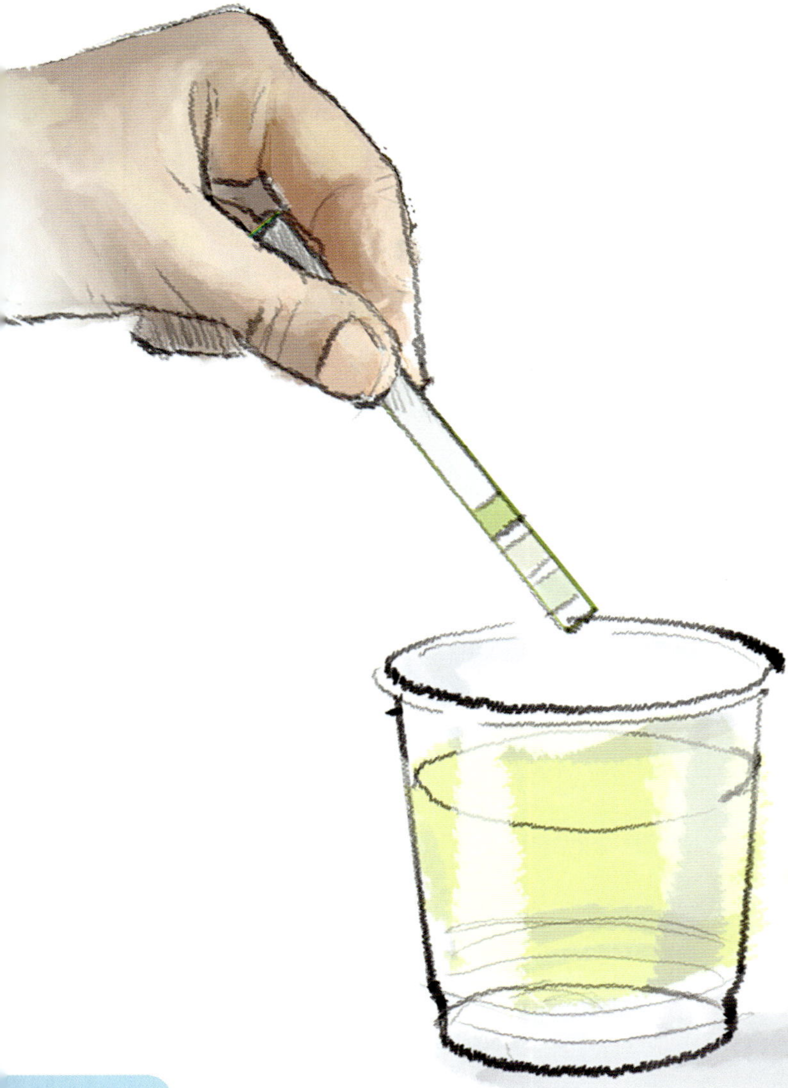

Treatment

Uncomplicated cystitis

If the test strip is negative for bacteria and there is no fever, it may be possible to wait a couple of days before starting antibiotics or consulting a doctor. Drink plenty of fluids (at least 1.5 litres per day) to flush the urinary tract and bladder. Even with a test strip positive for infection, antibiotics can often be delayed if symptoms are mild and there is no fever. Start antibiotics (tablet pivmecillinam 200mg, every 8 hours for 7 days) if the condition worsens.

Complicated cystitis

Seek medical attention for assessment and possibly a urine culture if antibiotic resistance is suspected, treatment is ineffective, the infection recurs frequently, or if there is high fever or suspected renal involvement. Up to one-third of women experience recurrent cystitis, defined as symptoms occurring at least twice within six months.

Far from help

If medical care is unavailable, antibiotics may need to be started without a preceding urine culture. A common choice is trimethoprim (200mg twice daily). For complicated cystitis with fever or suspected renal involvement, a broader-spectrum antibiotic, such as ciprofloxacin 500mg (1 tablet every 12 hours for 7 days), may be needed.

Prevention

- Drink plenty of fluids.
- Maintain careful hygiene. After using the toilet, wipe from front to back to avoid transferring bacteria towards the urethra.

Urinate in a glass container. Check urine for colour and smell. Use a test strip for nitrite or leukocyte esterase.

MYTH BUSTER

It is often suggested that cranberry juice or other substances that acidify urine can relieve symptoms and help prevent urinary tract infections. However, high doses are required, and there is no scientific evidence to support their use in treating an ongoing infection.

PYELONEPHRITIS (KIDNEY INFECTION)

Pyelonephritis often begins with typical cystitis symptoms that worsen. Bacteria ascend from the bladder through the ureter to the kidneys. Symptoms become more severe, and hospitalisation may be necessary. It is important to note that pyelonephritis can develop without noticeable urinary symptoms. The condition differs between women and men. In women it is normally an infection ascending from the bladder. In men it is associated with prostate enlargement, which causes problems emptying the bladder (see below).

Signs and symptoms

- General malaise
- High, fluctuating fever (temperature jumps between 38°C and over 40°C)
- Chills
- Pain and tenderness over the bladder
- Pain and tenderness in the kidney area
- Nausea/vomiting

With these symptoms, it is crucial to seek medical attention. Up to 30 per cent of women with cystitis and fever may have bacteria in their blood, indicating a risk of septicaemia.

Far from help

Pyelonephritis carries a risk of sepsis and rapid deterioration. Antibiotic treatment should be started immediately. We recommend ciprofloxacin 500mg tablets (1 tablet every 12 hours daily for 7 days). Seek medical advice as soon as possible.

Monitor renal function by tracking fluid intake and urine output.

Prevention

See the cystitis prevention section above (page 122).

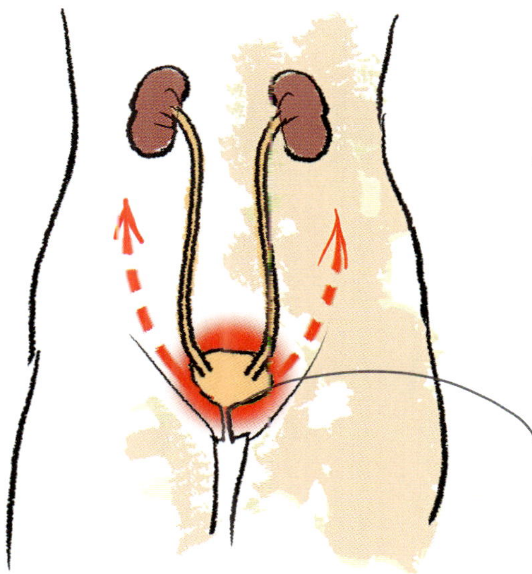

Pain radiation and tenderness in cystitis/pyelonephritis.

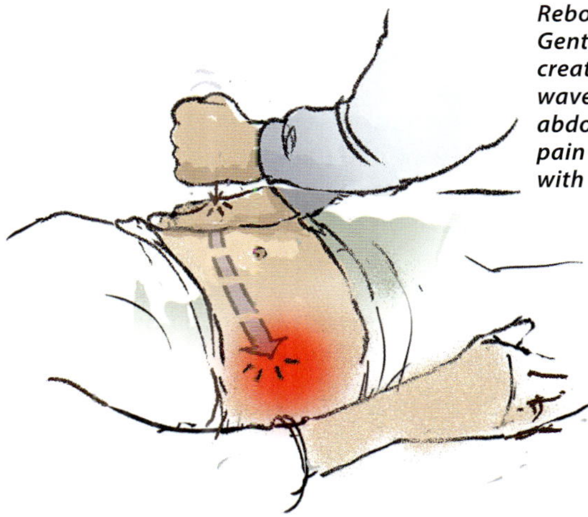

Rebound tenderness. Gentle thumping creates a slight wave moving in the abdomen, provoking pain around an area with inflammation.

URINARY TRACT INFECTION IN MEN

Cystitis and urinary tract infections are less common in men, particularly at younger ages. The most common urinary issues in men arise after the age of 50 to 60 and involve difficulties emptying the bladder (see below). The combination of voiding difficulties and infection presents a significant risk of bacteraemia and septic shock.

Normal urogenital anatomy in men. Note the distance to the anus, the length of the urethra, and the ureter passing through the prostate.

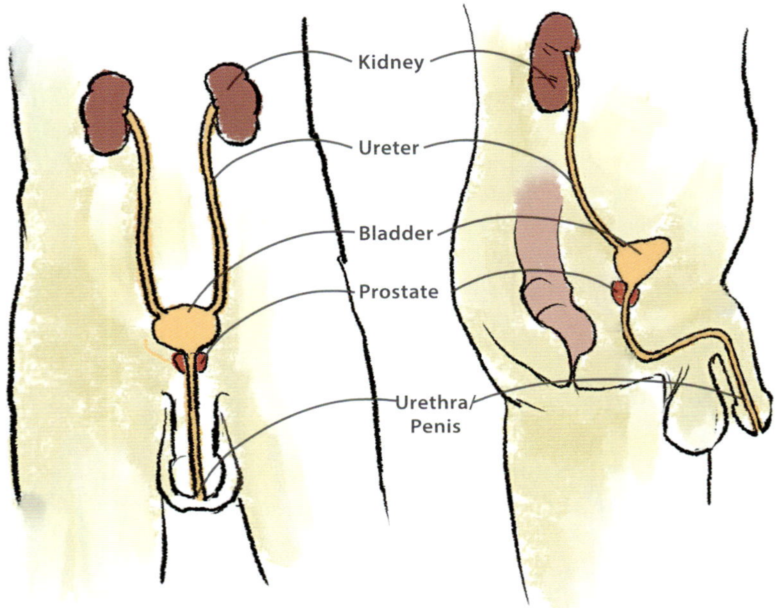

Signs and symptoms

Refer to the section above under 'Women/ Pyelonephritis' for common signs and symptoms. If an older man (60+ years) experiences chills, fever, general malaise, nausea or vomiting, with or without urinary symptoms, a urinary tract infection should be suspected until proven otherwise.

Treatment

Urgent medical attention is required for examination and treatment. It is not uncommon for this condition to progress rapidly, requiring intensive care.

Far from help

If a urinary tract infection is suspected and medical care is unavailable, the situation is potentially life-threatening. Diagnosis is based on symptoms, clinical signs, and possibly a urine test strip. Contact medical care for advice.

Initiating antibiotic treatment without a preceding culture is necessary. A broad-spectrum antibiotic with a longer treatment course is recommended, as the prostate is often also infected. Ciprofloxacin 500mg tablets (1 tablet every 8 hours daily for 10 days) is a common choice. If a large volume of residual urine is present, emptying the bladder via catheterisation may be life-saving (see below under 'Urinary retention').

Prevention

- Consult a urologist to determine the amount of residual urine left in the bladder after urination and whether bladder-emptying issues can be corrected.
- For additional prevention strategies, see the section on 'Urinary retention' below.

Urinary retention

This section focuses on men, as urinary retention is extremely rare in women. Between 60 and 80 per cent of men over the age of 60 experience prostate gland enlargement. This is often benign (age-related) but can occasionally be due to cancer. Symptoms, detailed below, usually increase gradually. Despite adaptations, they often become bothersome, creating a disabling need for easy toilet access.

A constant residual volume of urine in the bladder provides a favourable environment for bacterial growth. Additionally, there is a risk of the bladder overfilling (up to 1.5–2 litres), which can lead to the inability to empty the bladder entirely. This situation is painful and potentially damaging to bladder and kidney function. Normal residual volume after voiding is approximately 50ml.

Signs and symptoms

These symptoms are common in elderly men.

- Weak urine stream
- Difficulty initiating urination
- Prolonged urination time
- Dribbling after urination
- Frequent night-time urination

Progression to total retention can worsen symptoms, including:

- a feeling of heaviness and distension
- severe urgency and pain over the bladder
- frequent urination of very small volumes

MYTH BUSTER

Urine test strips for diagnosing urinary tract infections can yield false negatives, due either to insufficient bacteria or to bacterial strains that do not register on the strip.

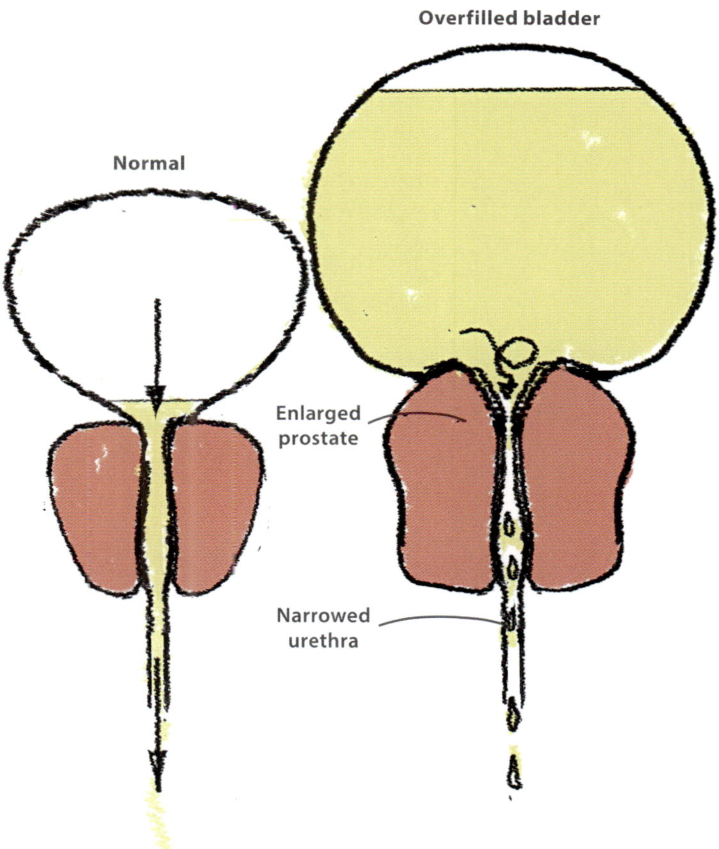

Schematic presentation of emptying problems with enlarged prostate. Left: Normal prostate and bladder emptying. Right: Enlarged prostate, narrowed urethra and emptying difficulties.

Urinary retention: over-distended bladder. Catheter in place, with the tip in the bladder and locking balloon.

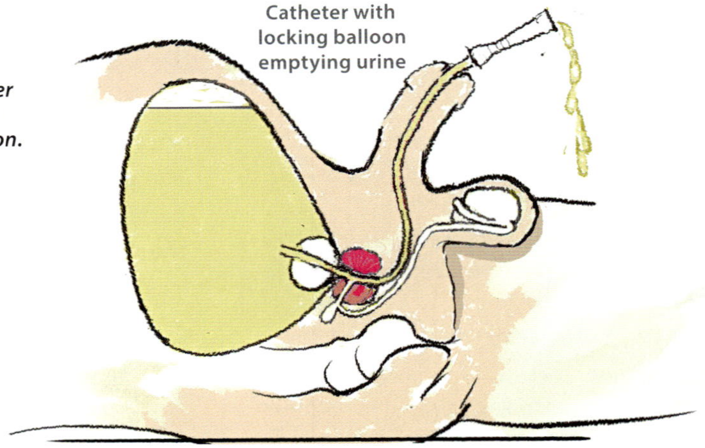

Treatment

Initially, attempt to create a calm environment, use relaxing medication (for example, diazepam 2mg tablets), and try auditory stimuli like the sound of running water. If these measures fail, the bladder should be emptied using a urinary catheter.

When in local waters, go to the nearest hospital for evaluation and treatment.

Far from help

Symptoms and physiological consequences will escalate rapidly. Immediate steps should include either arranging evacuation or inserting a urinary catheter and leaving it until consultation by a surgeon in the next port. If possible, seek guidance via radio or satellite phone.

Prevention

General guidelines:

- Be aware that certain medications, such as seasickness remedies (for example, Scopoderm), can affect bladder function and increase the risk of urinary retention.
- Allow sufficient time for urination; avoid rushing.
- Avoid excessive alcohol consumption.

If in doubt consult a urologist (see box below).

SPECIFIC MEASURES – CATHETERISATION

Before undertaking long ocean crossings of more than three to four days, a man with symptoms of prostate enlargement should consult a urologist. Depending on the severity of the condition, the urologist may recommend bringing catheterisation equipment. In such cases, a urotherapist will teach you how to use it.

Although most men find the idea of self-catheterisation daunting, it is manageable with the proper equipment and technique. There are examples of male sailors self-catheterising twice daily during Atlantic crossings. Young individuals with spinal cord injuries perform self-catheterisation daily for life, demonstrating that it is feasible.

If a catheter is inserted, it is advisable to leave it in place until reaching the next port with access to medical assistance.

KIDNEY STONES

Kidney stones are more common in men (10–20 per cent) than in women (3–5 per cent), with the highest prevalence occurring in individuals in their 40s. The incidence appears to be increasing, possibly due to dietary habits. Once a person has experienced kidney stones, the risk of recurrence is approximately 50 per cent.

Kidney stones form in the kidney and may dislodge, travelling with urine from the kidney into the ureter. This often occurs during urination, resulting in a dramatic and painful kidney stone attack.

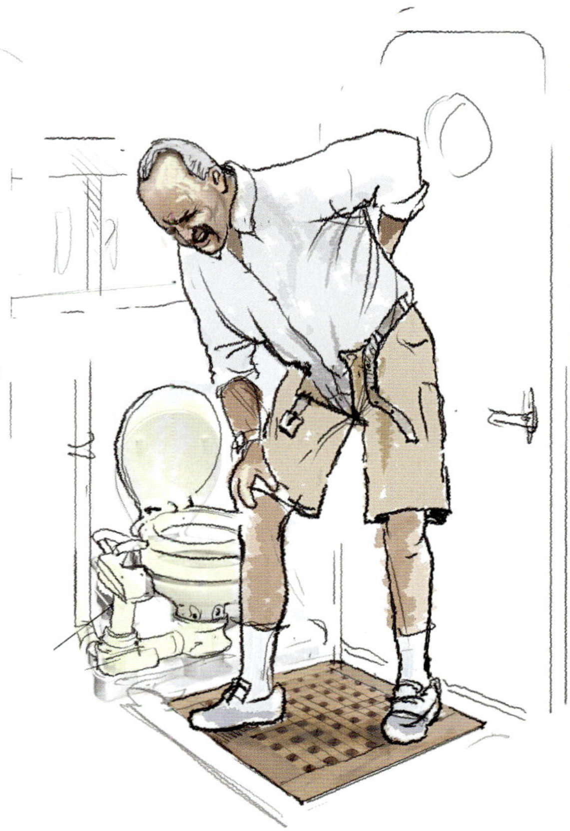

Acute kidney stone. Characteristically sudden onset of unbearable pain.

Signs and symptoms

The pain is severe and starts suddenly, described as a stabbing sensation, often occurring during urination. The pain is typically localised in the back, radiating to the groin and sometimes extending to the scrotum. Affected individuals are often restless, unable to find relief.

Pain episodes can last anywhere from half an hour to a day. Blood in the urine is common but not alarming in itself. About 80 per cent of kidney stones pass spontaneously through the ureter into the bladder, eventually being expelled during urination. However, stones larger than 5mm are unlikely to pass on their own.

Immediate action

The event is often dramatic. Focus on establishing a diagnosis and excluding other more serious causes. Providing pain relief is essential.

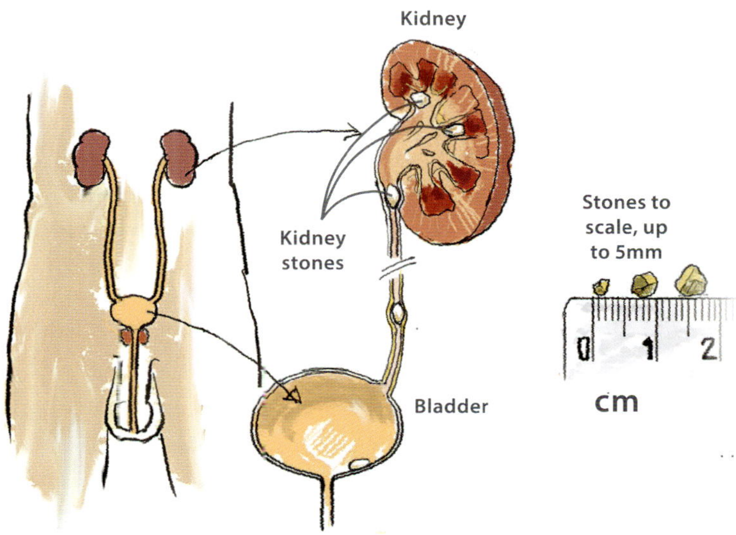

Formation, location and size of kidney stones.

Typical location of stabbing pain in acute kidney stone attack, often in association with urination.

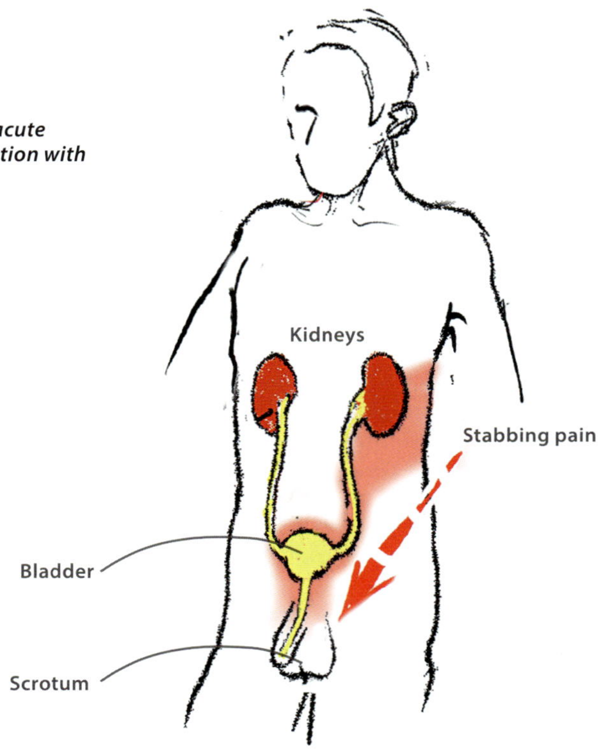

Treatment

- An anti-inflammatory medication (for example, NSAID, ibuprofen) is the first choice. Alternatively, combining with paracetamol can provide relief.
- If anti-inflammatory medication is available as a suppository, it will be more effective and act faster.
- Drink plenty of fluids, as increased urine flow enhances the likelihood of flushing out the stone.
- If the pain subsides, medical attention can be sought later for a follow-up upon returning home.

Contact or seek immediate medical attention if:

- the cause of the pain is uncertain
- the individual does not become pain-free
- there are repeated, severe pain attacks
- fever is present

Far from help

When far from medical care, the same recommendations apply. A doctor's visit is essential to confirm that the stone has passed and to ensure that the kidney has unobstructed drainage. This check-up should occur within two to three weeks.

An obstructed kidney will eventually sustain damage. Recovery to normal function is possible if the obstruction is relieved within about 14 days. If an infection develops, the risk of permanent kidney damage is significant, even in the acute stage.

Self-monitoring: You can check whether the stone has passed by urinating into a glass jar or container, which allows you to see the stone. Alternatively, filter the urine through a fine strainer or a piece of thin stocking.

ACUTE SCROTAL PAIN – TESTICULAR TORSION

This condition can occur in men of all ages but is most common in boys and younger men. Common causes of testicular pain include inflamed epididymis, cysts, or testicular torsion.

It is essential to rule out testicular torsion, as it is the focus here and can be detrimental to the affected testicle. Torsion occurs when the testicle twists around its own stalk (the spermatic cord), resulting in an acute interruption of blood circulation to the testicle.

Signs and symptoms

- Sudden, often dramatic onset of one-sided severe scrotal pain, frequently beginning during sleep.
- Swelling and tenderness of the affected testicle.
- Abdominal pain, nausea and vomiting may also occur.

Immediate action

In coastal areas, urgent transport to a hospital is required for examination and treatment.

Treatment

Testicular torsion must be treated surgically, ideally within six hours, to preserve testicular function. Due to the difficulty of clinical diagnosis, surgical exploration is often performed.

Far from help

In remote locations, an attempt to untwist the testicle manually may be necessary. Rotate the testicle gently in the specified direction. Seek medical attention as soon as possible, as surgical intervention is still required to prevent permanent damage.

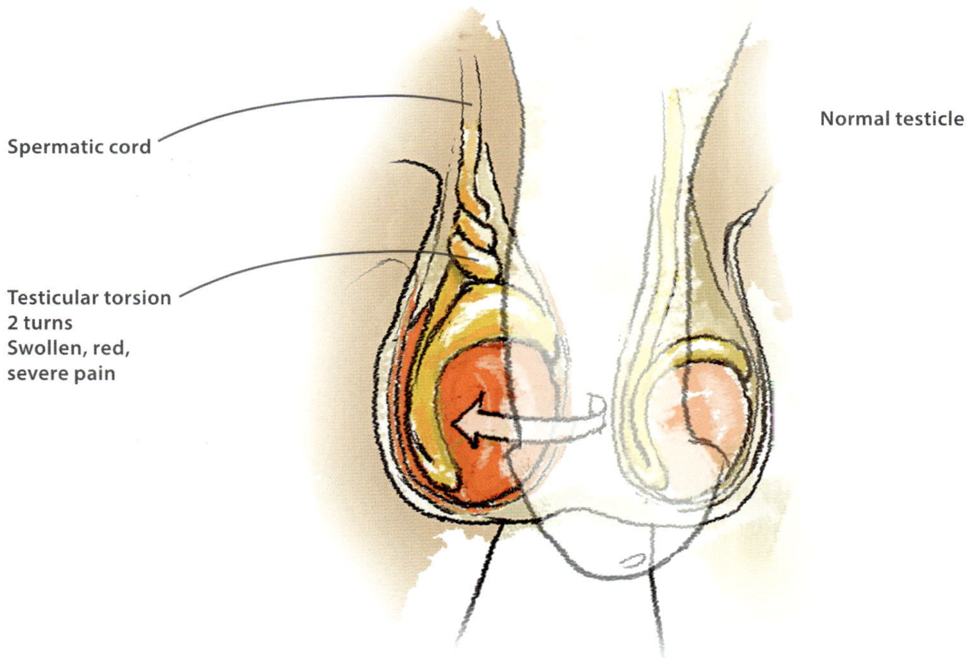

Twisted, swollen, ischaemic testicle. Attempt to untwist by rotating to the right. For the left testicle, untwist to the left.

16. HEAD INJURIES

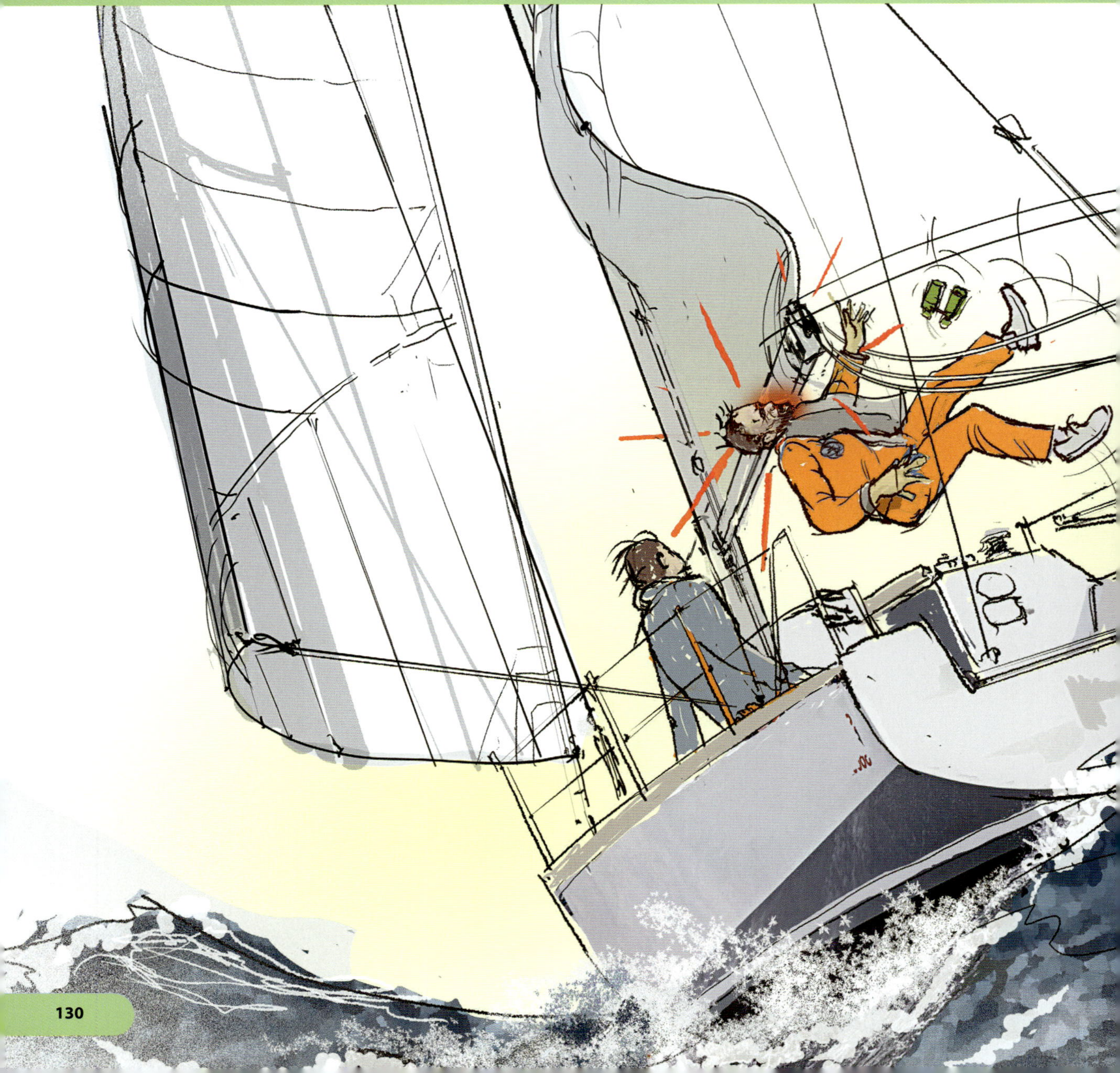

This section describes the various types of head injuries, ranging from scalp wounds to different levels of traumatic brain injury. It provides advice on how to manage these situations under the unique and challenging conditions encountered at sea, far from medical help.

IMPORTANT

All head injuries should be assessed by a doctor in a hospital. When at sea, it is particularly crucial to seek early medical advice in cases of head injury.

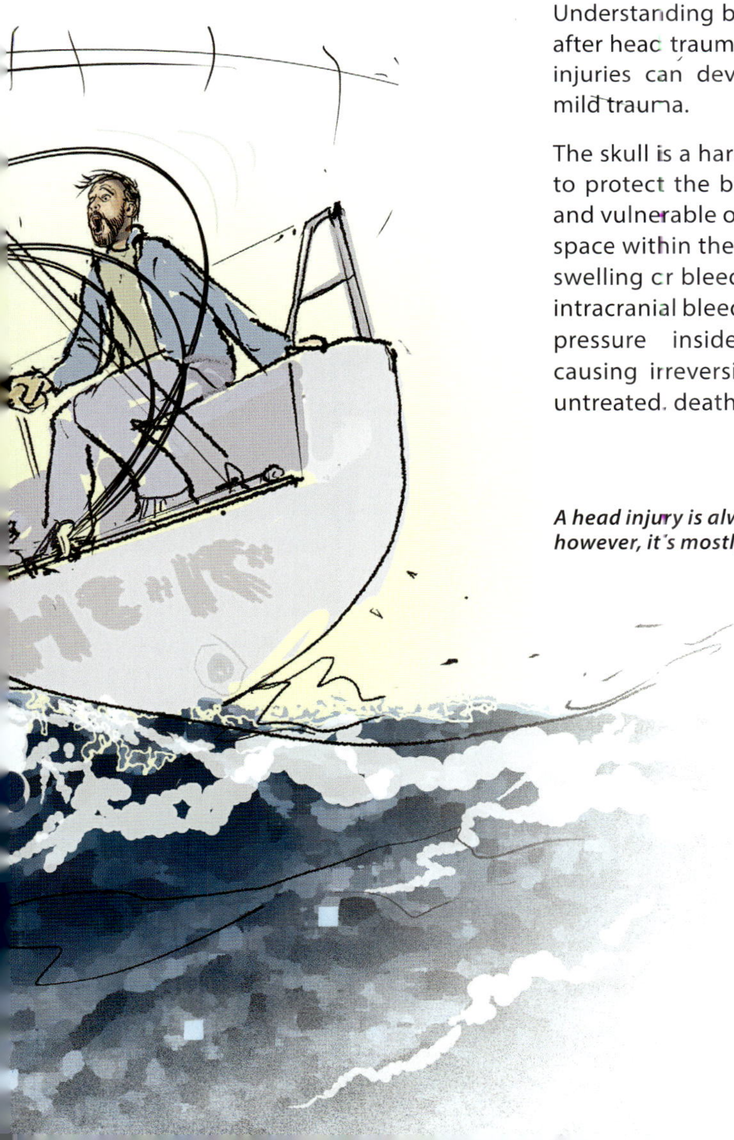

Minor head injuries resulting from falls or collisions are common during boat life. However, every such trauma must be thoroughly managed to exclude severe complications. There are well-documented cases of fatal accidents related to head injuries during ocean races and cruising.

Be aware! A scalp laceration often draws significant attention due to bleeding, but it is more important to evaluate the risk of an associated traumatic brain injury (TBI) and/or a neck injury. All persons with head trauma should be assessed by a doctor. At sea, you must obtain professional support via on-board communication systems.

Understanding brain injuries that may arise after head trauma is essential. Serious brain injuries can develop even after relatively mild trauma.

The skull is a hard, rigid structure designed to protect the brain – a vital but complex and vulnerable organ. However, the limited space within the skull allows little room for swelling or bleeding. Any brain swelling or intracranial bleeding will result in increased pressure inside the skull, potentially causing irreversible brain damage and, if untreated, death.

A head injury is always a potential disaster – however, it's mostly preventable.

INTRACRANIAL HAEMATOMA

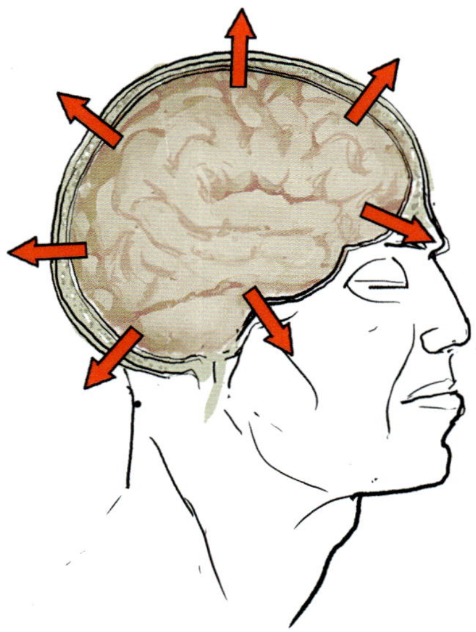

Elevated intracranial pressure caused by bleeding is directly transmitted to the brain due to the lack of extra space inside the skull. This endangers vital brain functions.

Symptoms and the clinical presentation of an intracranial haematoma vary depending on the location of the bleeding.

Epidural bleeding

- More common in younger individuals.
- Typically involves a period of unconsciousness following a head trauma.
- After regaining consciousness, the person may appear to improve and feel normal. However, if symptoms recur within 1 to 24 hours, this signals a life-threatening emergency requiring immediate evacuation and neurosurgery.

Subdural bleeding

- Often occurs in older individuals, especially those on anticoagulant therapy.
- The development of the haematoma and the resulting increase in intracranial pressure is gradual, with symptoms becoming apparent over several days.
- Treatment is surgical.

Intracerebral bleeding

- A profound and severe injury usually resulting in immediate unconsciousness and seizures.
- Prognosis is poor.
- Evacuation for treatment is necessary.

Anatomical location of intracranial bleeding.

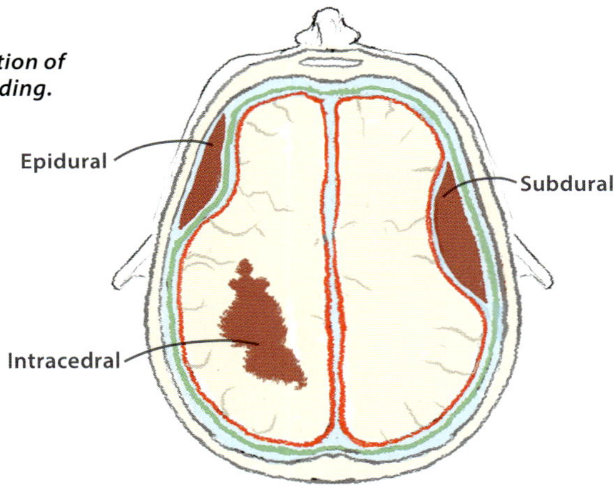

RISK FACTORS TO CONSIDER IN EVALUATING HEAD TRAUMA

- Age > 65 years
- Use of platelet inhibitors (for example, aspirin)
- Seizures following head trauma
- Paresis or loss of sensation
- Signs of skull fractures (impression or deformity) and skull base fracture see page 137
- Use of anticoagulants (for example, apixaban, warfarin, heparin)
- Haemophilia

ASSOCIATED SPINAL INJURY

The spinal cord is a direct extension of the brain, and head injuries are often accompanied by spinal injuries. It is essential to rule out fractures in the cervical vertebrae. A spinal cord injury at the cervical level can be profoundly disabling or life-threatening. Moving such a casualty is associated with risk for dislocation of a cervical fracture, worsening the spinal cord injury.

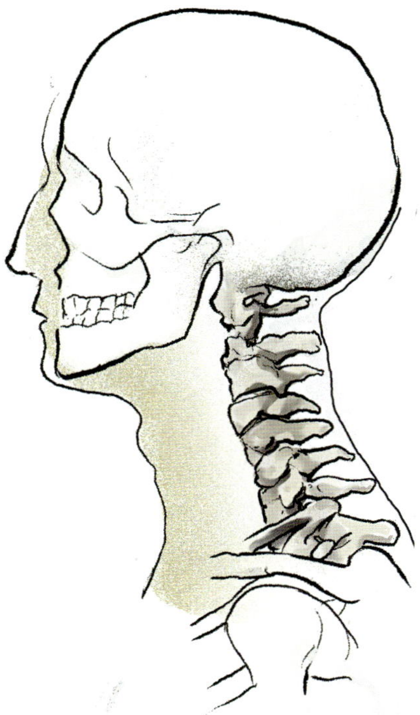

Our heavy head is mounted on thin and brittle cervical vertebrae. The spinal cord is in continuity with the brain.

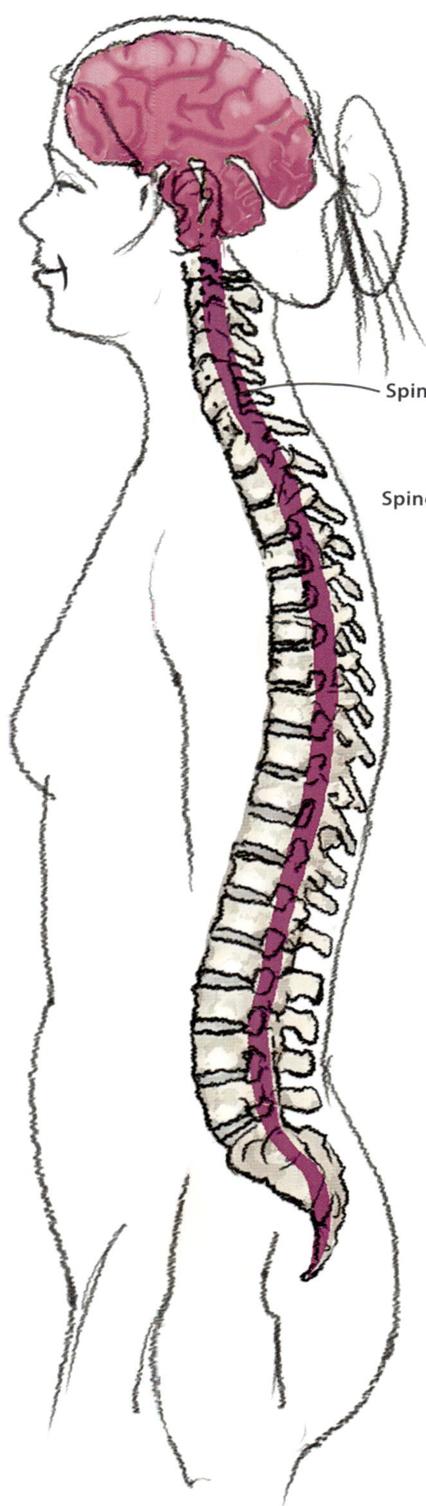

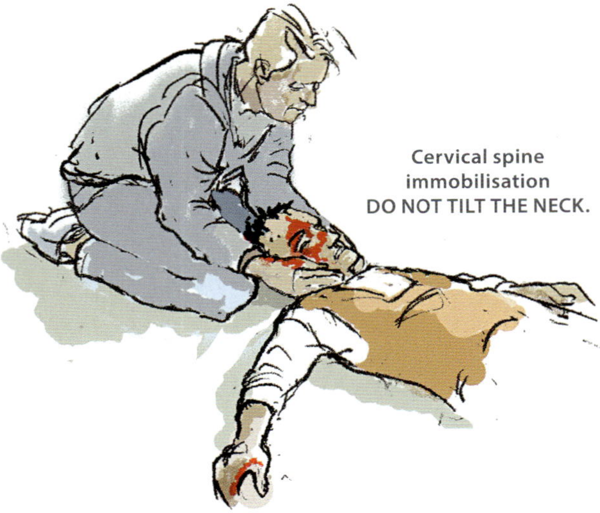

Cervical spine immobilisation DO NOT TILT THE NECK.

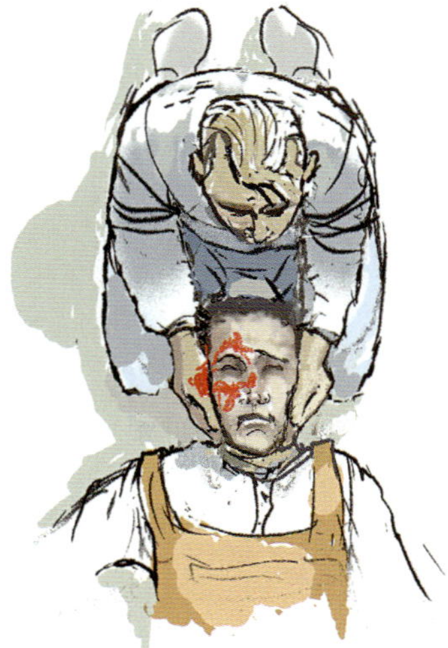

***CAUTION** – stabilise the neck also when the casualty must be moved. The person holding the head oversees this process. Stabilise the head and spine. Prepare for moving the casualty to shelter and away from danger.*

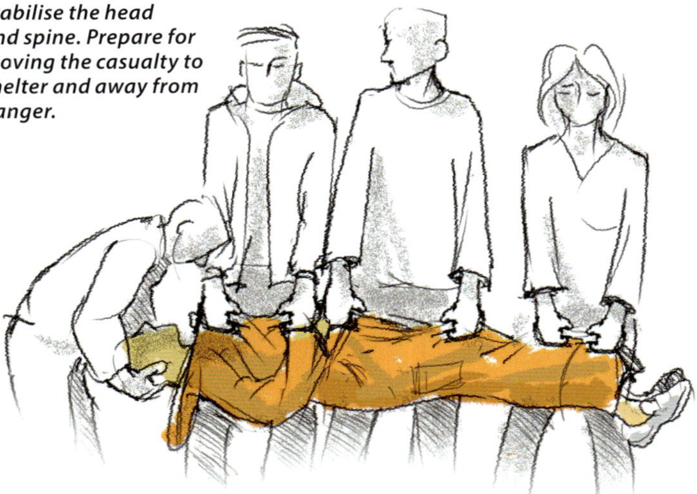

Detail – how to manually stabilise a neck.

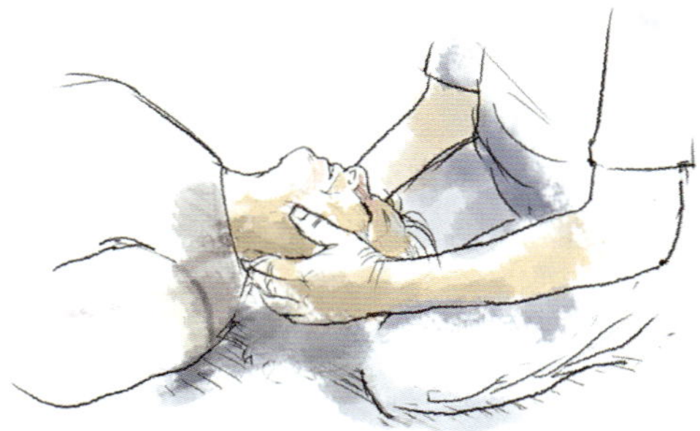

Immediate action

Stop and evaluate the situation. Scalp bleeding often gets lots of attention while other injuries are more urgent.

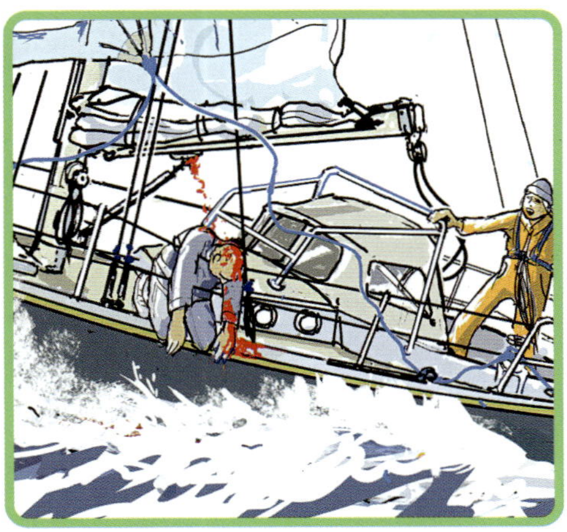

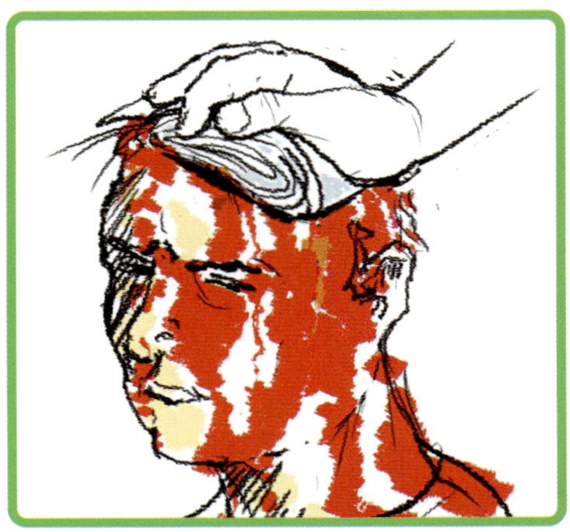

Primary survey (DRABC)

Follow the DRABC concept (see pages 12–13):

D – Danger	Identify and avoid dangers to yourself and the casualty; move to a safe place.
R – Response	Use the AVPU system to assess whether the person is conscious/responsive or unconscious/unresponsive. If unconscious, place them in the recovery position (see page 16).
A – Airway	Check and ensure a clear airway.
B – Breathing	Check and ensure breathing.
C – Circulation	Check for and stop major external bleeding; identify any signs of shock (see below and page 20).

The AVPU system provides a quick initial assessment of suspected head injuries:

A – Alert	Awake, oriented, and speaks spontaneously.
V – Verbal	Responds to verbal commands, may have slurred speech.
P – Pain	Diminished consciousness but reacts verbally or physically to pain stimuli (see page 13).
U – Unresponsive	Unconscious, no contact and unrousable.

Actions for the casualty

Move the casualty to shelter, preferably below deck, and allow them to rest under continuous observation and make a second survey.

- Make first GCS assessment (see below).
- Record baseline data: examine pupils, pulse, breathing and motor function (paresis).
- Note any periods of unconsciousness, seizures, vomiting or memory loss.
- Conduct a head-to-toe examination, checking for other injuries, including signs of skull base fractures (see below).
- Review the casualty's medical history and any risk factors.

TRAUMATIC BRAIN INJURY (TBI)

TBI is the standard term used for classifying head injuries in trauma care. The classification is internationally based on the Glasgow Coma Scale (GCS) protocol, which assesses the level of consciousness. The scale includes:

- eye opening
- verbal response
- motor response

After completing all three GCS steps, the scores are summed to provide a fair estimate of the severity of the injury. This score is valuable for communication with healthcare or rescue organisations. GCS assessments can also be repeated at different time intervals to monitor changes in an injured person's consciousness and general condition.

The GCS is a helpful tool, even for laypersons, in the challenging scenario of being far from medical assistance.

Classification of TBI

Minimal TBI, GCS 15: No risk factors, no loss of memory, no unconsciousness

Mild TBI, GCS 14–15: Suspected or confirmed short unconsciousness, vomiting > 2 times, memory loss of the incident

Moderate TBI, GCS 9–13: Confusion, difficulties in speaking, tiredness

Severe TBI, GCS 3–8: Unconscious

If GCS is less than 14 or if still unconscious/unresponsive, this is a profoundly serious situation, always an indication for urgent evacuation to hospital.

If GCS 14–15 with unconsciousness < 2 minutes and risk factors, do check-ups every 15–30 minutes with GCS for four hours and thereafter every hour for 24 hours. Establish contact with professional medical care or rescue organisation.

FACT

GLASGOW COMA SCALE (GCS)

Eye opening spontaneously (has open eyes): 4
On sound, demand ('Open your eyes!'): 3
On pain stimuli (see box page 13): 2
No eye opening: 1

Verbal response oriented (knows name, date, place): 5
Confused (response to questions not quite right): 4
Inappropriate words (random unrelated words): 3
Incomprehensible sounds (groans): 2
No response: 1

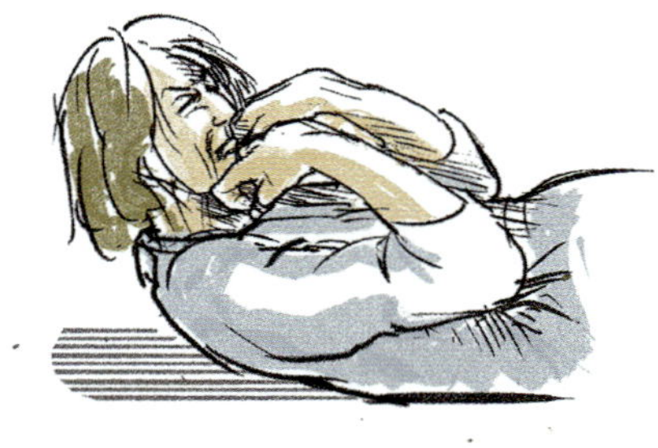

Motor response, responds to commands (move your arm, leg): 6
Localises pain: 5
Withdraws to pain: 4
Abnormal flexion response : 3
Abnormal stretch response : 2
No reaction: 1

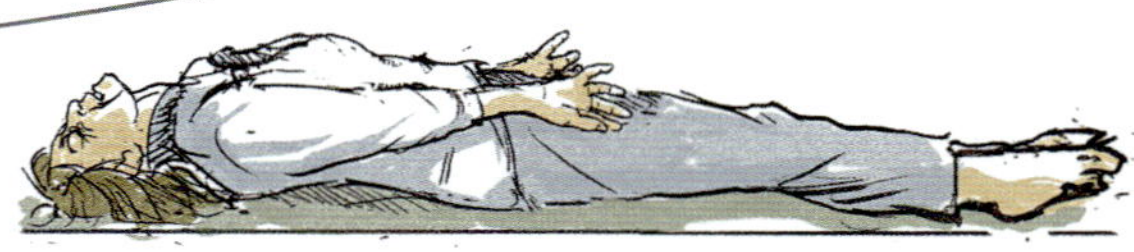

What to do on board

Early contact with medical expertise for advice is strongly recommended!

- Minimal TBI: Requires rest and observation on board for the first 24 hours. Ensure the person can be woken every two hours.
- Mild and moderate TBI: Corresponds to the former classification of 'concussion' and involves risks requiring regular checks, the extent of which depends on associated risk factors.
- Severe TBI: The person is unresponsive – this is easy to identify even for a layperson and always necessitates urgent evacuation. While waiting for evacuation, place the person in the recovery position (see page 16) and monitor their airway and breathing.

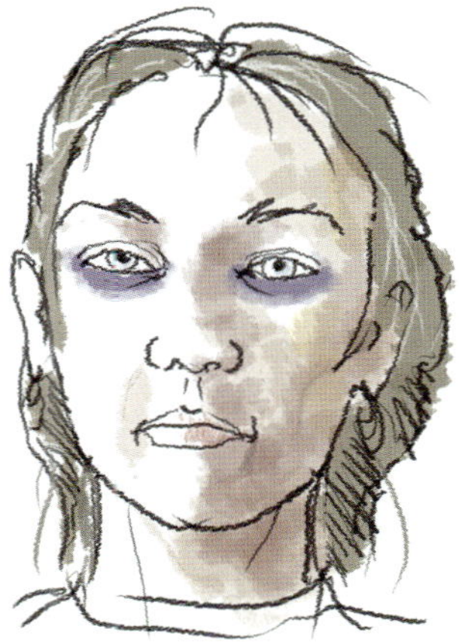

Signs of a skull base fracture include raccoon eyes (periorbital haematoma), blood-stained discharge from the nostrils and/or ears, and bruising behind the ears. By definition, this is an open fracture – start antibiotics (e.g., phenoxymethylpenicillin 1g every 8 hours).

Key checks while on board

General appearance

If the person must be kept on board, it is important to check general appearance. Look for the following symptoms:

- difficulty waking up
- headache, nausea or vomiting
- seizures
- loss of strength in arms or legs
- confusion or blurred vision
- signs of a skull base fracture

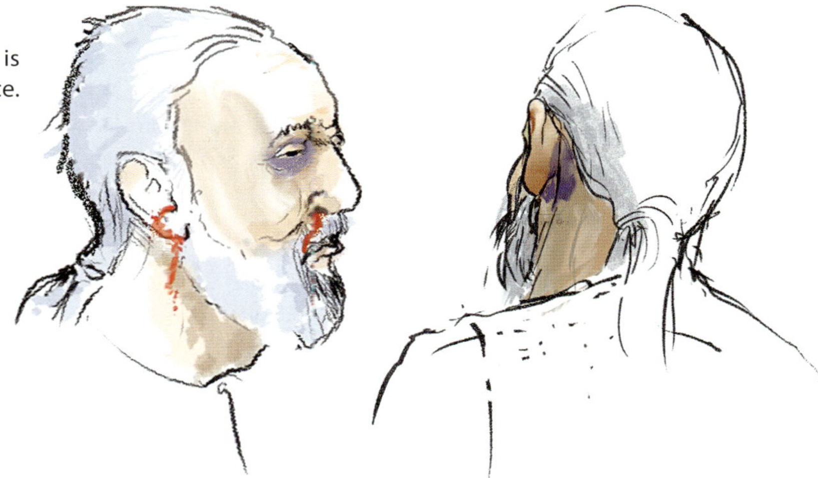

Consciousness

- Use the Glasgow Coma Scale (GCS) protocol to assess the casualty at least every 30 minutes for the first 4 hours post-trauma, then every 60 minutes for the next 4 hours, and at regular intervals for up to 24 hours.
- Lowered consciousness is the first sign of increased intracranial pressure. A drop of > 2 points on the GCS is a serious warning sign.

Paresis

Test for strength in the arms and legs.

To test arm strength, ask the casualty to hold both arms straight out in front of them for one minute. Weakness will cause one arm to drop.

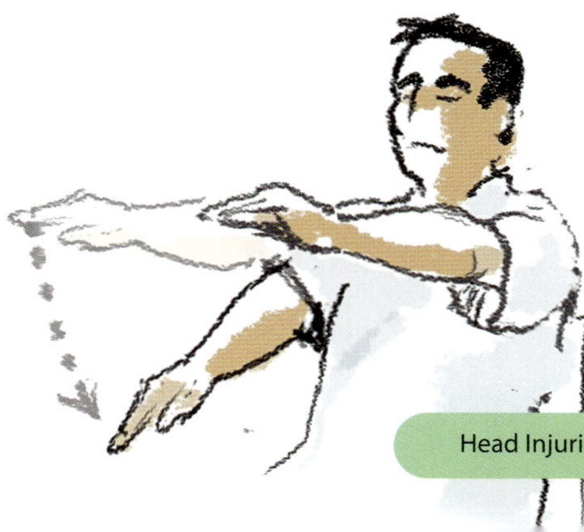

Pupil size and reaction to light

A wide pupil that does not react to light suggests high intracranial pressure.

> **PRACTICE TIP**
>
> Some individuals naturally have pupils of different sizes or atypical light reflexes. Familiarise yourself with your crew's normal pupil reflexes using a flashlight to establish a baseline.

Pulse

A slowing pulse and increasing blood pressure are ominous signs.

Breathing

Increased and irregular respiratory rates may indicate rising intracranial pressure.

Managing a serious TBI at sea is extremely challenging. Deteriorating parameters – such as reduced consciousness, abnormal pupil reactions or irregular breathing – indicate a severe TBI. Evacuation to a hospital is critical if possible. Conduct an initial GCS assessment (see box) and monitor for changes.

Treatment of pain

- First choice: paracetamol.
- Avoid: aspirin and NSAIDs (for example, ibuprofen, diclofenac) due to their negative effects on blood coagulation.
- Avoid combinations with sedatives, as they can impair consciousness.

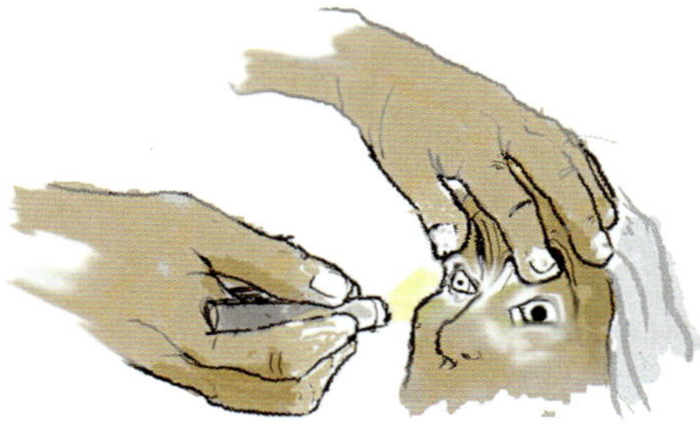

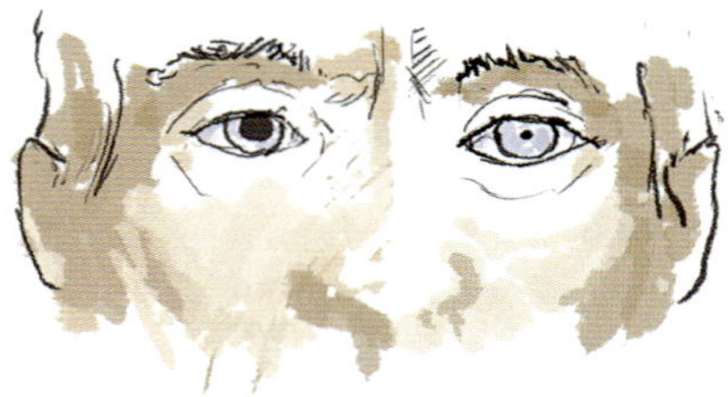

If pupil sizes become unequal, use a torch to check light reaction by shining the light into each eye individually. Normally, the pupil will contract on both sides. A dilated pupil that does not react indicates brain injury. Practise!

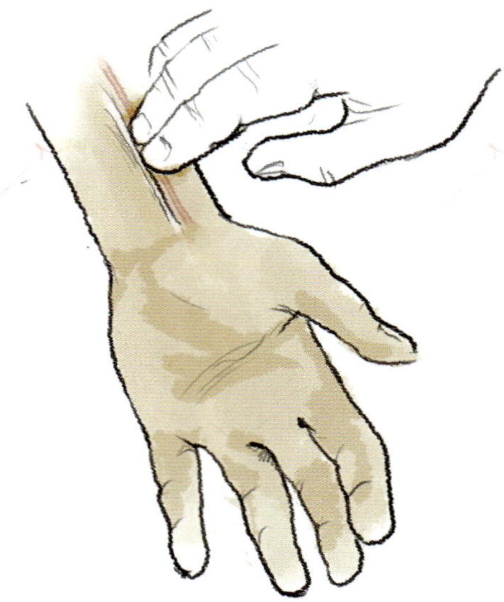

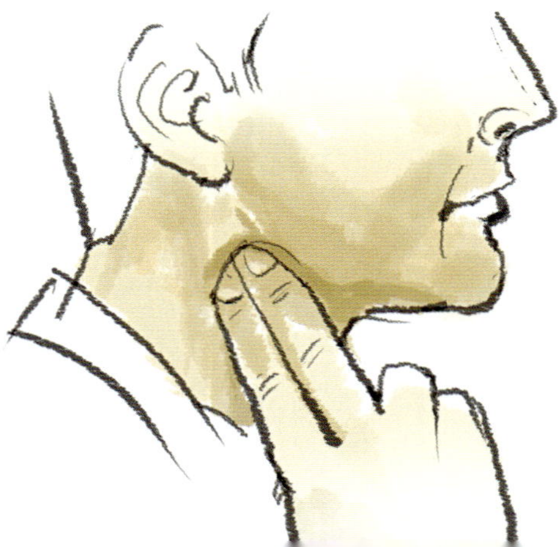

Check the radial or carotid pulse. Practise!

SCALP LACERATIONS

The scalp is rich in small blood vessels with limited contractile ability, which often leads to significant bleeding. If not managed properly, bleeding may require transfusions. However, the hard bony base of the scalp offers an advantage when controlling bleeding. Pressure applied firmly against the skull bone will usually stop the bleeding, even at sea. Once bleeding is controlled, decisions regarding wound management can be made.

FACT

A layperson with NO access to syringes and needles can provide some local anaesthesia using a lidocaine solution. Soak a compress with lidocaine solution (prescribed by a GP for inclusion in the first aid kit) and place it over the wound and surrounding skin. After 20 minutes, some, but not perfect, anaesthesia will occur. See also page 26, 'Wounds'.

Steps for managing scalp lacerations

- Cut or shave the hair around the wound.
- Clean the wound thoroughly with soap and clean water or physiological saline solution.
- Inspect the wound: Lift any flaps if the wound is curved. Check for cracks or fractures in the skull bone.
- Close the wound: Cover the wound entirely with scalp tissue and secure the edges using sutures or suture tape (see below).

An extensive scalp laceration with profuse bleeding. Bleeding should stop within 10 to 15 minutes with local pressure unless the person is on antithrombotic or anticoagulant therapy (for example, aspirin, warfarin, apixaban), in which case it will take longer. A pressure bandage must be secured in two directions to accommodate the shape of the head

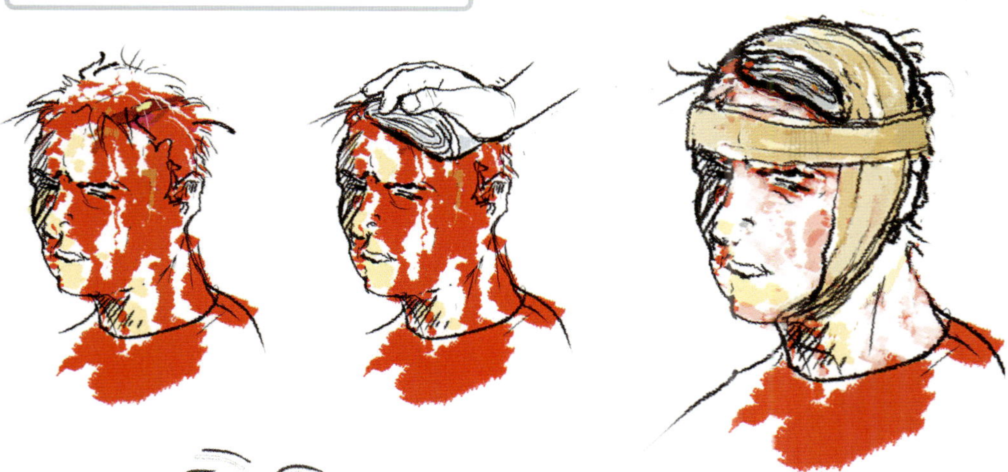

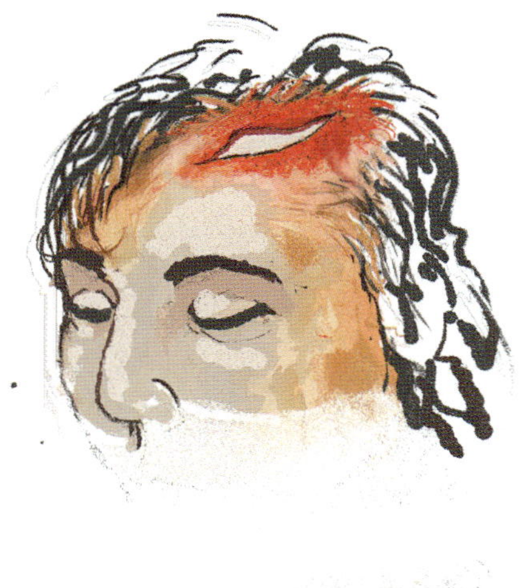

A scalp laceration with the skull bone visible. The bone appears undamaged. Bleeding has stopped, and hair has been removed. The wound has been cleaned thoroughly and must be closed to protect the bone surface.

Methods to close the wound

Suture tape:

- Easy to use for a layperson.
- Limitations: Remaining hair stubble may reduce adhesion. Ensure hair is removed 3–4cm around the wound.
- Reinforcement: Apply special skin glue (for example, Liquiband or Dermabond) along the wound edges.

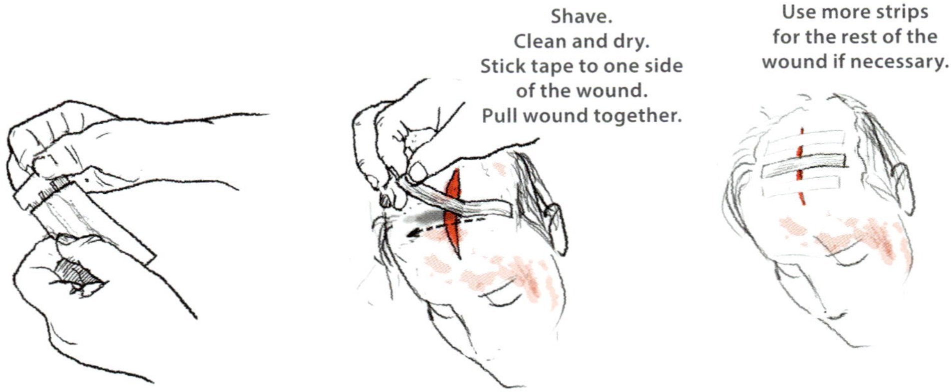

Self-adhesive wound closure strips

Suture tape is a convenient option for laypersons. Skin glue can be used to reinforce the adhesion.

Surgical sutures:

- Requires needle and thread.
- Special surgical instruments are ideal, but a haemostatic clamp may suffice.
- Suturing is easier with prior practice. Allow at least 20 minutes for oral painkillers or topical anaesthesia to take effect.

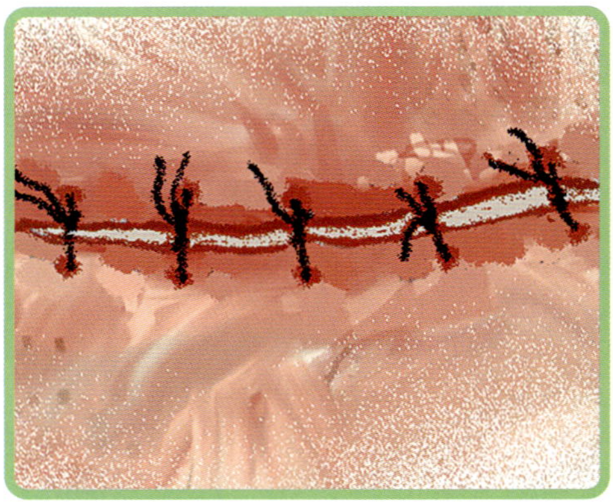

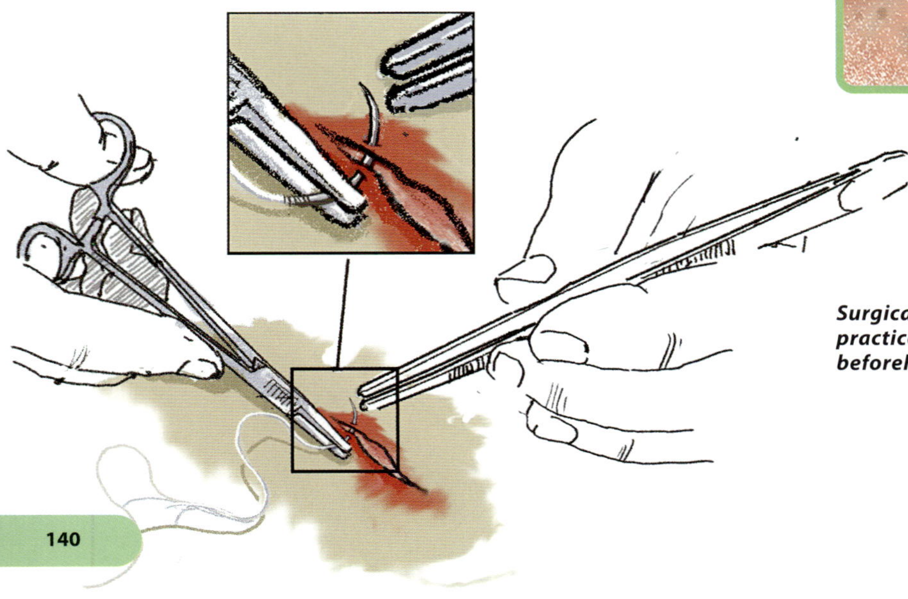

Surgical sutures require preparation and practice. Ensure adequate anaesthesia beforehand.

Suture stapler:

- A specialised tool for quick wound closure.
- Training is recommended.
- A specific tool is required to remove the clips after healing.

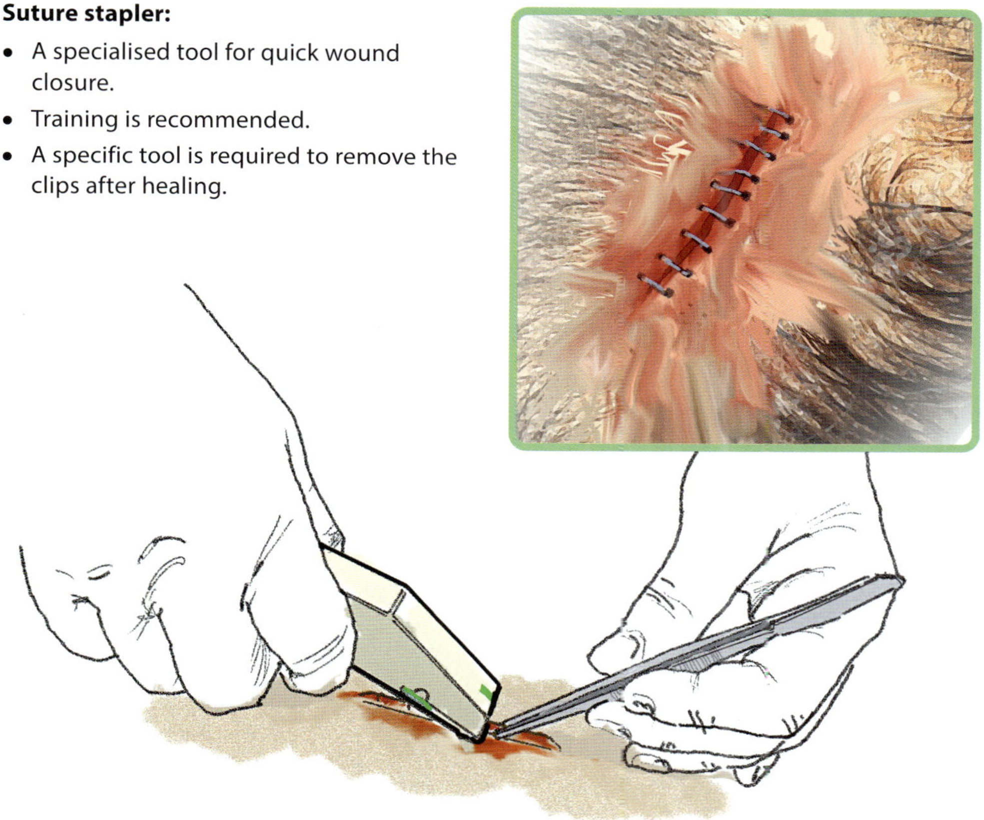

A suture stapler is a fast option for wound closure, but requires training to use.

Last resort – hair bundling:

- Long hair can be tied in small bundles to hold wound edges together.
- Take care to avoid leaving hair inside the wound, as this may impair healing and increase the risk of infection.

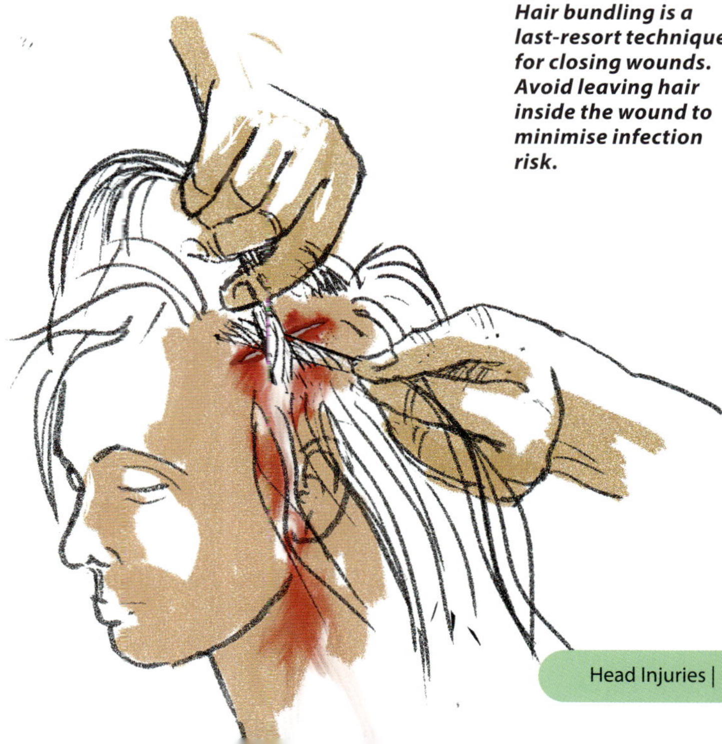

Hair bundling is a last-resort technique for closing wounds. Avoid leaving hair inside the wound to minimise infection risk.

SKIN GLUE

Different types of skin glue exist on the market, for example, Histoacryl, Dermabond and Leukosan. They are expensive but can be used to close minor wounds or lacerations (3–4cm) and, as suggested, to reinforce closure with surgical suture tape.

17. FACIAL INJURIES

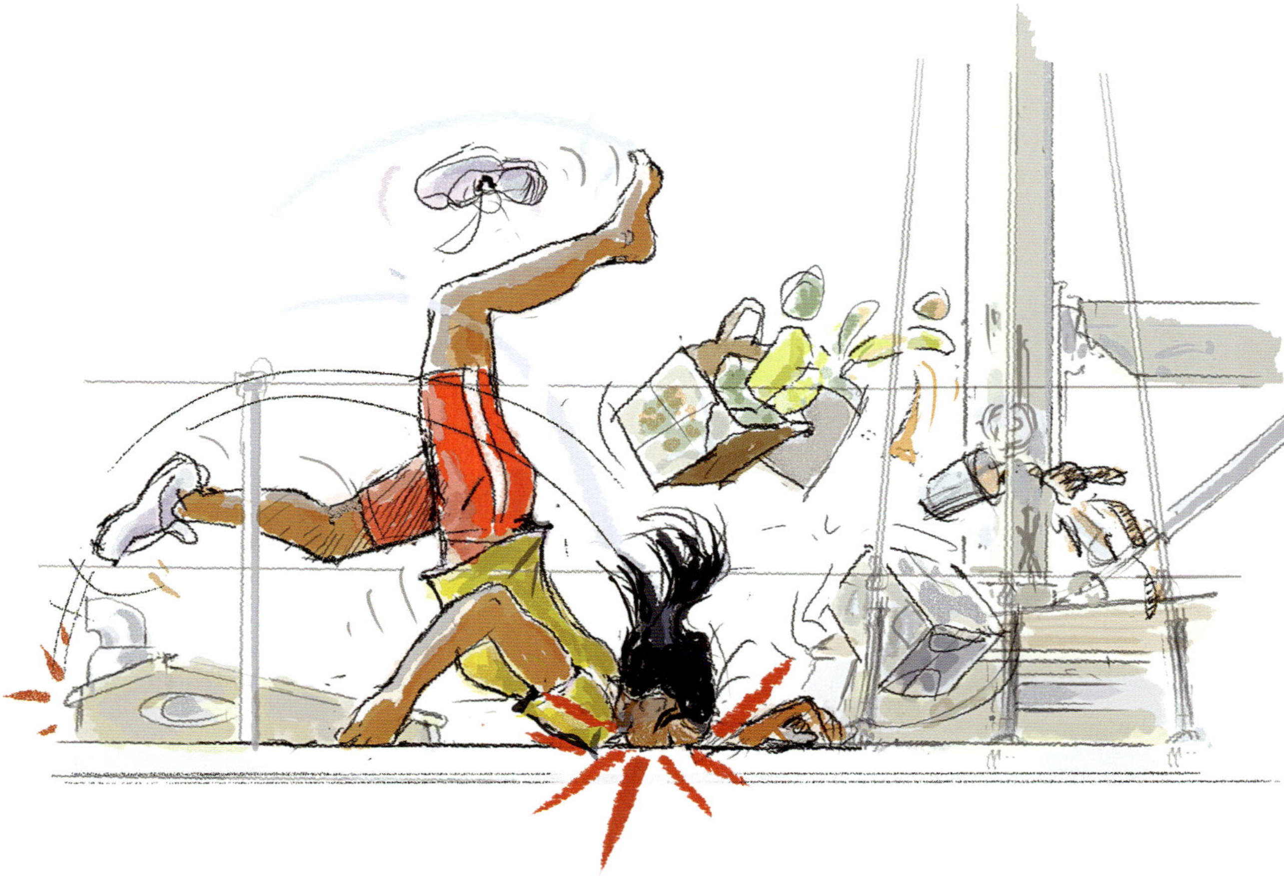

Tripping and injuring your face can bring different sorts of complications.

This section covers facial wound injuries, nosebleeds and fractures as well as tooth-related problems.

WOUNDS

Facial wound injuries can result in cosmetically unattractive scars. It is essential to provide careful wound care to prevent infection, which can complicate healing.

Immediate action / Treatment

Mechanical cleaning should always be the first step. Small wounds with straight edges can often be managed with special suture tape (see equipment list) as demonstrated, see image. Larger wounds, especially those that are complex with elements of crush injury and contamination, should, if possible, be treated by a doctor to minimise the risk of infections and unnecessary scars. Remaining dirt, especially in abrasions, often appears as bothersome tattoos after healing!! Aside from cosmetics, most facial wounds can be successfully managed on a leisure boat, even if you are far from medical care. Be aware of the importance of lining up eyebrows and lip contour when they are dislocated by the wound.

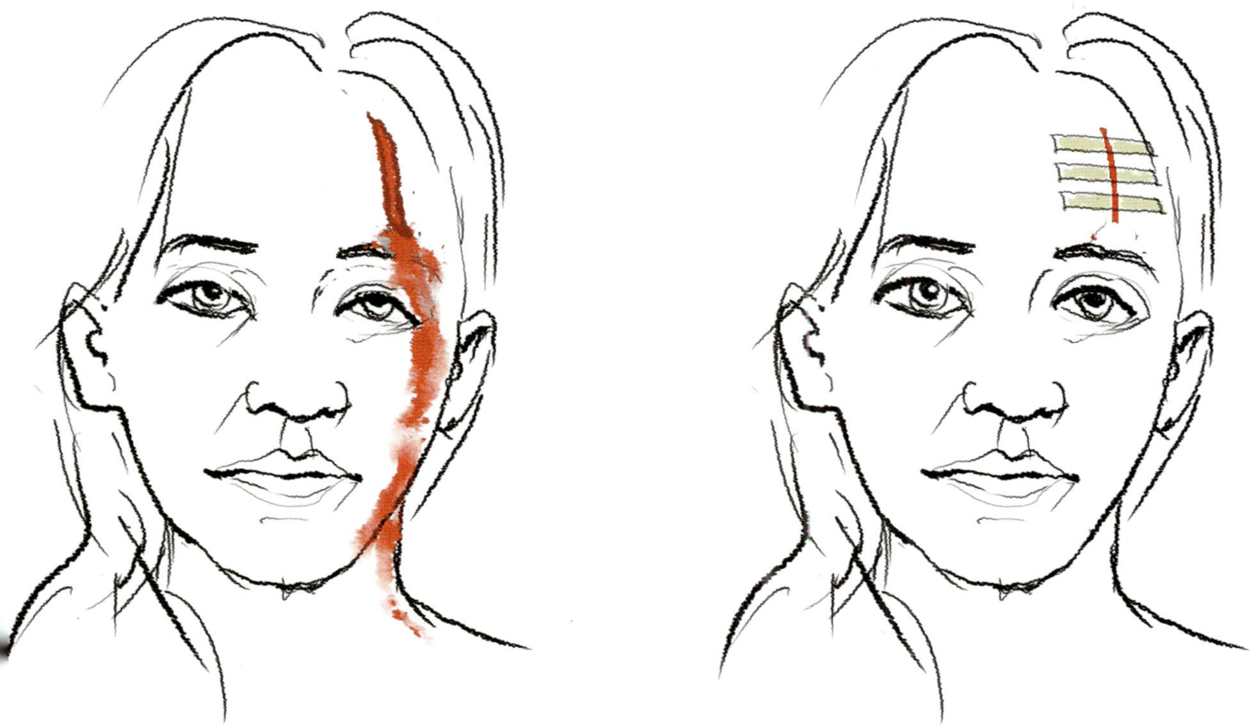

A wound with straight edges closed with suture tape after thorough cleaning.

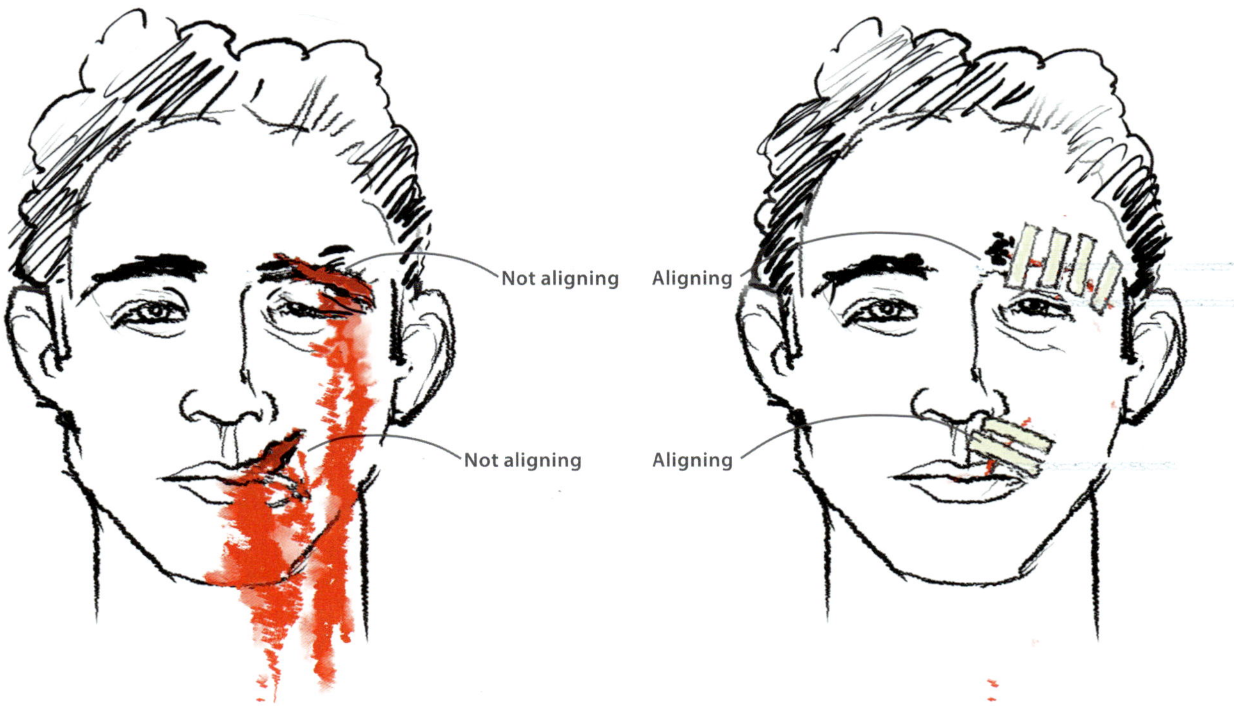

For wounds on the lip or eyebrow, be careful to match the skin/mucous membrane on the lip and maintain the line of the eyebrow.

NOSE FRACTURE

Falls or blows to the nose can cause a fracture of the nasal bone. Significant dislocation may result in one nostril becoming blocked. A nasal fracture can also have notable cosmetic implications and alter one's appearance.

Immediate action

If the nose is hit and potentially broken or shattered, seek medical attention on the same day if possible. If the nose is significantly deviated, affecting airflow through the nostrils, it may be necessary to attempt straightening it. This should be performed by an ear, nose and throat specialist.

Far from help

If you are far from medical assistance, it is not a major risk to wait several days for repositioning. While the procedure is easiest immediately after the injury, it can still be successful even after a delay of several days. Straightening the nose is painful but not dangerous. In urgent cases, anyone in the crew can carefully use a thumb-and-forefinger grip to attempt straightening it immediately after the injury.

If the fracture is accompanied by an open wound, antibiotics (for example, phenoxymethylpenicillin) should be considered. As always, if in doubt, use your communication equipment to seek medical advice.

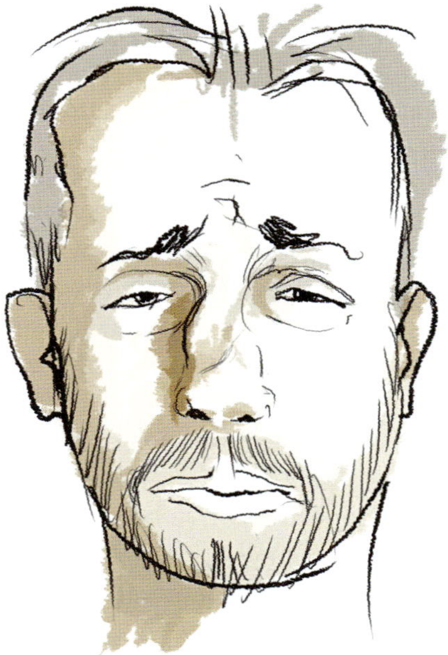

If a nostril is blocked – try to reposition the nose.

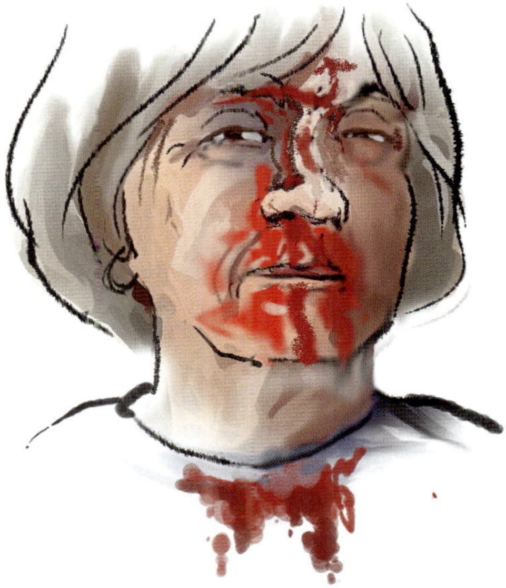

Nose fracture with an open wound.

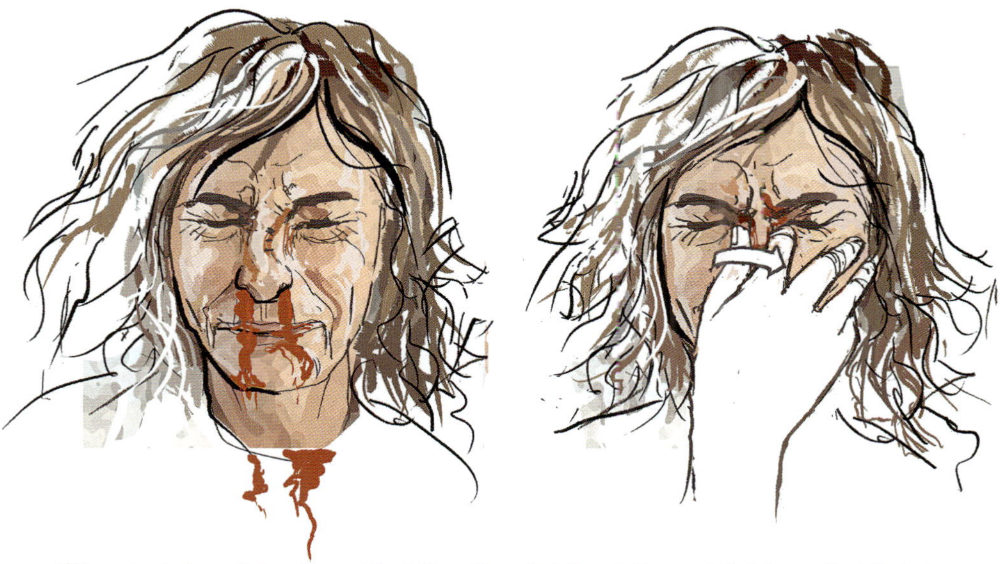

If there is obvious dislocation with obliteration of airflow in the nostril, it is worthwhile to try reducing the dislocation.

NOSEBLEEDS

The majority of people experience a nosebleed at some point in their lives. Some cases may require medical attention to stop the bleeding.

Most nosebleeds (90–95 per cent) are anterior (frontal), occurring in the soft part of the nose. These are typically caused by dry mucous membranes, nasal congestion, colds, trauma or other irritations. Anterior nosebleeds are easily accessible and can usually be stopped by pinching the soft part of the nose.

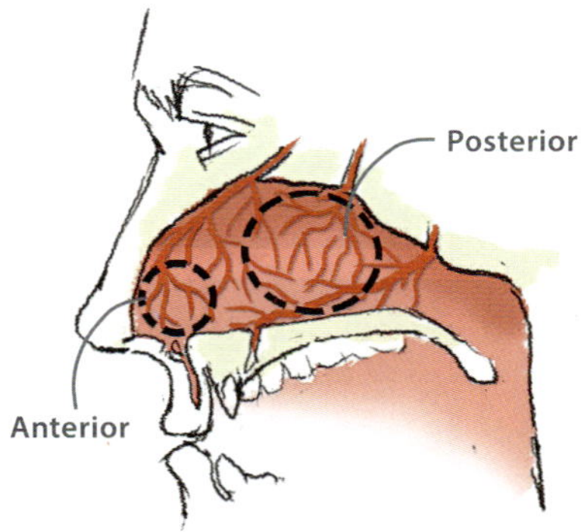

Anterior vs. posterior nosebleed. The latter is more challenging.

Posterior nosebleeds, while less common, are more challenging to treat. These involve bleeding from vessels further back in the nasal cavity and may require medical intervention.

Immediate action / Treatment

Nosebleeds can usually be managed with simple measures, as described below:

1 Have the person sit upright – lying down increases head pressure and worsens the bleeding. Lean the person forward to prevent swallowing blood. Firmly pinch the soft part of the nose for at least 15 minutes. Avoid blowing the nose, as it may dislodge clots and restart bleeding. If bleeding continues, maintain pressure for another 15 minutes.

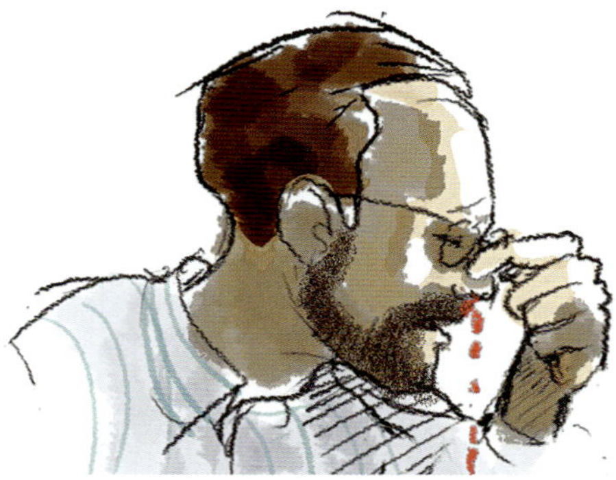

Sit upright and pinch the nose to stop nosebleed.

Large cotton ball compresses blood vessels in the frontal soft part of the nose.

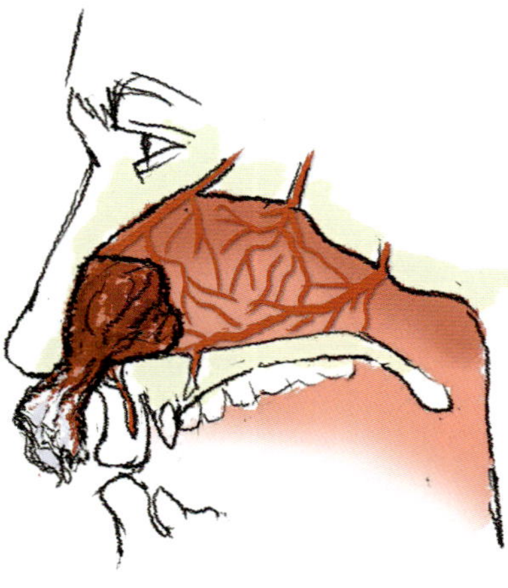

2 If the bleeding persists, blow out blood clots gently and insert a large cotton ball soaked in olive oil or nasal spray. Pharmacies offer ready-made cotton or compresses with clot-promoting substances, which are useful to keep on hand. Leave the cotton in place for at least 30 minutes and repeat if necessary.

3 Try melting an ice cube in the mouth and pressing it against the hard palate near the back of the nose. Cold constricts blood vessels and may reduce bleeding. Alternatively, apply an ice pack to the exterior of the nose. However, excessive cold can negatively affect blood clotting, so balance is essential.

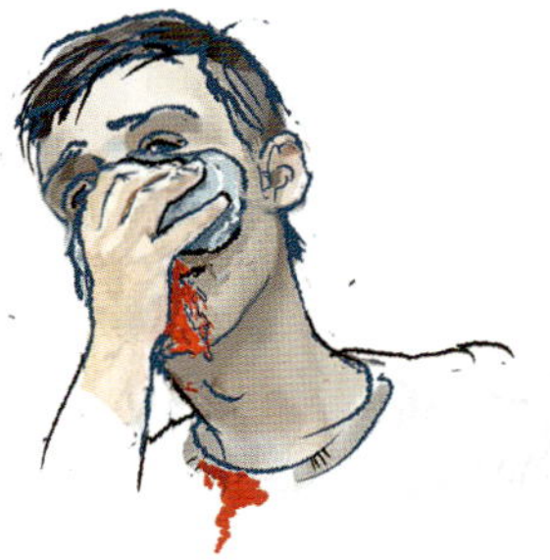

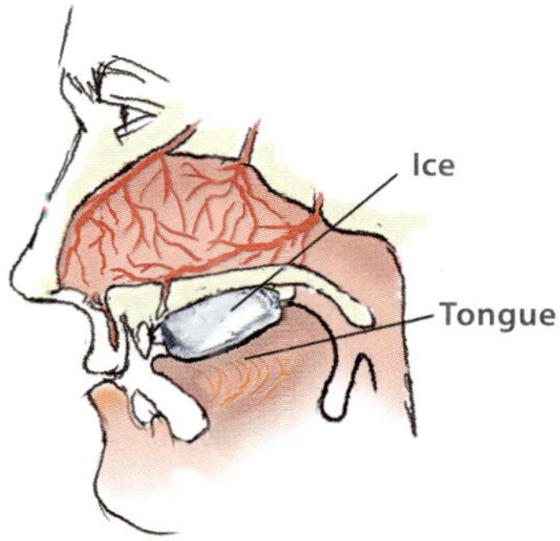

Try cooling with ice if the nosebleed will not stop.

Far from help

For severe, persistent bleeding that is unresponsive to the above methods, an anterior nasal tamponade may be required:

- Pull out a roll of gauze and tear or cut it into a narrow strip approximately 2cm wide and 1m long.
- Coat the gauze generously with Vaseline.
- Using tweezers, gradually insert the gauze into the affected nostril, packing it until no more space remains. Leave a small tip hanging out for easy removal.

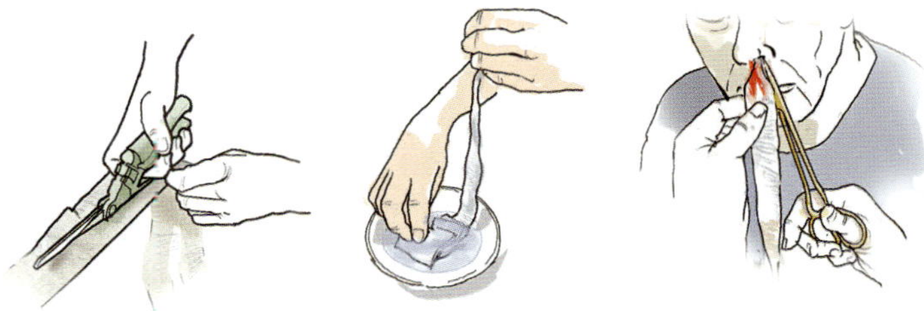

Pull out a roll of gauze, tear or cut it into a narrower strip about 2cm wide and 1m long. Coat it generously with regular Vaseline.

If this method is ineffective and the person experiences significant blood flowing backwards into the throat, this may indicate a posterior (rear) bleed. Posterior nosebleeds are more serious, especially in older individuals, and may require hospital treatment to prevent complications like circulatory shock. Seek advice. Evacuation might be needed.

Anterior nasal tamponade.

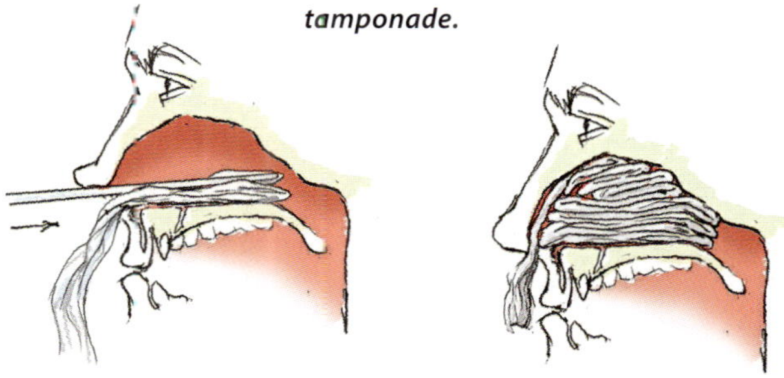

Prevention

To prevent nosebleeds, especially if you are prone to them, maintain soft, moist and healthy nasal membranes. Use nasal oil sprays and avoid picking your nose. Instead, rinse the nasal cavity with water or saline solution.

JAW FRACTURE

Falls or blows to the face can also affect the jaw and cause fractures in various locations. Common sites for jaw fractures.

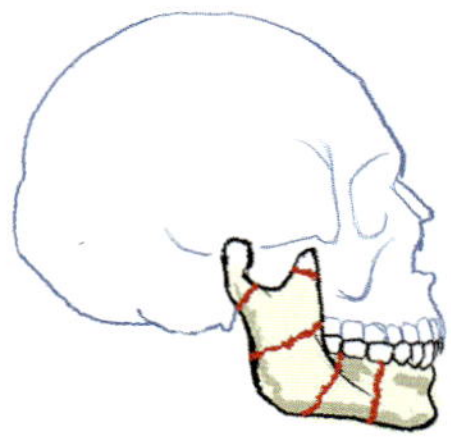

Signs and symptoms

As with all skeletal injuries, a jaw fracture will cause swelling and tenderness around the site. The injured person may recognise the condition themselves, as it is very painful to bite down and the teeth no longer align properly.

Treatment

Ideally, seek medical attention on the same day. However, if you are far from help, manage the condition by taking painkillers and switching to soft, mashed or liquid food until you can reach the next port. If the suspected fracture is located in the part of the lower jaw containing teeth, it is considered an open fracture. In such cases, antibiotics are crucial. Administer amoxicillin-clavulanate 875/125mg, every 12 hours for 10 days.

If the injury is caused by a strong impact or involves significant dislocation, especially with other facial injuries, it may require urgent evacuation if medical care is several days away.

DENTAL INJURIES

The visible part of a tooth consists of an outer enamel layer that covers the dentin, which makes up the tooth structure. The root of the tooth is embedded in the jawbone. Inside the root is a closed cavity (the pulp), housing the nerve and blood vessels.

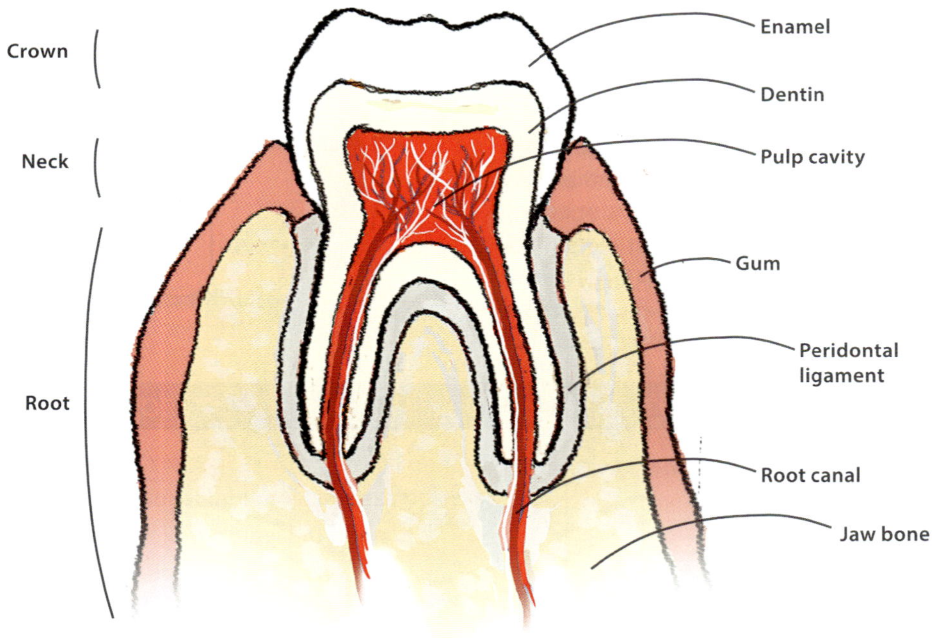

Fissure / Fracture

Symptom is that the tooth becomes sensitive to temperature and painful when exposed to air or when tapping the tooth. Treatment is to switch to soft foods that do not require chewing until a dentist can be consulted.

Damage to the enamel and dentin can be left untreated if you are far from a dentist. If there are very sharp edges, you can try to round them off with a nail file if necessary.

A piece of enamel is gone. Round off sharp edges.

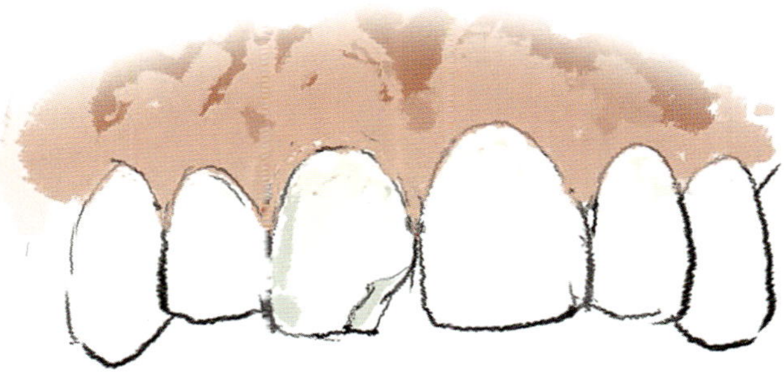

If the crown of the tooth is broken and the nerve is exposed (visible as a small red spot), the pain will be significant. In such cases:

- Immediate action: Cover the nerve with 'dental cement' such as Cavit. Maintain good oral hygiene by rinsing with an antiseptic solution.
- Long term: Seek dental care as soon as possible for further treatment.

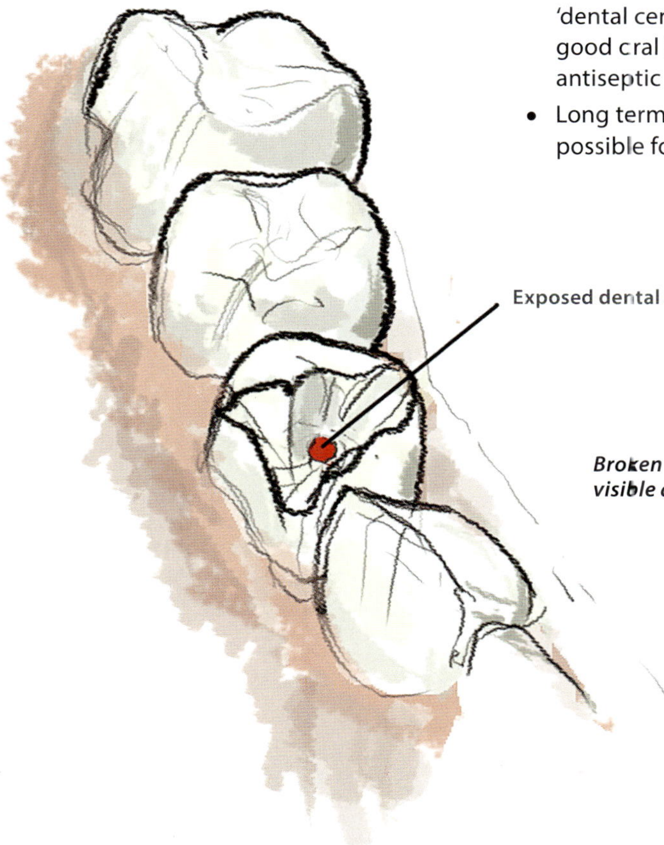

Broken tooth crown with exposed nerve visible as a red spot.

Knocked out

If the tooth is loose but still in place, avoid chewing on that side and maintain good oral hygiene (for example, rinse with an antiseptic such as Corsodyl). Loose teeth often heal if left undisturbed.

If the tooth is completely knocked out:

- Visit a dentist the same day, if possible.
- Rinse the tooth gently in water without scrubbing.
- Reinsert the tooth into its socket if possible. If not, keep it moist by storing it in the mouth (for example, under the tongue or in the cheek) or in saline solution until you can see a dentist.

Knocked-out baby teeth are usually not reinserted, but a dental check-up is still essential to avoid damage to the underlying permanent tooth.

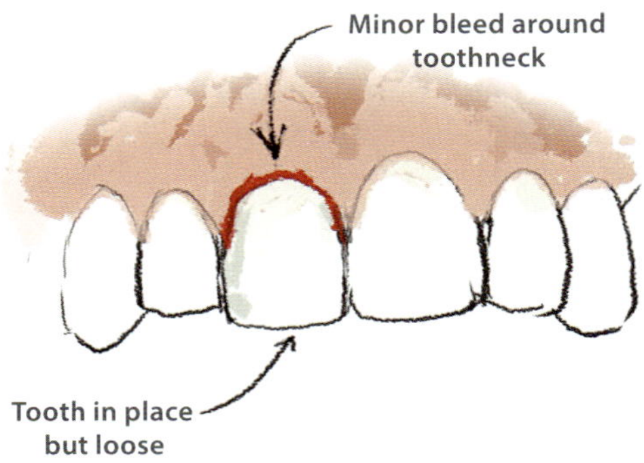

Loose tooth, wobbly, but still in place. Minor bleed round the tooth neck.

#1 Knocked-out tooth. #2 When cleaning, hold only the crown and never the root, as it can be damaged and hinder healing. Suitable cleaning is rinsing in plain water. #3 After cleaning, you can put it back in its original place. #4 Keep it in place by biting on a compress or a gum eraser.

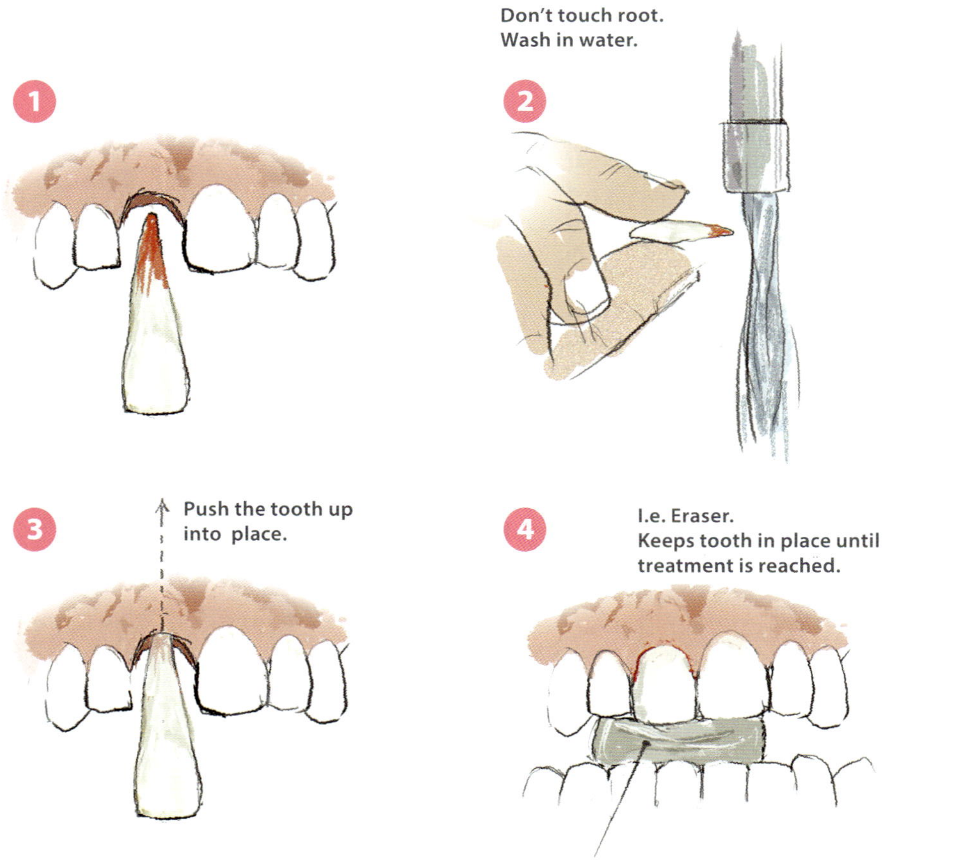

TOOTHACHE

Signs and symptoms

An infected tooth is usually caused by bacteria affecting the nerve, tooth root and surrounding structures, i.e. the jaw. The root of the tooth is enclosed in the pulp, a closed cavity in the tooth. This condition can be extremely painful due to increased pressure inside the tooth.

- Intense pain, tenderness and swelling in the affected area.
- Fever and an abscess near the root tip (which may drain into the mouth or skin).
- In rare cases, the infection can spread to the throat, causing life-threatening swelling and airway obstruction.

Immediate action

Visit a dentist urgently for treatment (for example, restoration, extraction or antibiotics).

Far from help

- Provide strong pain relief (for example, full-dose paracetamol, possibly combined with codeine or morphine).
- If there is swelling or fever, administer amoxicillin-clavulanate 875/125mg every 12 hours for 10 days.

Prevention

- Regular dental check-ups, especially before long trips.
- Be cautious with hard foods to avoid dental injuries.
- Good oral hygiene: use an electric toothbrush, interdental brushes, dental floss and toothpicks

Toothache.

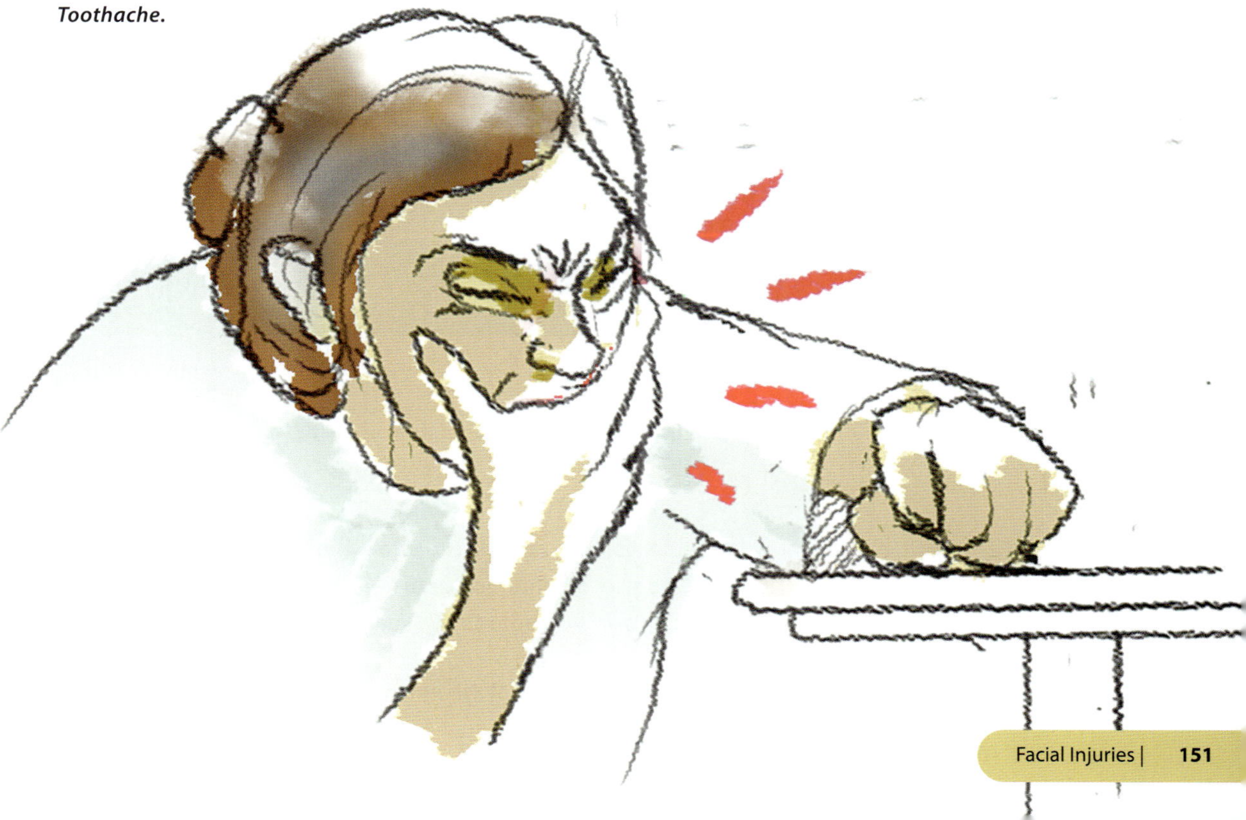

18. CHEST AND ABDOMINAL TRAUMA

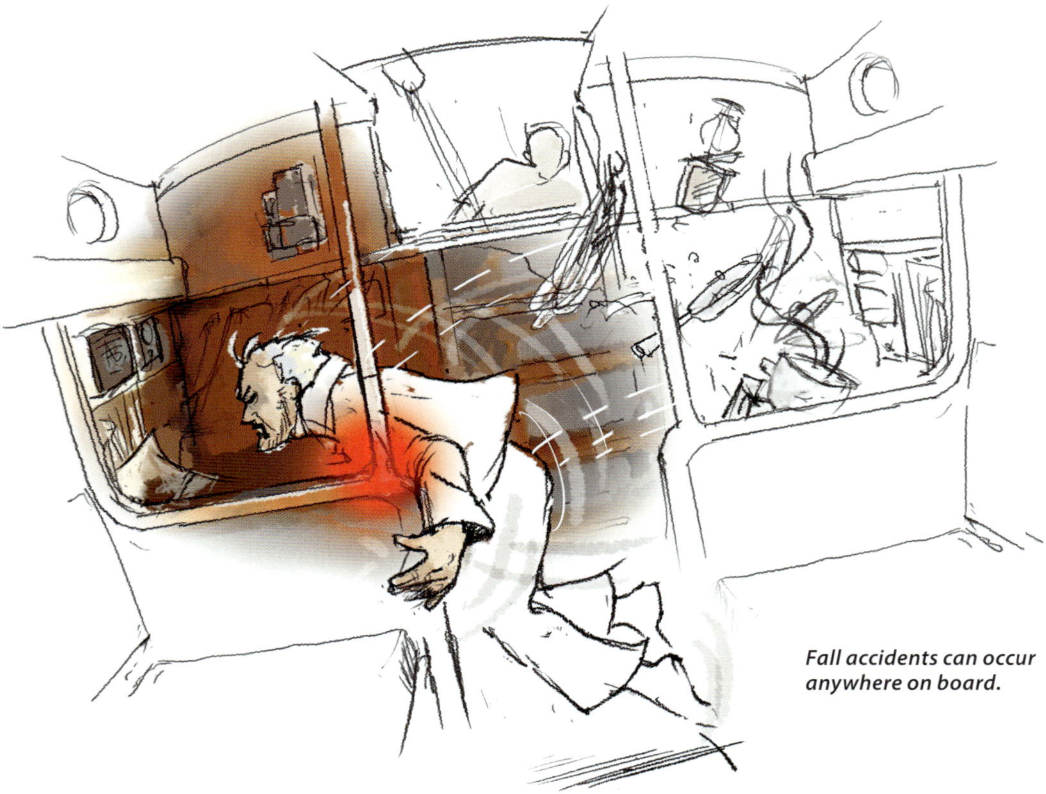

Fall accidents can occur anywhere on board.

Trauma to these body parts is challenging due to the risk of injury of vital organs hidden in the thoracic and abdominal cavities.

RIB FRACTURES

The chest protects several internal organs (heart, lungs, major blood vessels, spleen and liver), which can be affected by injuries to the ribs and chest. Rib fractures are common and typically occur after falls on to the chest, blows or collisions. During boating activities, a common cause is when someone working in the galley is suddenly thrown backwards, colliding with the interior on the opposite side of the boat. Many navigation tables and ribs have been fractured in this manner.

The primary concern is not the number of fractured ribs but whether lung complications, such as bleeding (haemothorax) or air leakage (pneumothorax), occur within the pleural cavity, as described below.

Signs and symptoms

Intense, immediate pain that typically worsens during the first week and may persist for around four weeks. Pain is exacerbated by movement and breathing, making deep breaths particularly painful.

Local direct tenderness: press directly on the site of impact.

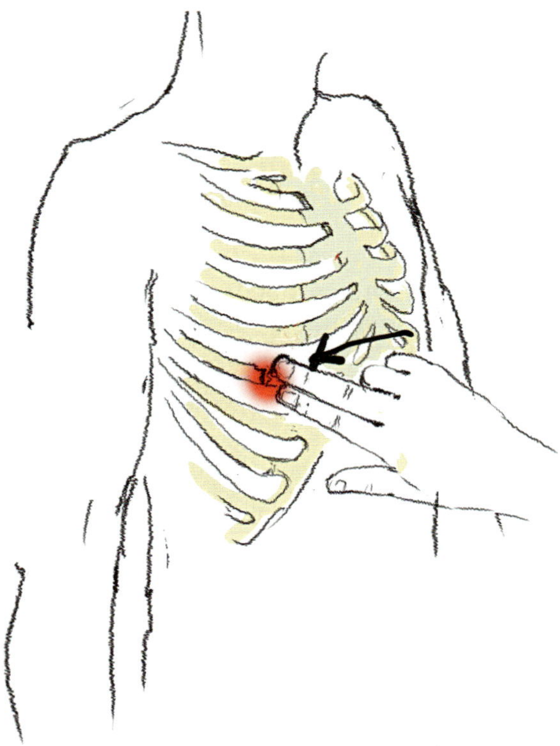

Indirect tenderness test: press, for example, on the breastbone, far from the painful area, to check chest springing.

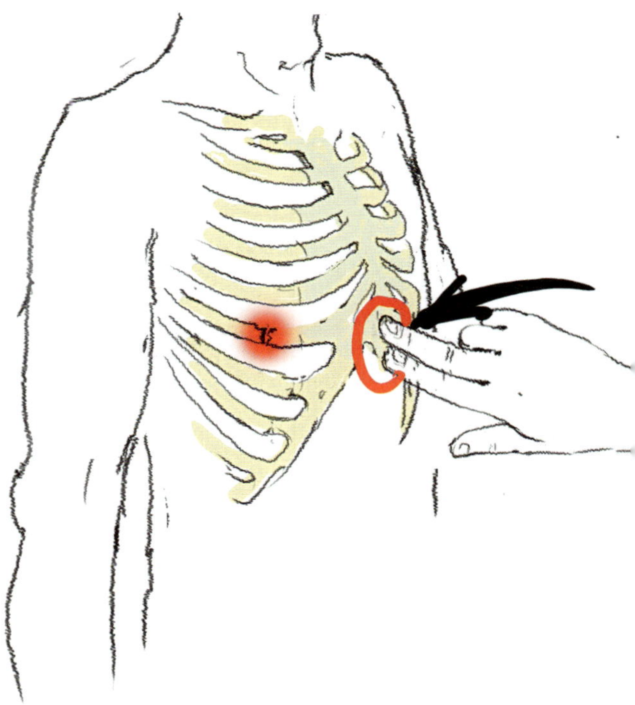

Direct and indirect tenderness indicates a fracture; direct tenderness alone suggests muscle injury.

Immediate action

- Provide pain relief.
- Help the injured person find a position that allows calm and less painful breathing movements.

Treatment

Significant pain relief is essential; more than just paracetamol may be required (see page 248).

Encourage deep-breathing exercises as much as the pain allows to reduce the risk of lung complications, such as pneumonia.

Monitor the person closely for signs of deterioration and seek immediate medical attention if:

- shortness of breath increases
- severe coughing develops
- nausea occurs
- cold sweats appear
- signs of shock are evident

At the hospital, the focus will be on assessing lung complications, such as lung collapse or bleeding into the pleural cavity. The risk of complications increases with the number of fractured ribs.

Far from help

In most cases, the situation can be managed as described above. However, in cases of severe trauma, pronounced shortness of breath or signs of shock, the situation becomes critical and evacuation may be required for rapid hospital intervention.

COMPLICATIONS OF RIB FRACTURES

Bleeding (haemothorax) and leakage of air inside the pleura (pneumothorax) resulting from a fractured rib puncturing the pleura or the lung are complications that may become serious. Minor haemo- or pneumothorax are common and resolve spontaneously. However, these conditions can escalate and require immediate evacuation and treatment.

Haemothorax

Signs and symptoms

A large bleed into the pleural cavity is a classic example of internal bleeding. This bleeding is not visible externally and is only realised when the situation is getting worse. The person may display signs of haemorrhagic shock as well as respiratory impairment:

- rapid breathing and pulse
- cold sweats
- pallor and cyanosis (bluish skin)

Pneumothorax

- A small pneumothorax is a common finding in association with rib fractures.
- A large pneumothorax occurs when the lung collapses like a deflated balloon, ceasing to function. With only one functioning lung remaining, the person experiences severe shortness of breath, circulatory issues and signs of impending shock, including rapid breathing and pulse, cold sweats, pallor and cyanosis.
- A specific and severe variation is a tension pneumothorax, which can occur in both blunt and penetrating trauma as well as spontaneously. A tissue valve forms at the site of injury, causing a one-way flow of air into the pleural cavity. This leads to increasing pressure within the thorax, eventually displacing the heart and major blood vessels. If untreated, this condition poses an immediate threat to life.

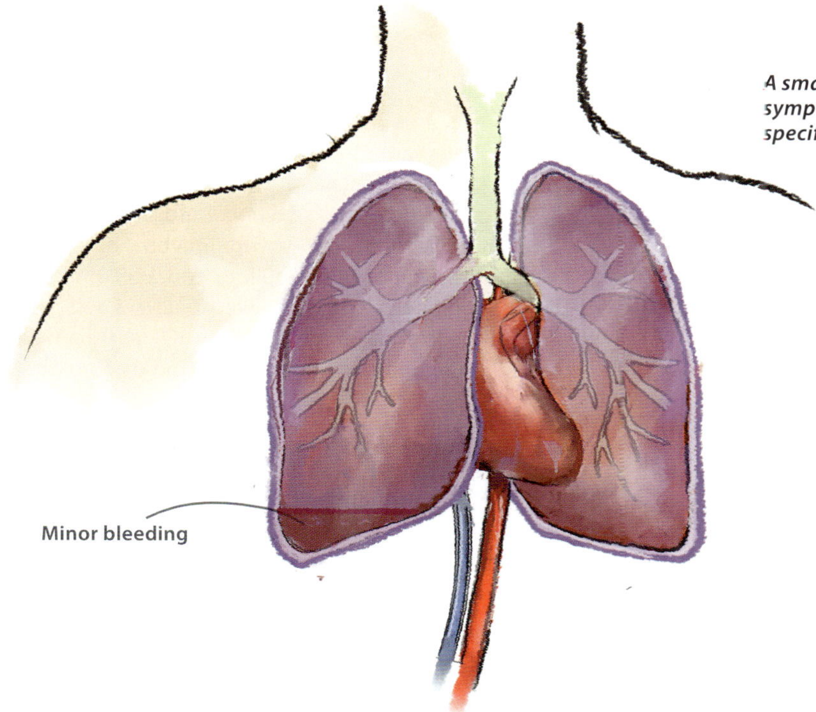

A small bleed in the right thorax causing no other symptoms than the rib fracture and requiring no specific treatment.

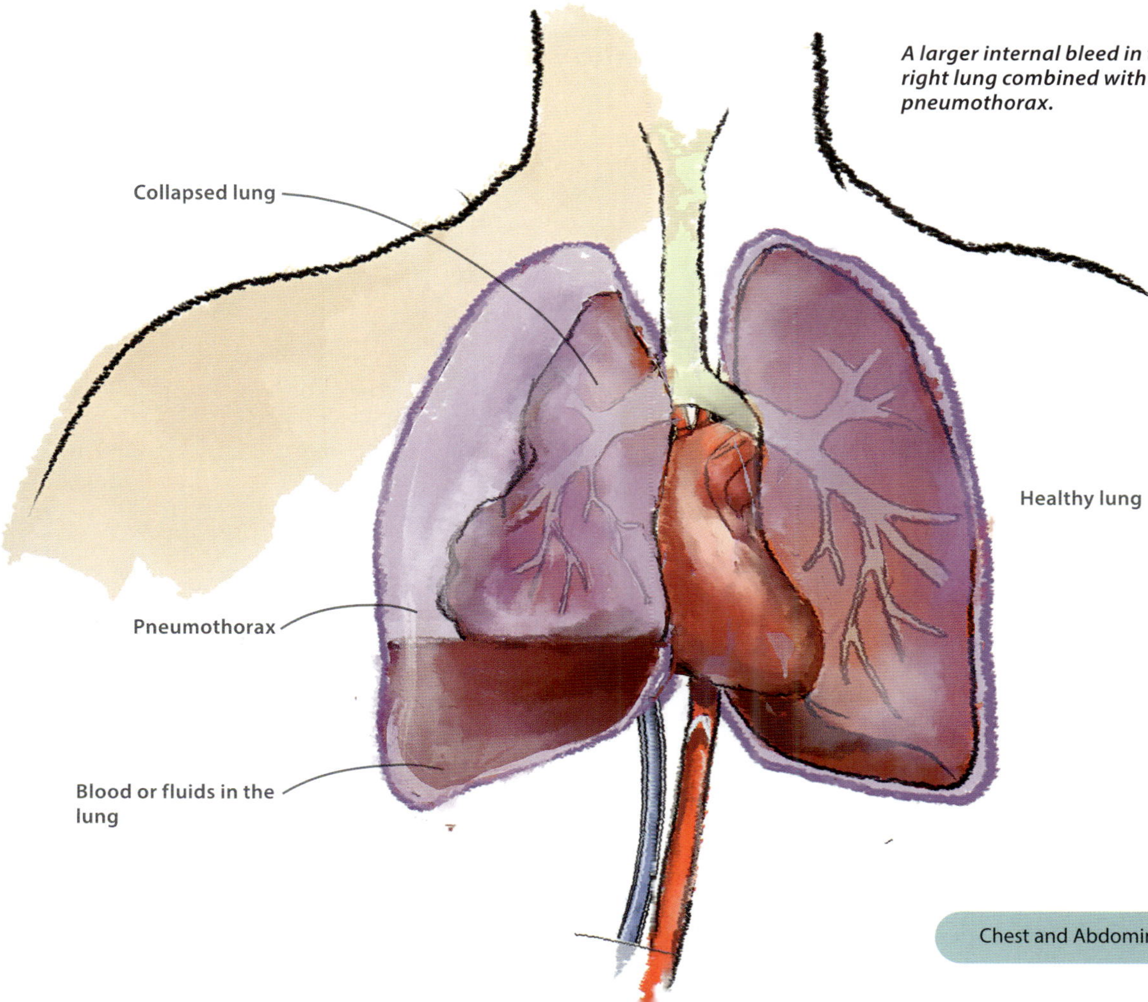

A larger internal bleed in the right lung combined with a pneumothorax.

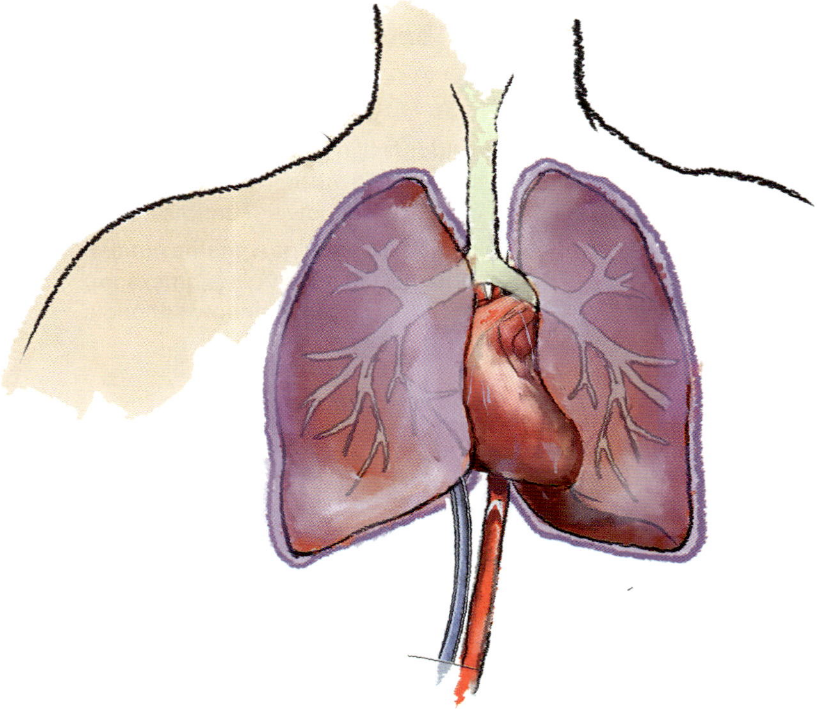

Above: Normal anatomy of lungs and heart. Below: Lung fully collapsed by tension pneumothorax, displacing the heart and major blood vessels.

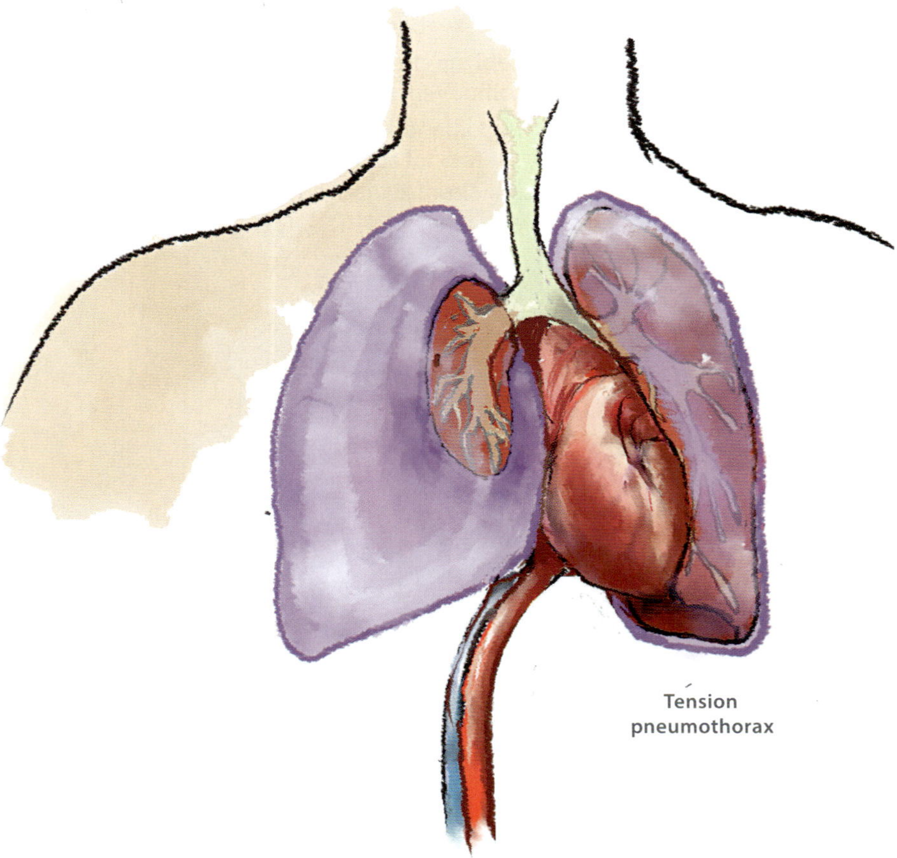

Immediate action / Treatment

In cases of chest injury with suspected lung complications, prompt medical examination is needed. Arrange transport to hospital. Position the person with the injured side down to facilitate breathing and optimise lung function. Give potent analgesics, possibly in combination with a sedative. In hospital, a decision is made about draining blood and air with a thoracic tube or other surgical procedure.

Far from help

Careful monitoring of general appearance and breathing. Find the best position for the casualty. Administer potent pain relief and prepare to evacuate. With a tension pneumothorax, a very serious and life-threatening situation is faced with no radical help to give.

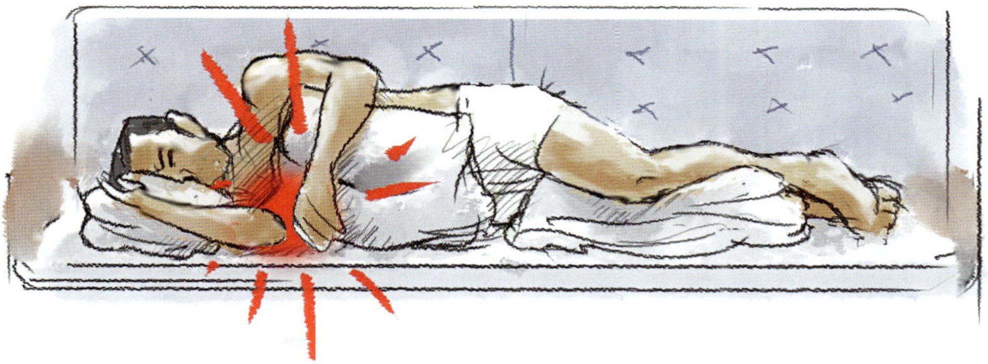

Position with the injured side down after chest trauma.

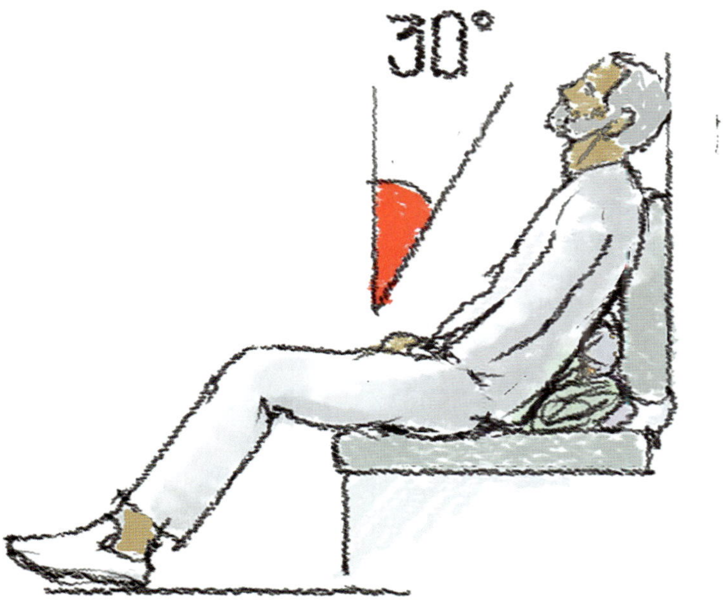

A sitting position often provides comfort after chest injury.

PENETRATING CHEST INJURY

Severe penetrating chest injuries from sharp objects or gunshots are fortunately rare but remain highly challenging. Such injuries require rapid transport to a hospital.

Signs and symptoms

- A 'sucking' sound during breathing
- Presence of a penetrating thoracic wound
- Increasing signs of shock and cyanosis

Immediate action

While awaiting medical attention, apply a thin plastic film as a flutter valve – a simple and potentially life-saving measure.

Penetrating chest injury with a 'sucking' sound during breathing. Principle of a temporary valve: after cleaning the wound, firmly tape a thin plastic film over it, leaving one side open to act as a flutter valve.

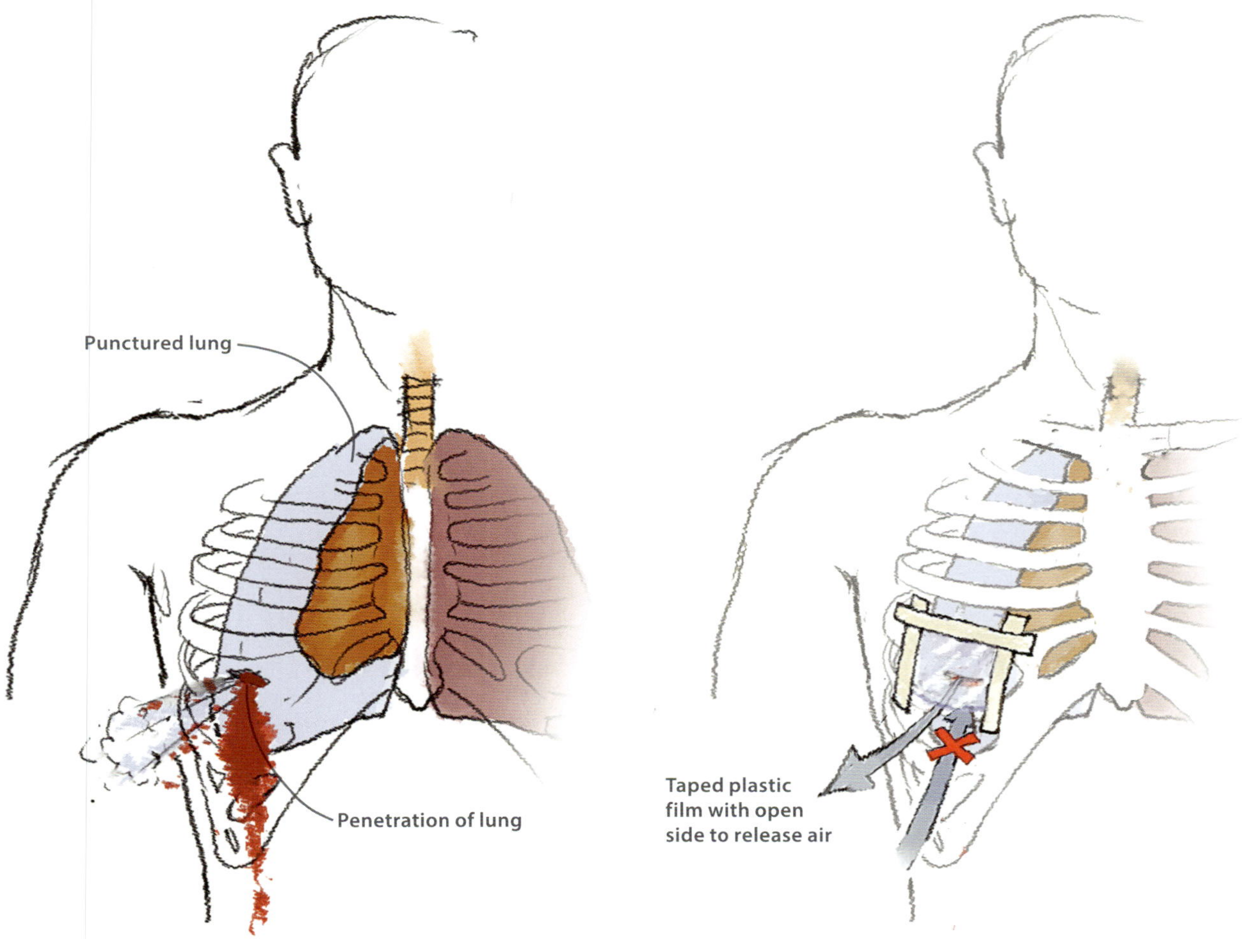

BLUNT ABDOMINAL TRAUMA

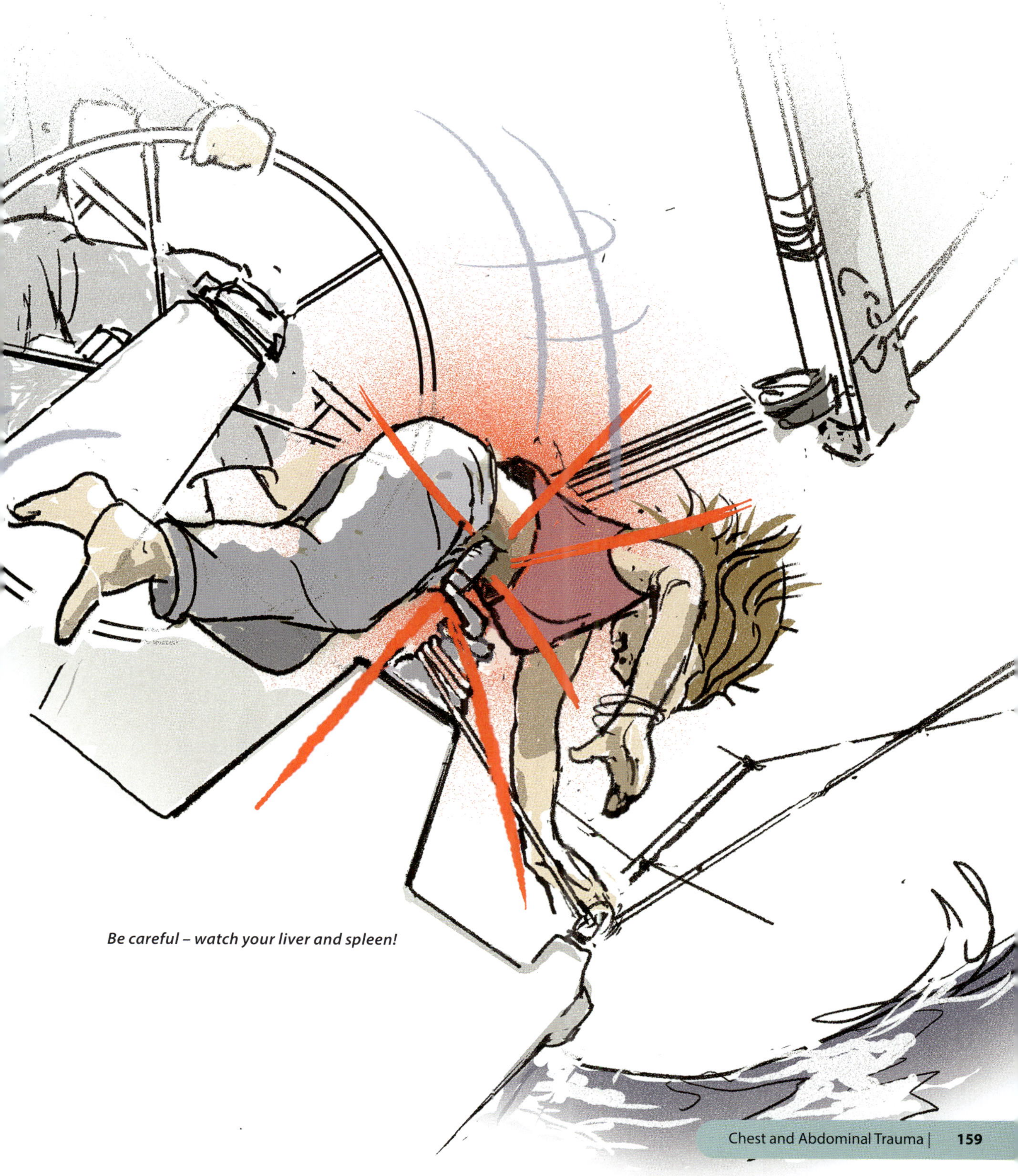

Be careful – watch your liver and spleen!

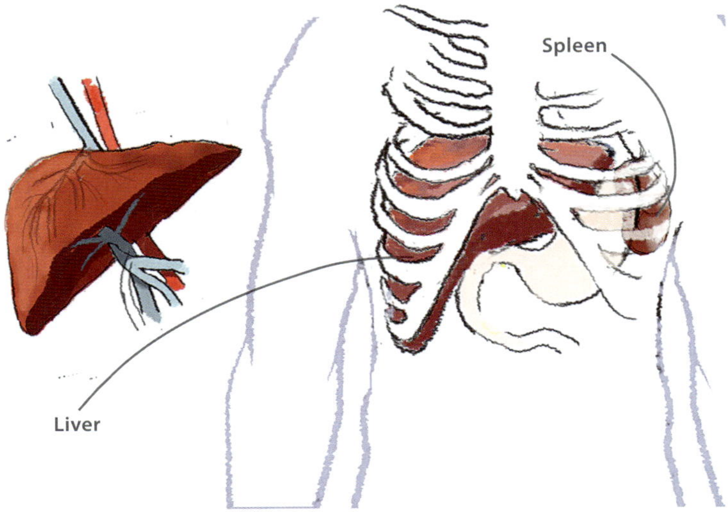

The liver and spleen are protected by the ribcage but have fragile structures.

Blunt abdominal trauma is relatively common in outdoor activities and is often mild. However, after direct impact to the liver or spleen, there is a risk of significant injury. Unfortunately, the threshold of force required to cause serious damage is difficult to define.

Signs and symptoms

Be cautious if an injured individual describes their accident but appears unaffected. The injury may worsen over hours or even days due to slow or increasing bleeding. Symptoms include:

- increasing abdominal pain
- signs of haemorrhagic shock, such as rapid breathing, rapid pulse, pallor and cold sweats

Liver injuries often cause referred pain in the upper right shoulder, while spleen injuries may cause pain around the left shoulder.

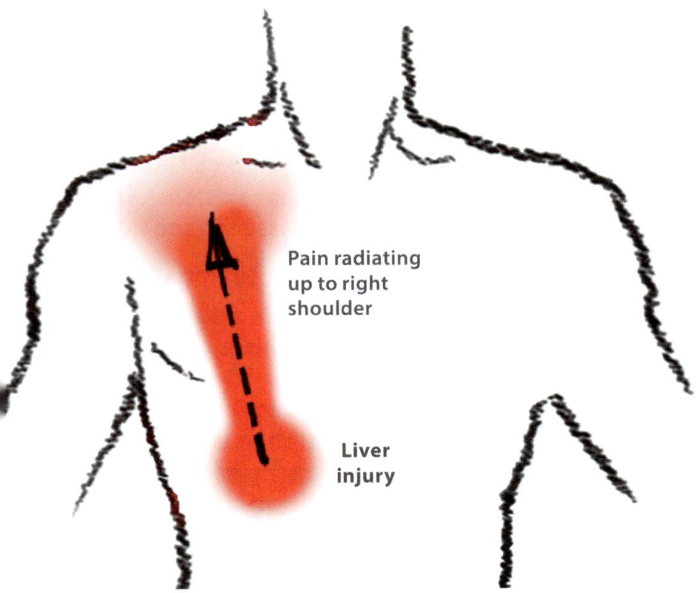

Pain distribution in liver injury.

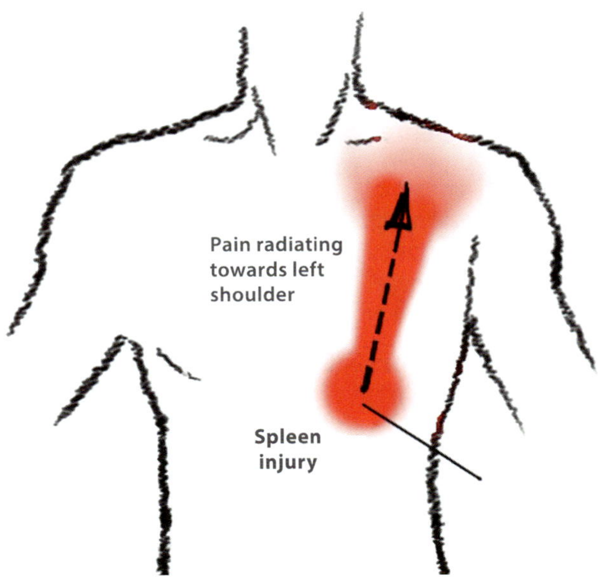

Pain distribution in spleen injury.

Immediate action

Anyone complaining of abdominal pain or pain extending to the shoulder after trauma should be taken directly to a hospital for examination, observation or surgery.

Treatment

Severe internal abdominal bleeding is a significant danger and requires hospital treatment.

Far from help

This is a challenging situation involving a potentially life-threatening injury. Take the following steps:

- Ensure the person rests.
- Administer analgesics (e.g., paracetamol, codeine or morphine) but avoid NSAIDs due to the risk of exacerbating bleeding.
- Monitor pulse, breathing and, if possible, blood pressure.
- Work diligently to arrange evacuation and seek external medical support.

Prevention

The fundamental principle is prevention. Instruct your crew about the risks and stress the importance of being proactive in both thought and action to avoid such injuries. Do not forget the dangers ashore, especially for children.

Be preventive also when ashore!

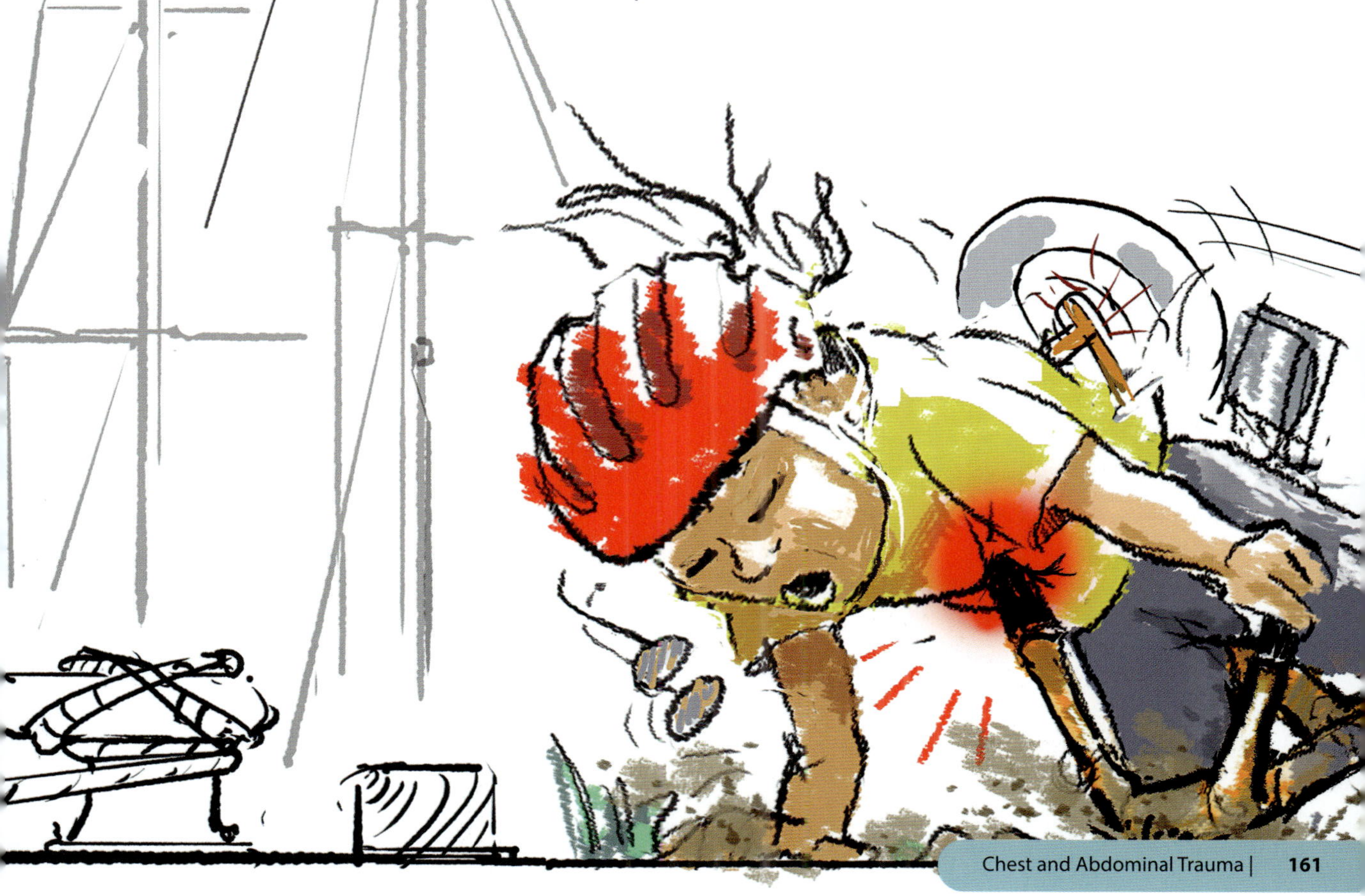

19. ORTHOPAEDICS – GENERAL

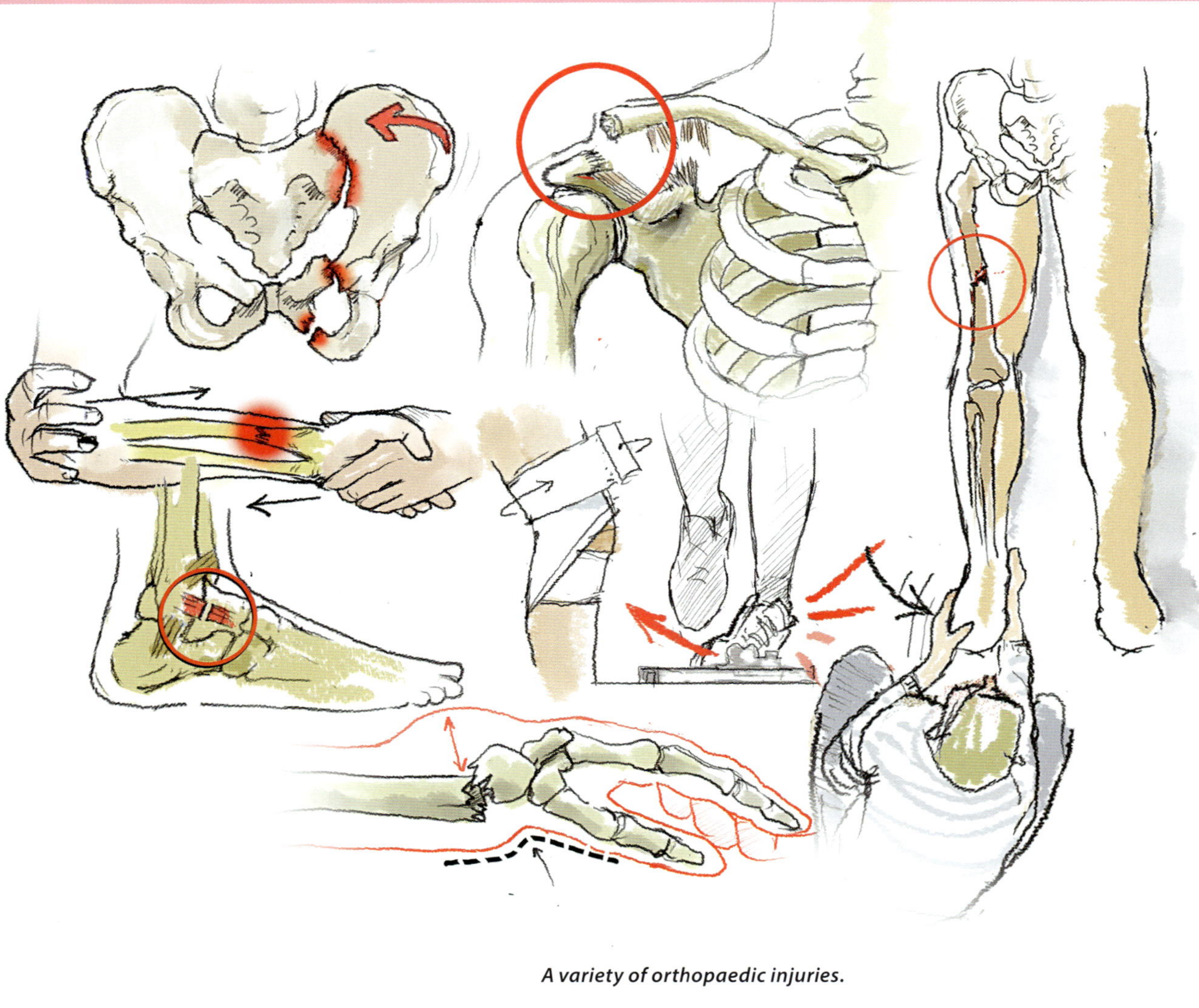

A variety of orthopaedic injuries.

Sprains, dislocations and fractures are relatively common injuries associated with trauma during boating, often resulting from falls, collisions or impacts on a specific body part. These injuries range from simple sprains to limb- or life-threatening fractures. For a layperson, it can be challenging to distinguish between these types of injuries, and hospitals frequently use X-rays to confirm whether it is a fracture or a sprain.

The primary goals are to:

- identify suspected or clear fractures
- assess which fractures require urgent transport to a hospital.
- determine which injuries, after initial first aid, allow for continued sailing to the next port
- identify injuries that can potentially be managed independently, such as sprains and simple fractures

How can a layperson determine whether it is a fracture or a sprain?

What is a sprain?

A sprain occurs when a joint is forced beyond its normal range of motion, stretching or tearing the ligaments and joint capsule while leaving the bones intact. Sprains can occur in virtually any joint. Surgery or casting is rarely required, regardless of severity.

What is a dislocation?

Dislocation (luxation) happens when the joint surfaces lose contact with each other. This always involves tearing one or more ligaments.

What is a fracture?

A fracture occurs when one of the skeletal parts breaks or develops a serious crack.

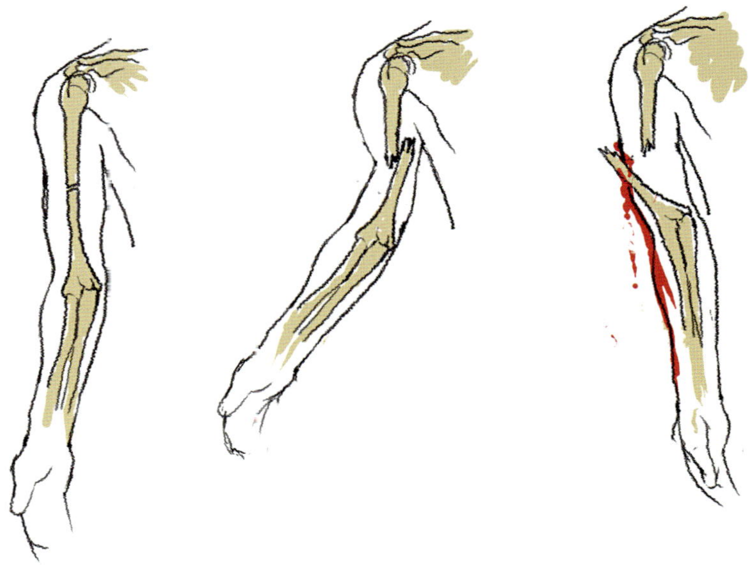

Types of fractures: Far left: Crack (fissure) with no dislocation. Middle: Dislocated fracture. Far right: Open fracture with a wound near the fracture site.

In the case of an open fracture, meticulous wound care is essential, and antibiotics should be administered from the ship's dispensary if far from a doctor (see page 249).

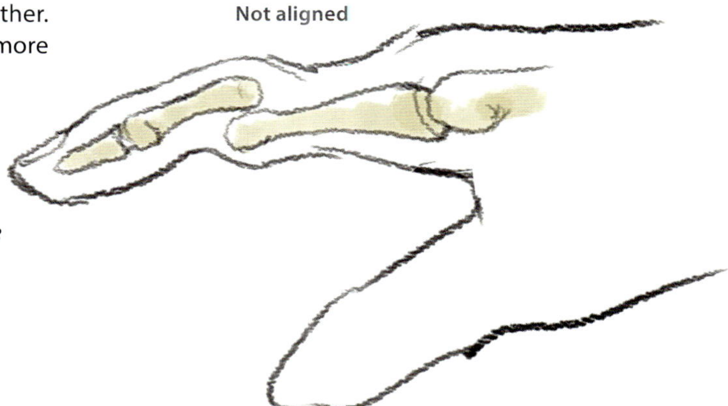

Example of dislocation in a finger where the joint surfaces no longer have contact.

Signs and symptoms

The common signs of sprains and fractures are similar, making assessment challenging, but fractures usually present more pronounced symptoms:

- pain
- direct tenderness
- indirect tenderness
- swelling around the injury

Clear signs of a fracture include:

- misalignment/dislocation
- open fracture with skin damage and exposed bone
- pathological mobility (bending a limb where there is no joint)
- 'fracture scrape' (audible and palpable grinding when fractured parts move)

Direct tenderness (pain when pressing directly on the affected area) combined with indirect tenderness (pain in the area when compressing the limb lengthwise) suggests a possible fracture or a fissure.

The biggest challenge arises with joint injuries, as they may involve a combination of ligament and skeletal damage. In contrast, fractures in long bones, such as the upper and lower arms, thighs and shins, are generally easier to assess.

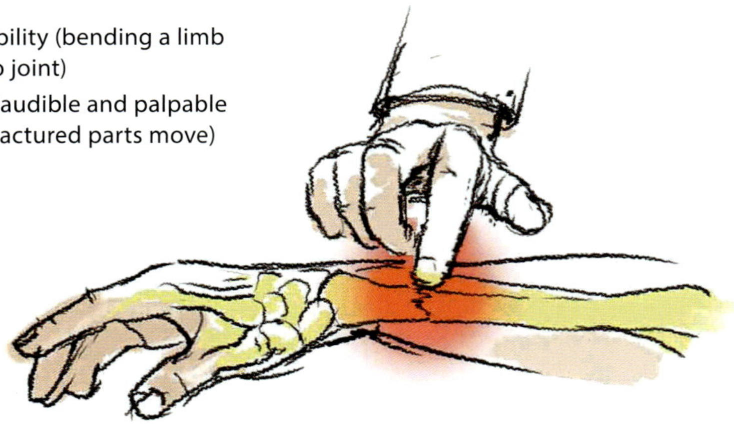

Top: Direct tenderness.
Bottom: Indirect tenderness.

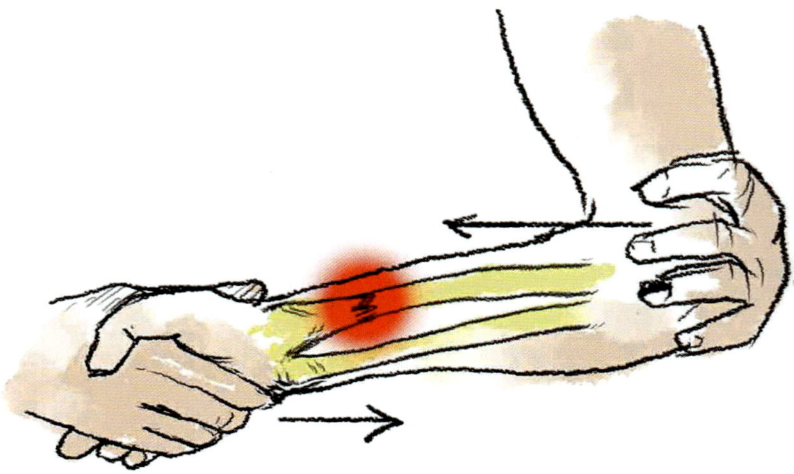

DISTAL STATUS

Fractures in the limbs (arms, thighs, shins) can risk vascular and nerve injury. Always check distal status – the condition of the limb below the fracture site – to identify signs of vascular or nerve damage. Immediate hospitalisation is required if impairment is detected.

Assessing distal status

- Circulation: Check pulse, capillary refill and temperature.
- Sensation: Lightly touch fingers/toes and ask how it feels.
- Mobility: Ask the person to move their fingers or toes.

Examination of distal status

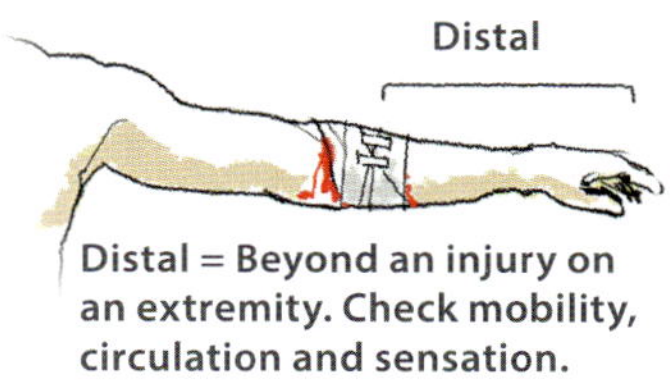

Definition of 'distal' – the part of an arm or leg beyond the injury. Always compare with the uninjured side.

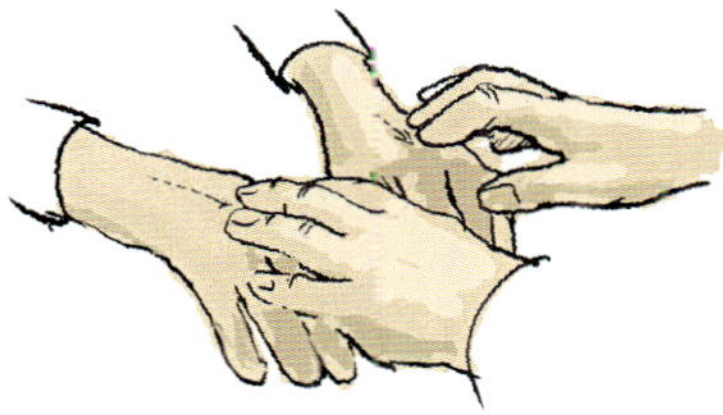

Assess sensation by gently touching the injured person's hands and fingers, or the top of the foot and toes if it is a leg injury, using your own fingertips. Ask them how it feels. Compare sides.

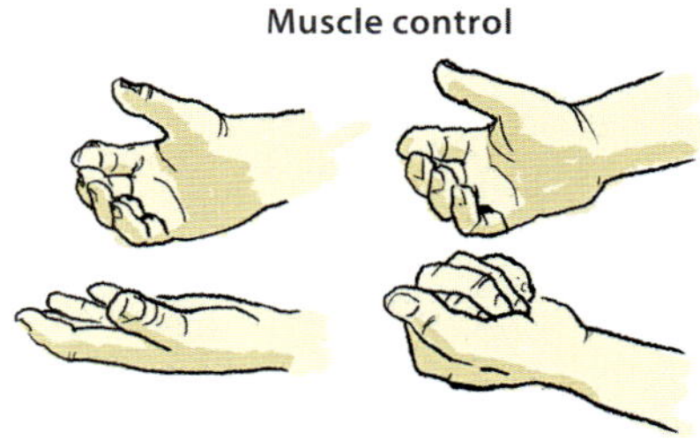

Assess mobility by asking the person to open and close their hands. Left hand: Normal mobility. Right hand: Reduced or no mobility.

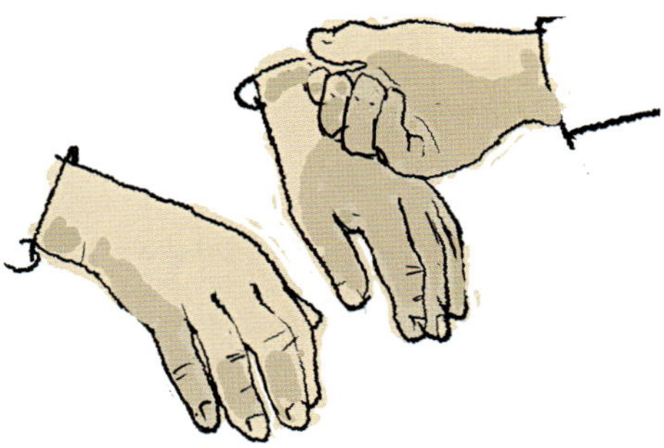

Assess temperature by checking whether the area feels warm or cold. Use the back of your own hand, which is most sensitive to temperature.

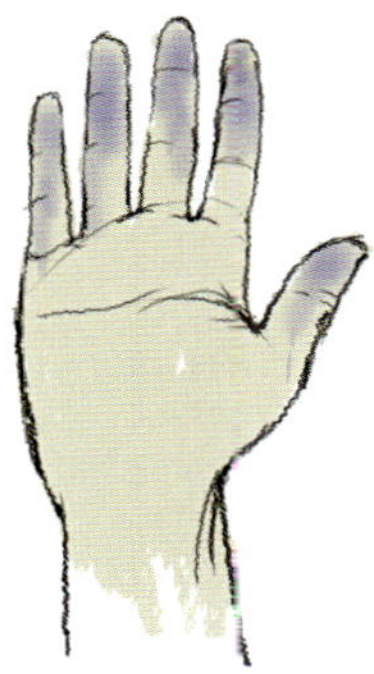

Assess oxygenation, by checking skin colour: is it pale, blue or normal?

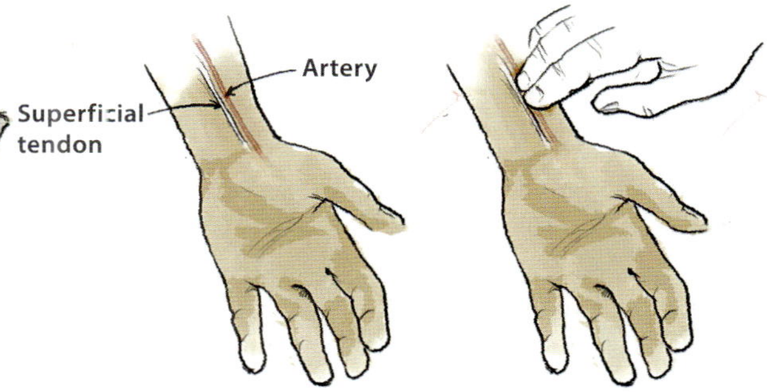

Is the pulse still present? See page 20.

Reduced sensation and mobility indicate nerve injury. This can be caused by direct trauma to the nerve but, most importantly, by acute circulatory impairment due to a vascular injury. Always compare with the healthy side!

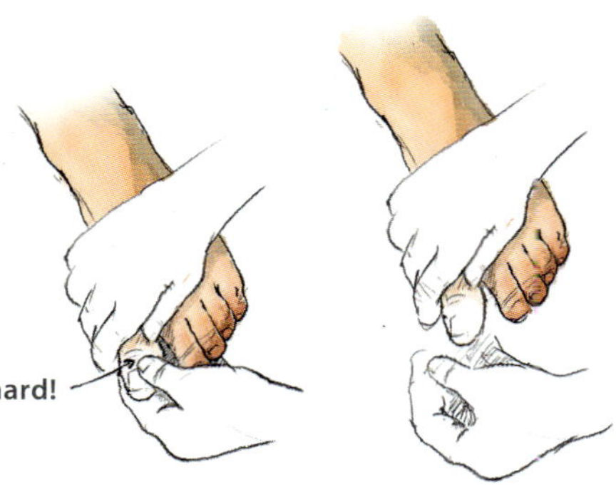

Check 'capillary circulation' by pressing firmly with your thumb and index finger on a fingertip or toe tip, then quickly releasing it. The area will turn white (bloodless). With normal circulation, it will quickly return to the same colour as the healthy side. If circulation is impaired, recovery will take much longer!

COMPARTMENT SYNDROME

Injuries or fractures of the lower leg, forearm or thigh bone carry the risk of severely impaired circulation within an hour to a day due to a condition called compartment syndrome. In these body parts, the muscles are organised into compartments surrounded by a strong and rigid muscle membrane. Blood vessels and nerves have limited space within these compartments. Significant bleeding or a fracture can cause the pressure inside the confined space to rise so high that blood vessels and nerves are damaged.

Signs and symptoms

Compartment syndrome should be suspected if the initial pain and swelling caused by the injury increase and become severe. In the foot or hand, signs of circulatory or nerve impairment, as described in the distal status section (see page 165), may develop.

The ultimate consequence of untreated compartment syndrome is significant functional impairment or loss of the limb. In extreme cases, it can even become life-threatening. The time frame ranges from shortly after the trauma to up to a day.

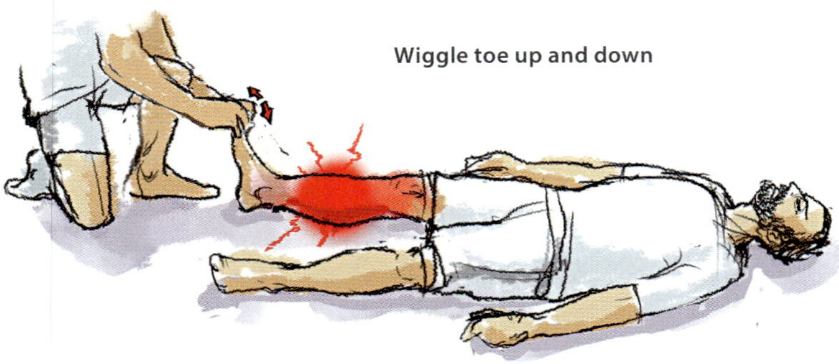

Lower leg with significant swelling after injury. A simple test for suspected compartment syndrome is extremely severe pain in the calf when the big toe is gently pulled upwards.

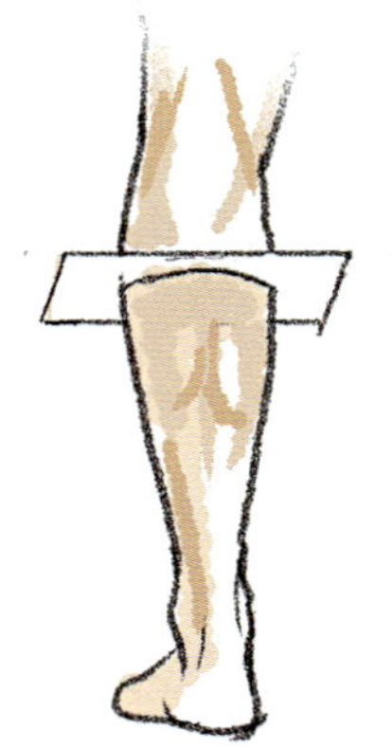

Cross-sectional anatomy of the calf showing muscle compartments, nerves and blood vessels. Increased pressure in a compartment may block circulation and cause nerve injury.

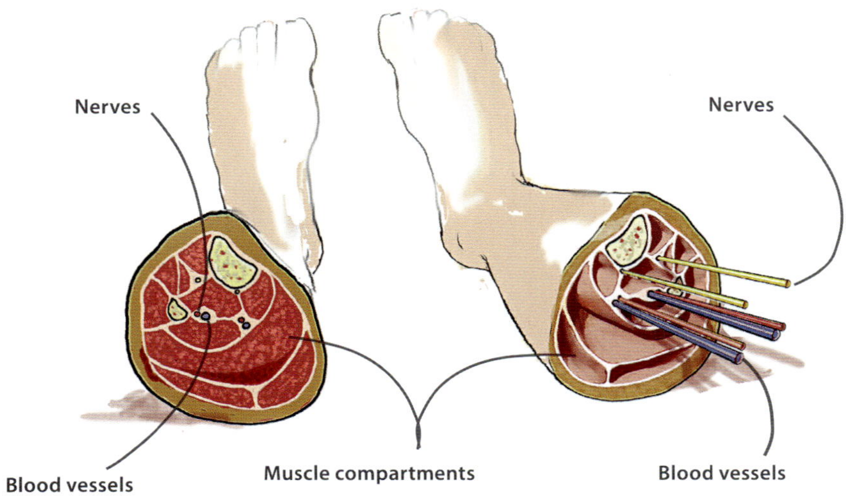

Immediate action / Treatment

An injury at risk of causing compartment syndrome requires urgent medical attention. If increased pressure is suspected, immediate medical evaluation is essential. Administer strong analgesics while waiting for the ambulance. Stabilise fractures. Treatment is surgical.

Far from help

Even if the primary injury appears manageable for a day or more on board, the development of compartment syndrome can lead to serious consequences. This situation constitutes a clear reason for urgent evacuation rather than waiting until the next port. Repeatedly assess distal status and monitor the condition closely, as the situation can rapidly become unbearable.

SUPPORTIVE, STABILISING BANDAGES

Elastic bandage

Regular elastic bandages are often sufficient for minor injuries. We recommend a slightly heavier type (for example, Dauer bandage), with wider bandages (10–12cm) for knees and feet and narrower ones (8–10cm) for hands and arms. Stabilising the bandage with a splint can also be helpful.

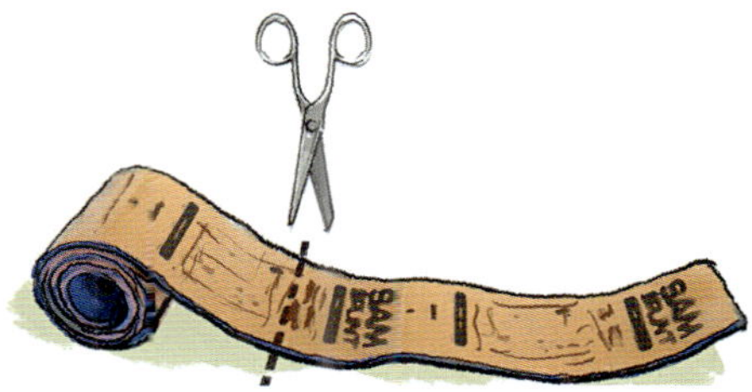

Malleable foam-covered aluminium splint.

Aluminium splint

A foam-covered, formable aluminium splint is an excellent addition to medical equipment and is available under various brands. These splints are approximately 1m long and 15cm wide but can be cut to fit different parts of the arms or legs. It is advisable to wrap the injured limb with a soft bandage to protect the skin before applying the splint, which can then be secured with elastic bandages.

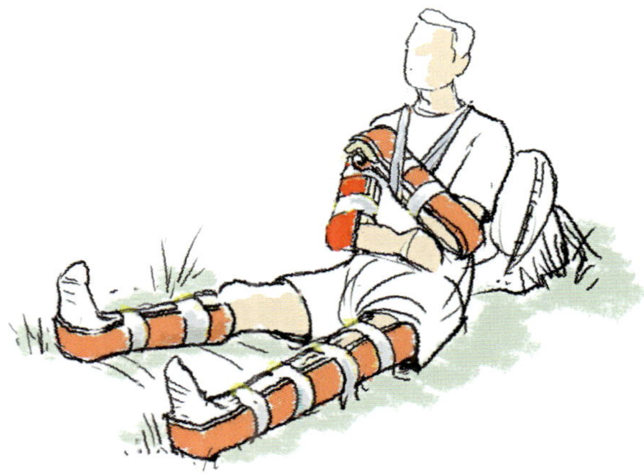

Examples of using aluminium splints.

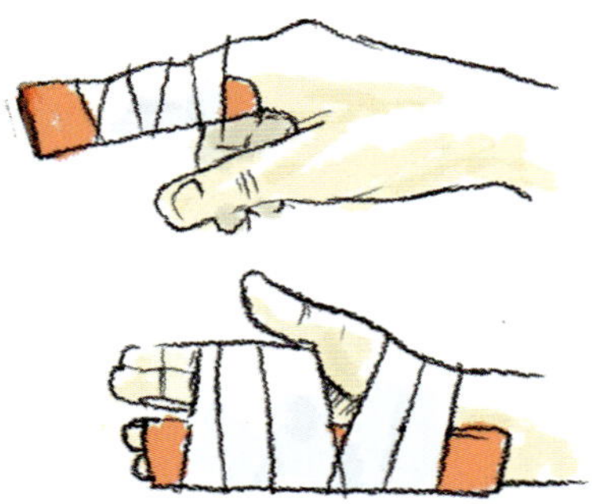

The longitudinal stability of the aluminium splint is achieved by folding it as shown.

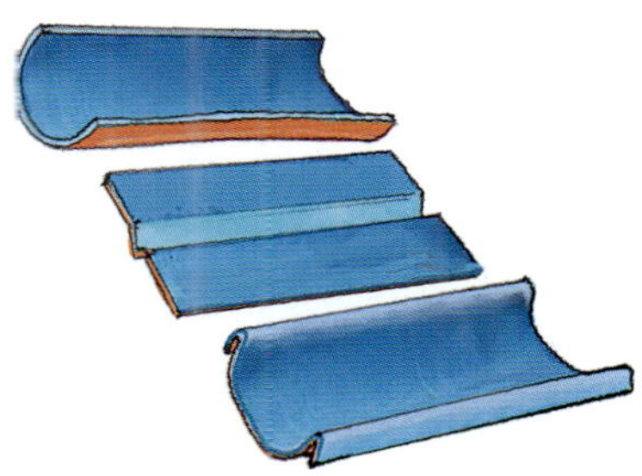

Plaster splint (plaster of Paris)

Another option, especially for hand and arm injuries, is to apply a plaster splint. Plaster bandages are available at some pharmacies. See plaster techniques for hand and arm injuries on page 201.

Is it sensible to bring plaster? For longer sailing trips, we recommend considering it. At the very least, have a malleable aluminium splint on board. The main advantage of plaster is that it moulds comfortably to the shape of the limb and provides excellent stabilisation as long as it remains dry. It is particularly useful for hand or wrist injuries, which are common.

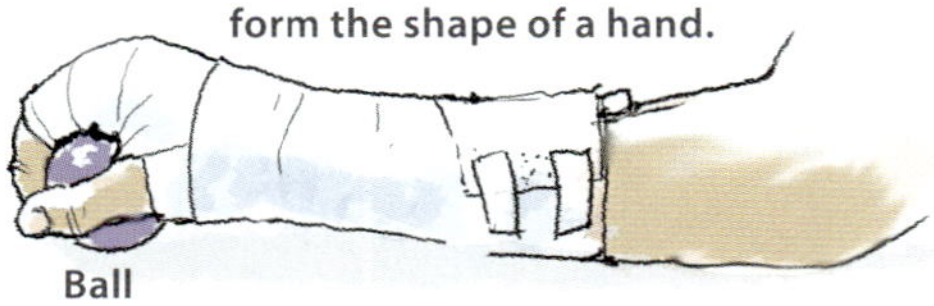
Hold the ball in the hand to form the shape of a hand.
Ball

A well-fitted plaster splint on an injured wrist. Hold a tennis ball to position the hand while the bandage is applied.

Drawbacks of plaster splints:

- Vulnerability to water: plaster becomes soft if it gets wet.
- Comparison with aluminium splints: aluminium splints are water-resistant but cannot provide the same tailored fit as plaster.

If no plaster or aluminium splints are available, use improvised materials. For example, cut up a fender, chop a board, or use an oar to create a makeshift splint.

IMPORTANT!

As a layperson, never apply a circular plaster bandage around a limb. Swelling around the injury can impair circulation. Instead, apply a splint – that is, a plaster plate that covers only half the limb's circumference, which is safe and effective.

'Collar and cuff'/Sling

For shoulder and upper arm injuries, a 'collar and cuff' is often preferable to an arm sling (triangular bandage). Its advantages include:

- providing a good, elevated position for the hand, reducing the risk of bothersome swelling
- allowing the weight of the arm to provide gentle traction along the upper arm
- enabling free movement of the fingers

To create a collar and cuff:

1. Use a scarf or a wide strip of fabric, ideally with soft padding, to form a loop around the neck.
2. Adjust the length so the hand is elevated high on the chest. Secure the loop with a cable tie.
3. Create a second, comfortable loop for the wrist, securing it with another cable tie.

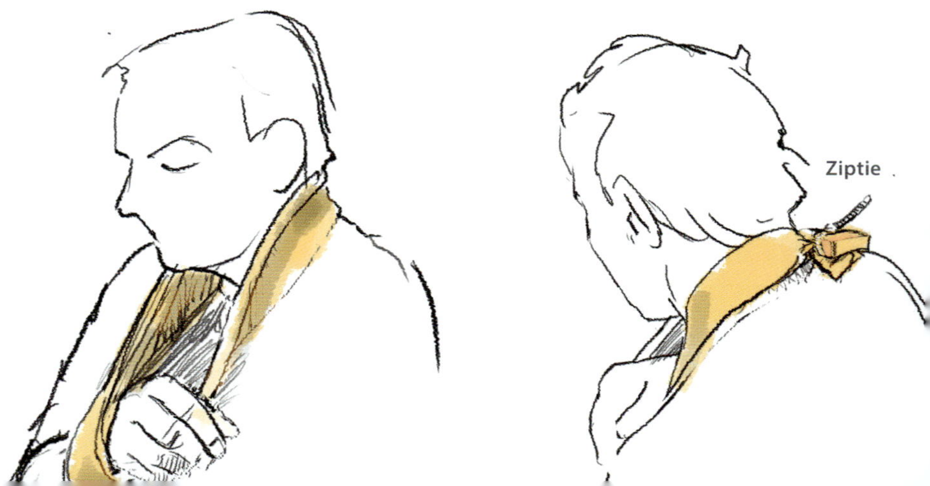

Collar and cuff.

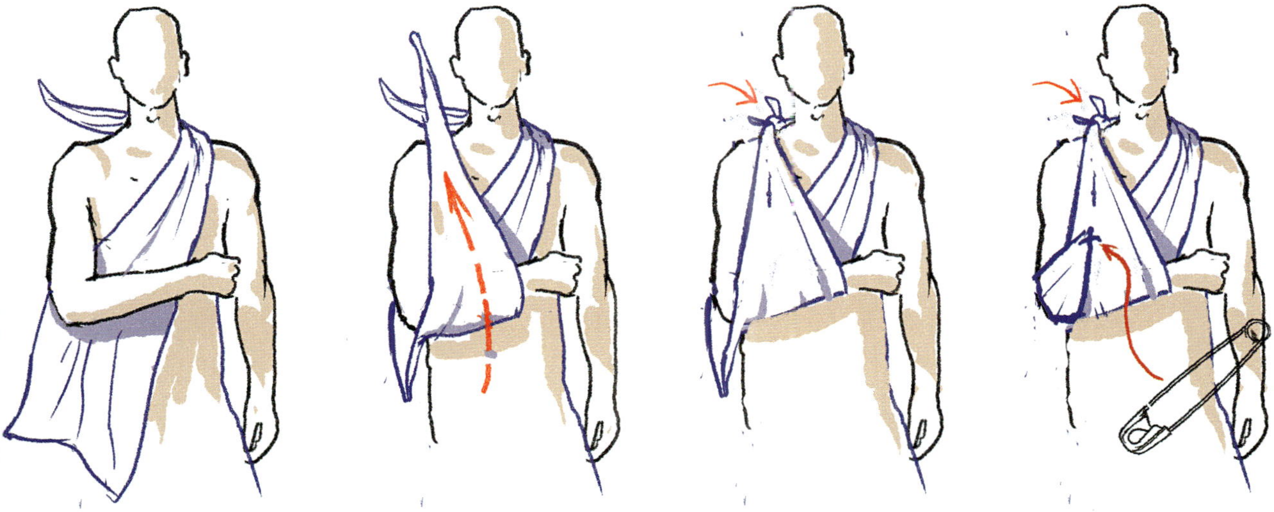

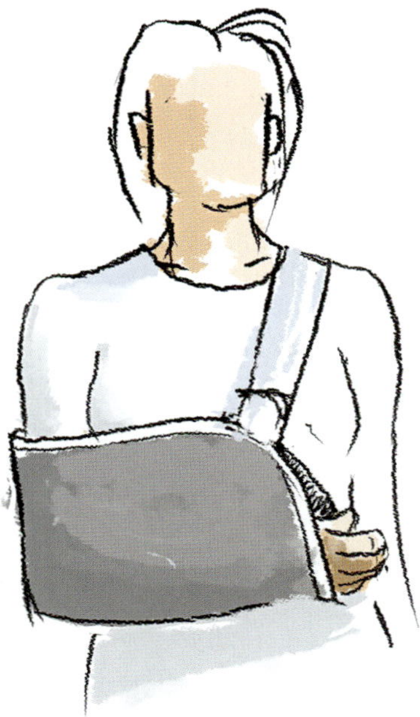

A classic arm sling (triangular bandage) can replace a collar and cuff but is particularly effective for forearm and wrist injuries. To the left: a pre-made arm sling.

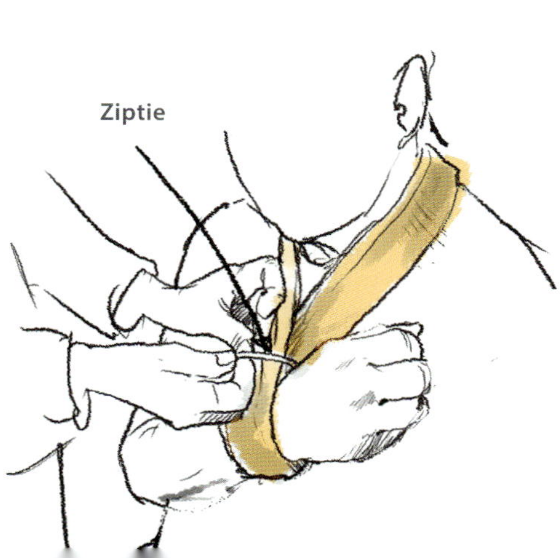

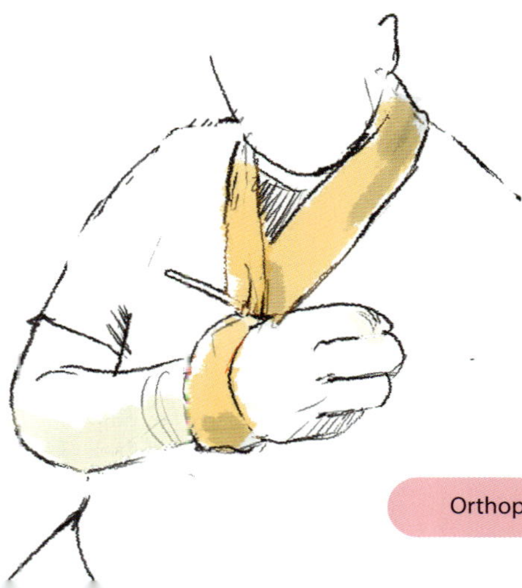

FRACTURE STABILISATION

When stabilising a fracture, it is important to immobilise the joints on both sides of the fracture; otherwise, the injury will not be properly stabilised. For example, in the case of a thigh bone fracture, both the hip and knee joints should be immobilised. Remember to protect the skin by using cushions.

A femoral fracture stabilised by a temporary splint made from cushions, a boathook and elastic bandages.

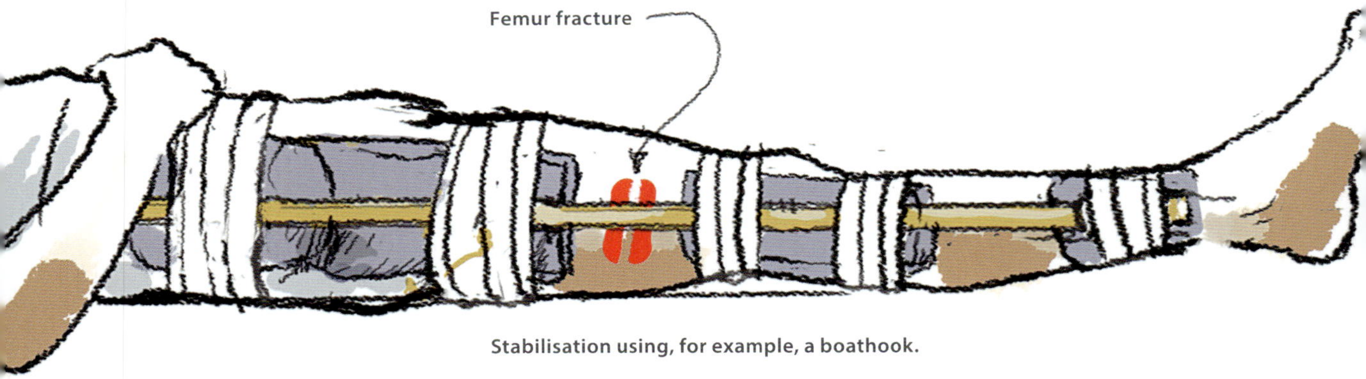

Stabilisation using, for example, a boathook.

Prompt reposition

Prompt reposition involves pulling a severely dislocated broken arm or leg into a better position immediately after the accident. It is crucial to check distal status both before and after the intervention. Of course, the need for prompt reposition is reduced if you are near medical care with rapid ambulance transport available, unlike in situations where professional help may be delayed by a day or more.

NEVER attempt prompt reposition for elbow or knee joint fractures without professional consultation!

When to consider prompt reposition

As a rough guideline, you should consider repositioning a severely dislocated fracture under the following circumstances, particularly when far from medical assistance:

- signs of impaired distal status (see above)
- femoral fractures (see page 214)
- significant misalignment
- expected long evacuation time
- open fractures with exposed bone (important to reposition the bone and cover it with muscles)
- severely angulated ankle fractures

Remember to stabilise the repositioned fracture using pillows, splints or any other appropriate materials.

FAR FROM HELP

- When far from help – the advice from a professor in orthopaedic surgery!
- Remember to observe how symptoms develop over time after orthopaedic injuries. A haematoma in a hip can initially be as painful as a fracture or a fissure. Have the person rest in a comfortable supine position and give an analgesic. If the person gets better and can bear weight on the leg or use the arm within 12 to 24 hours, this suggests a benign injury.

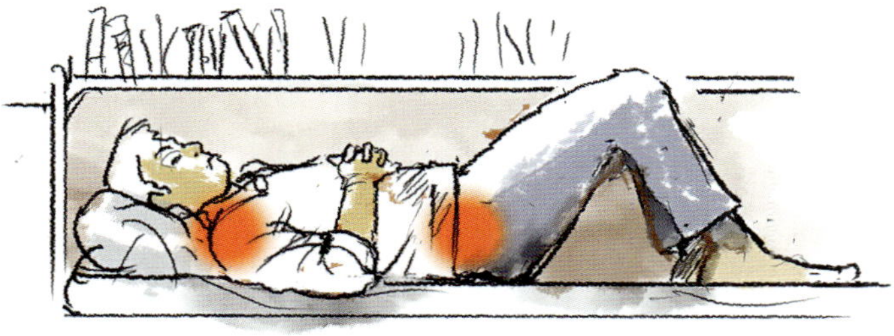

It is reassuring if rest and painkillers help!

PAIN MANAGEMENT IN ORTHOPAEDIC INJURIES

Paracetamol (1g every 4–6 hours, maximum 4g in 24 hours) is an effective baseline medication for adults. If this is insufficient, combine it with an anti-inflammatory medication like ibuprofen (400mg every 8 hours). For fractures and more serious injuries, stronger pain relief may be required, such as opioids like codeine combined with paracetamol or morphine for severe pain.

Prompt reposition of a severely dislocated femoral fracture. Gentle but firm traction.

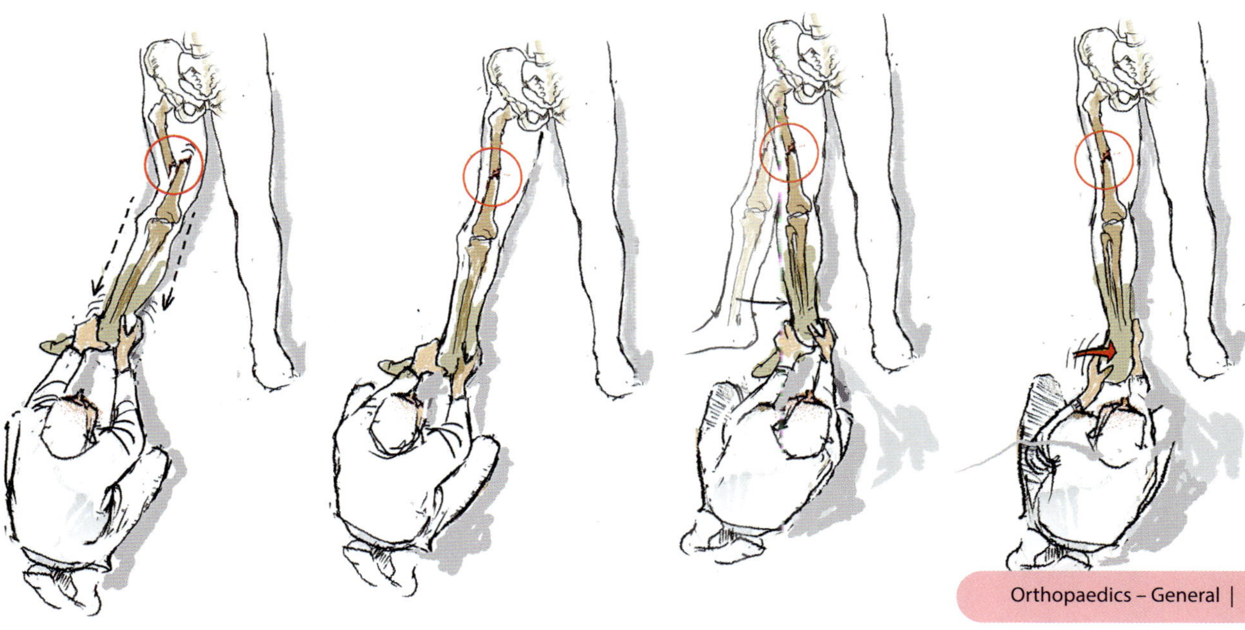

20. SPINAL INJURIES

There are many situations involving a risk for back or spinal injuries.

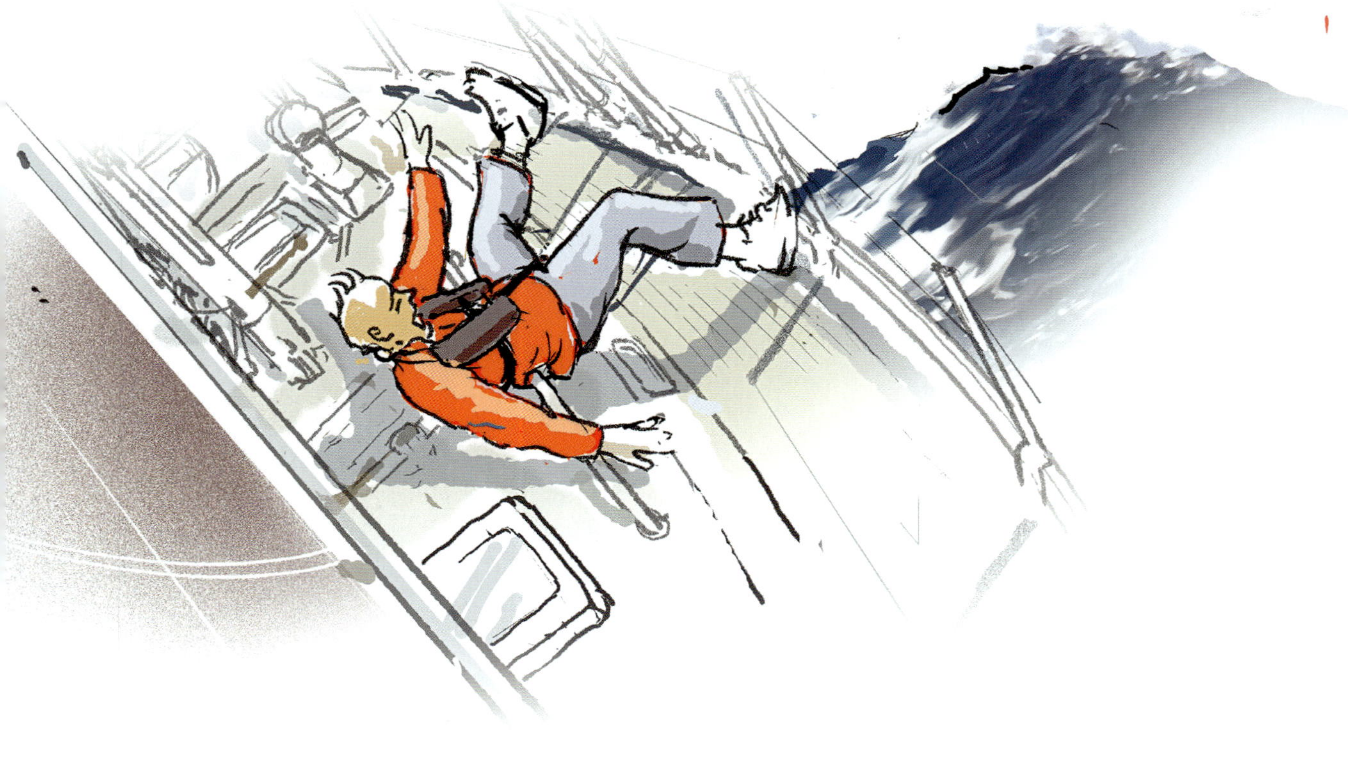

A layperson typically has limited ability to examine and diagnose spinal injuries. However, this overview of common types of injuries may help with the initial assessment on board.

The risk of nerve injury following spinal trauma can range from none to severe, involving fractured vertebrae that may damage the spinal cord and nerves, potentially causing loss of mobility and/or sensation below the injury site as well as respiration loss.

The vertebrae collectively form a protective yet partially movable skeletal tube, the spinal canal, which surrounds the spinal cord – an extension of the brain.

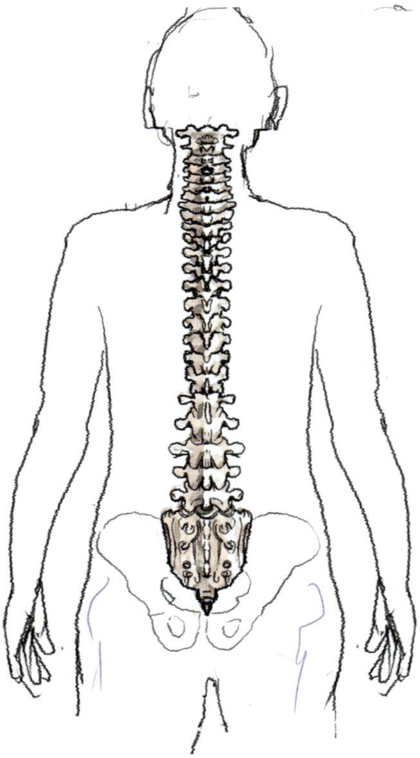

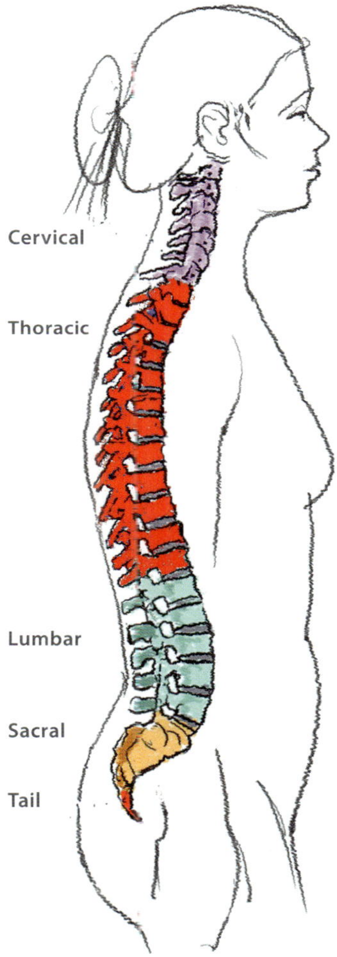

The spine is composed of 26 vertebrae (7 cervical, 12 thoracic, 5 lumbar plus sacrum and coccyx), along with muscles and ligaments. The vertebrae protect the spinal cord, which is in continuity with the brain.

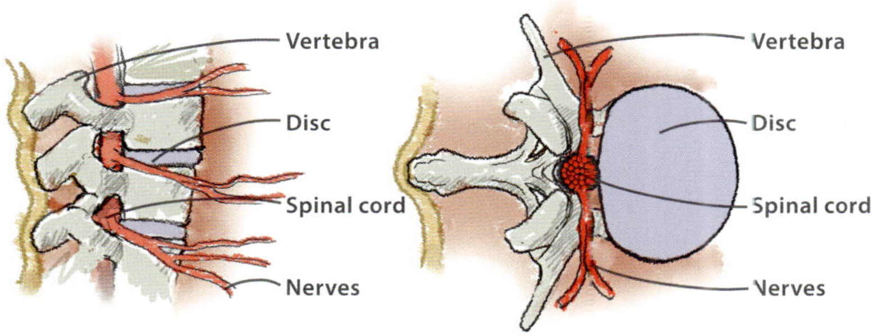

The spinal cord has significant nerve branches (both sensory and motor) that extend between the vertebrae, which are cushioned by discs.

VERTEBRAL COMPRESSION FRACTURE

Vertebral compression: landing on the buttocks can transmit force along the spine, causing compression of one or more vertebral bodies.

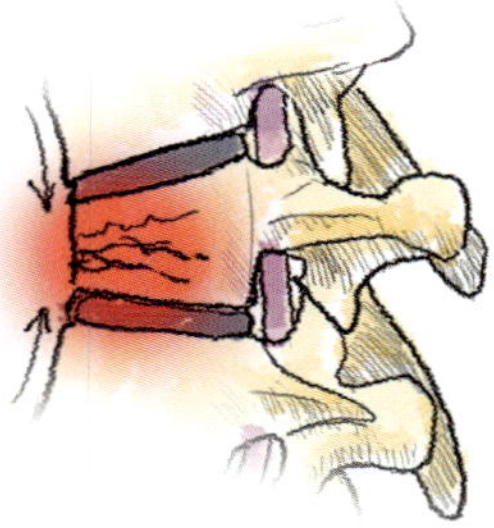

Compressed vertrebal body

The most common type of spinal injury involving a fracture is vertebral compression, typically occurring in the thoracic or lumbar spine. This injury can happen even after relatively mild trauma, such as sitting hard on the buttocks or experiencing strong jolts while riding a fast motorboat in rough seas. These forces compress the vertebral body.

This injury is most common in individuals with weakened bones, particularly older women, but it can occur at any age following significant accidents.

Signs and symptoms

- Acute pain and tenderness over the affected vertebra
- Possible radiating pain down the legs or around the chest
- Nerve damage is less common with vertebral compression fractures

Immediate action

If on a motorboat, avoid further injury by reducing speed and follow the seas.

Treatment

Seek medical attention for proper examination. Administer paracetamol and/or ibuprofen for pain relief.

Far from help

A vertebral compression fracture can be managed during a longer crossing, provided there are no signs of nerve involvement. The course of action depends on the type of trauma, pain pattern and symptoms (for example, loss of sensation or motor function in the legs). See the section below on unstable fractures. Treatment involves pain relief and gentle movement exercises.

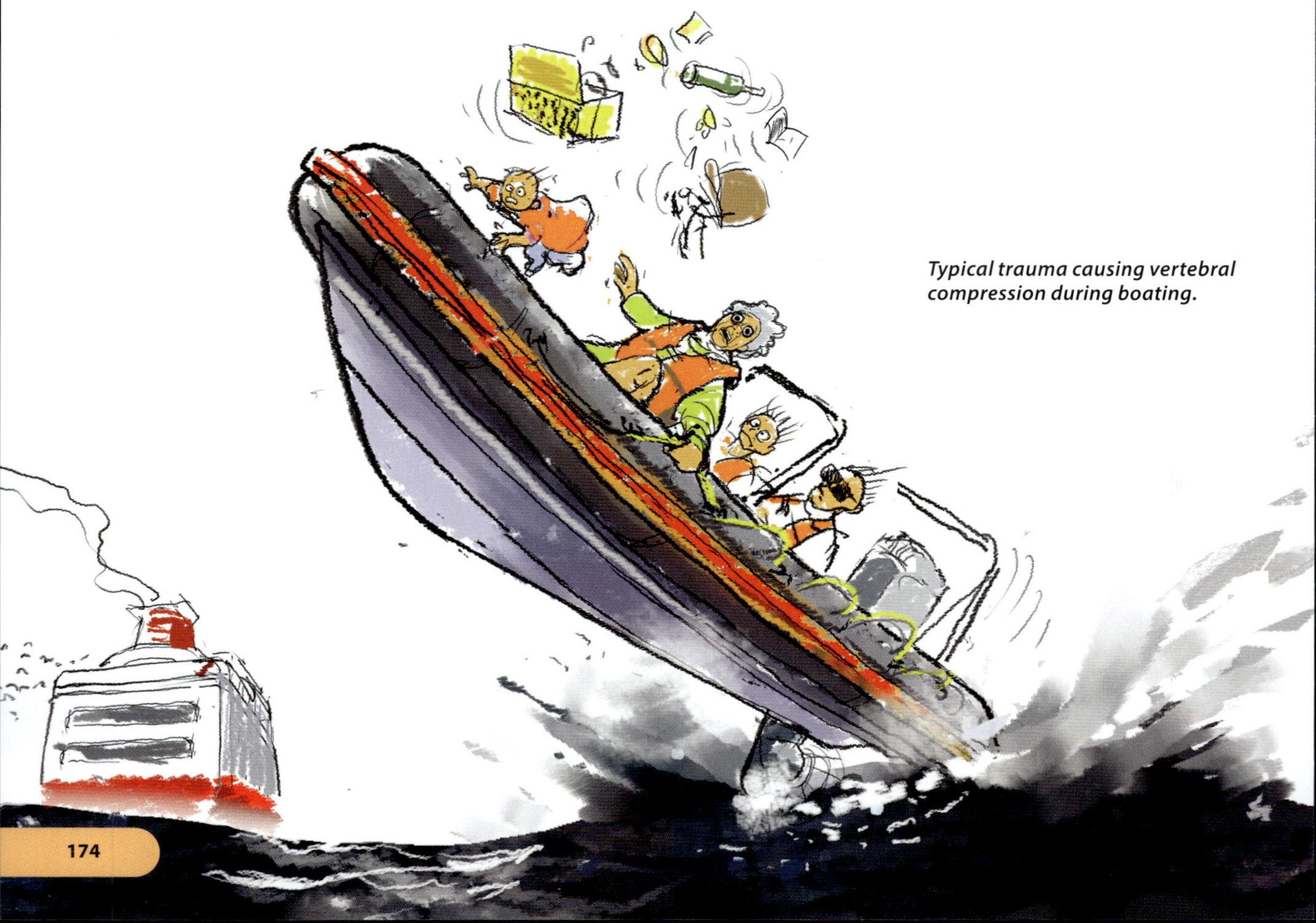

Typical trauma causing vertebral compression during boating.

FRACTURE OF A SPINAL PROCESS

Another common and generally harmless spinal injury is a fracture of a spinal process. This can occur after a fall or a direct blow to the spine. The dorsal bony projection of the vertebra may fracture or crack, as illustrated.

Signs and symptoms

- Localised pain and tenderness over the affected projection when palpating the back
- No risk of nerve involvement, as the rest of the vertebra remains intact

Immediate action

- Stop activity.
- Rest.

Treatment

- Seek medical assessment and examination.
- Provide pain relief.
- Encourage gentle movement and exercises.

Far from help

Confirm that the injury is uncomplicated and does not involve nerve damage. Administer pain relief and encourage gentle movement.

The spinal processes are the protrusions along the exterior of the spine. An isolated fracture of a spinal process does not affect the spinal cord.

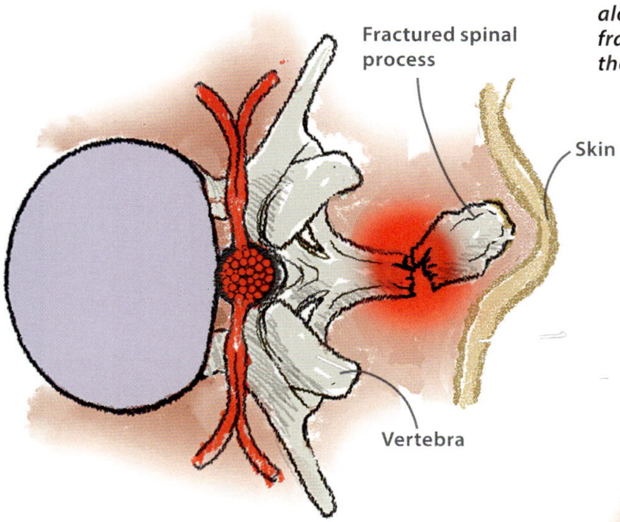

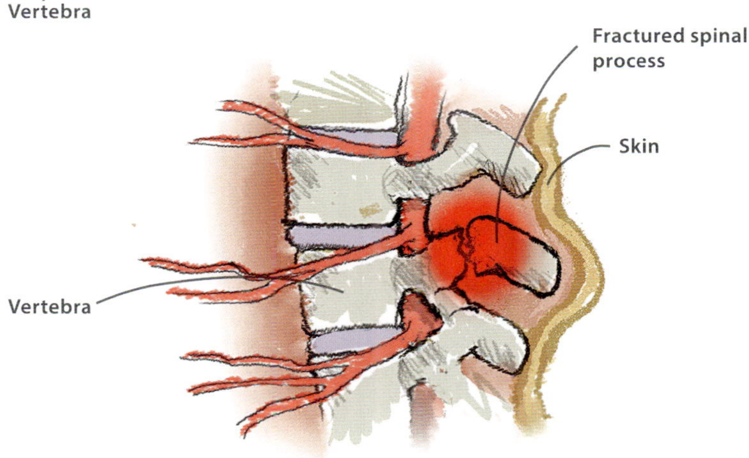

CERVICAL SPINE INJURY

These dramatic and often severely disabling injuries, involving unstable fractures and nerve damage, typically occur during diving accidents but can also result from severe falls, cycling or motorcycle accidents. Tragically, they often affect young individuals.

Compared to other vertebrae, the cervical vertebrae are slender and more fragile, making them particularly susceptible to injury. A common scenario involves a person diving head first into shallow water, resulting in paralysis from the shoulders down and leaving them floating in the water, requiring immediate rescue.

Signs and symptoms

Suspect a cervical spine injury if the following are observed:

- a typical injury mechanism, such as diving head first
- pain or tenderness in the neck
- weakness or paralysis in the arms and/or legs
- numbness in the arms and/or legs
- reduced sensation in the fingers and toes
- if the uppermost vertebrae are affected, risk of respiratory muscle impairment

CAUTION!

Even after milder head or spinal trauma, it is crucial to rule out this type of injury due to its potentially serious consequences.

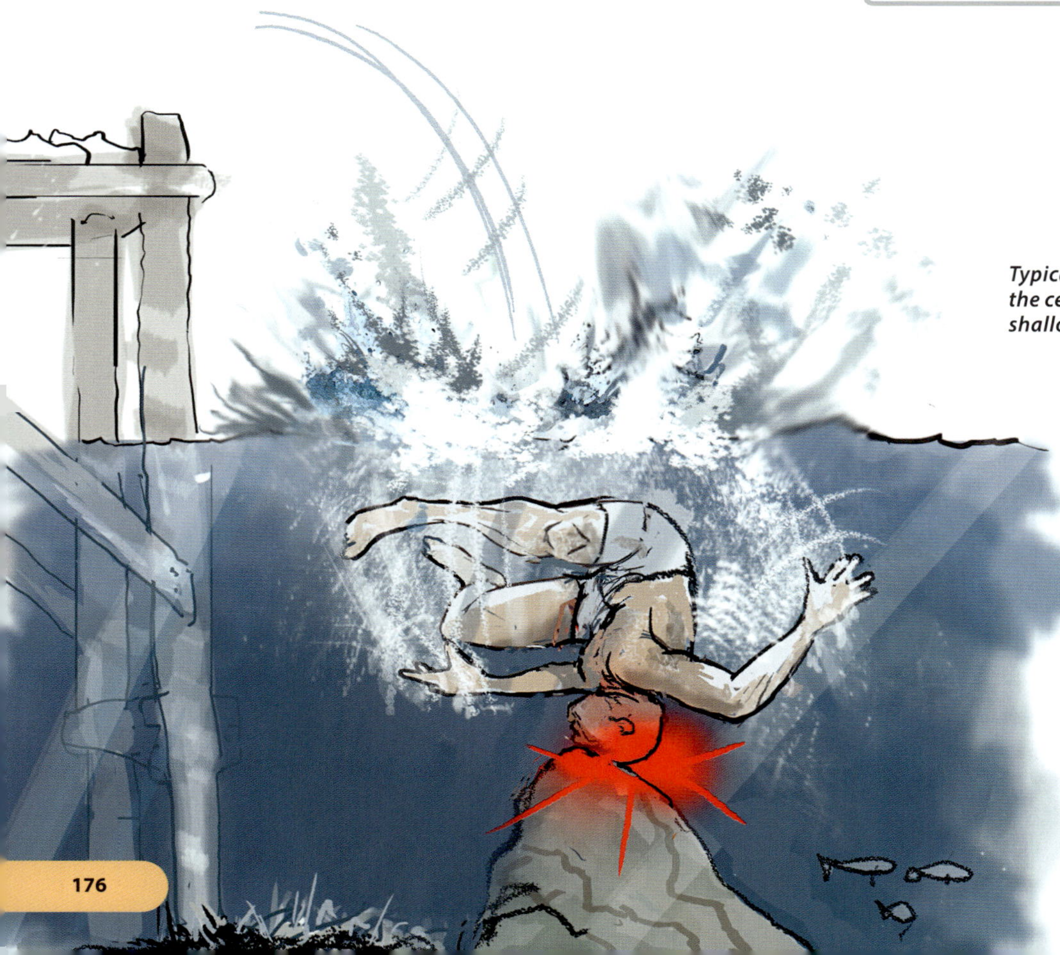

Typical trauma causing injuries to the cervical spine. Never dive in shallow or unfamiliar waters!

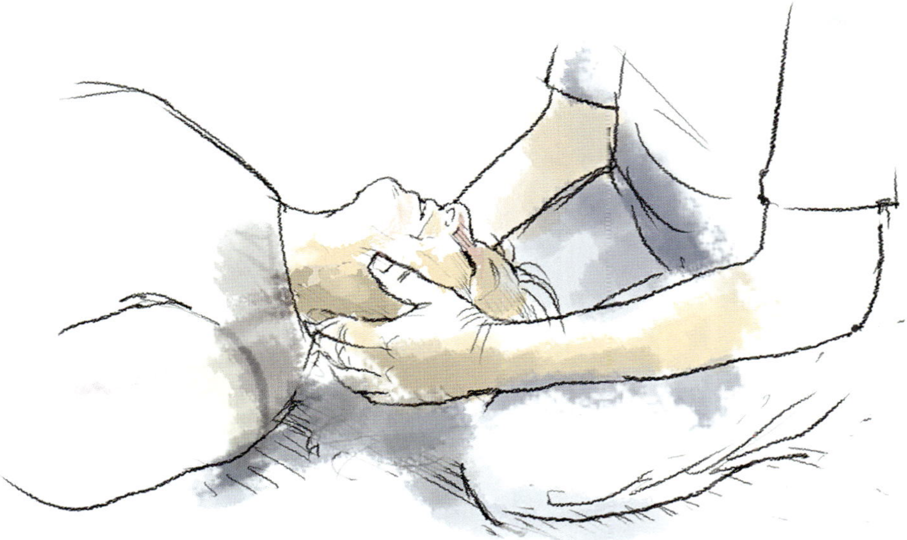

Manually stabilise the cervical spine by placing one hand on each side of the head, with fingertips gently gripping under the jaw and palms resting over the ears.

Immediate action

- Rescue the individual from the water.
- Call for evacuation and transport to a hospital.
- Manually stabilise the injured neck using your hands, as shown in the illustration. Maintain this position until an ambulance arrives. For longer waits, consider using tightly wrapped bandages and pillows to prevent inappropriate movements of the cervical spine.
- Check for an open airway. If the person is not breathing open up the airways by performing a jaw-thrust manoeuvre whilst keeping the neck immobilized. The jaw is pulled forward without tilting the head as in chin lift.

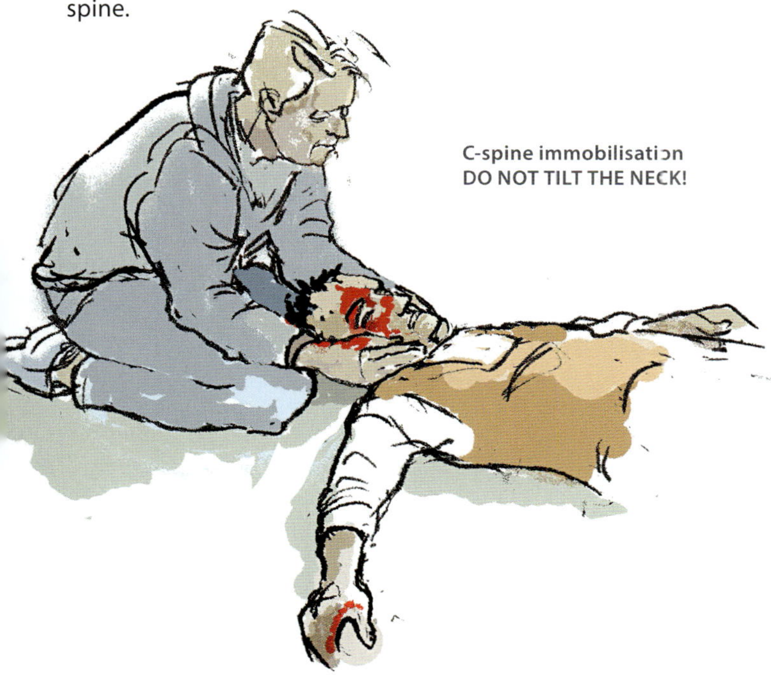

C-spine immobilisation
DO NOT TILT THE NECK!

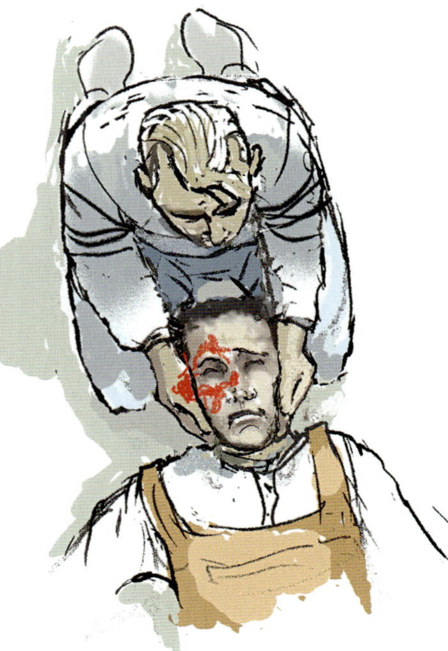

> **NOTE!**
>
> In cases of high cervical spine injury, breathing muscles may become paralysed, posing an immediate risk of hypoxia and further complications. Rescue breaths may serve as a temporary solution.

Treatment

Refer to the steps outlined above under 'Immediate action'.

Far from help

Managing cervical spine injuries in remote locations is extremely challenging due to the high risk of respiratory issues. Evacuation is critical, and delays can worsen the situation.

- Make the individual as comfortable as possible.
- Stabilise their neck with pillows or blankets.
- Keep them warm.
- Administer pain relief (analgesics) and possibly a sedative.
- If the person must be moved, proceed with extreme caution and avoid any unnecessary movements of the spine. Always seek medical advice.

Prevention

Cervical spine injuries are preventable! Strictly prohibit crew members from diving head first. Always enter the water feet first, regardless of its depth.

CAUTION! Be cautious when moving someone with a suspected spinal injury. Avoid spinal movements. If lifting is necessary, use the individual's clothing and coordinate as a team. The person stabilising the head must lead the action.

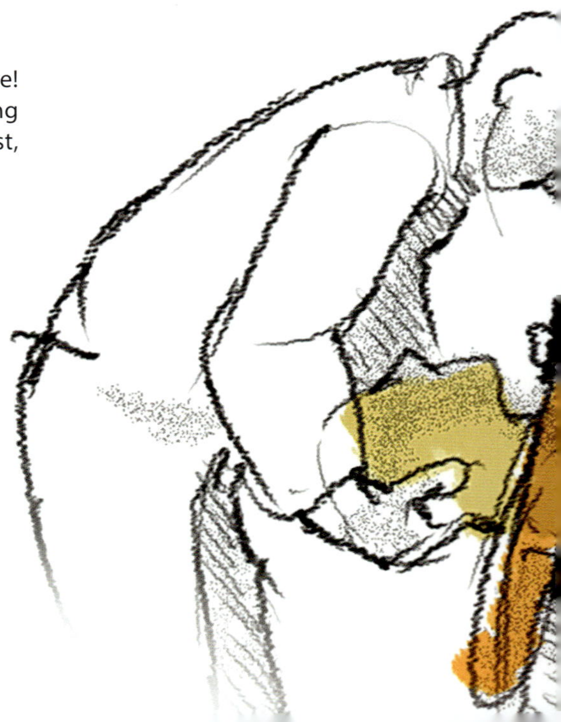

Use rolled-up blankets or towels for stabilisation, and secure with elastic bandages or strong tape, such as Gorilla/ gaffer/duct tape.

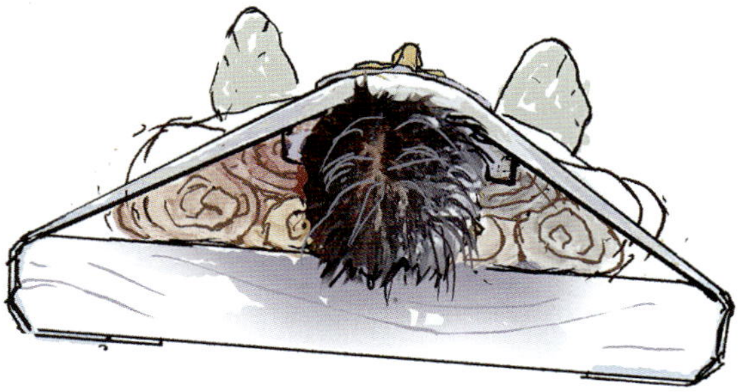

Stabilisation of neck awaiting transport to hospital.

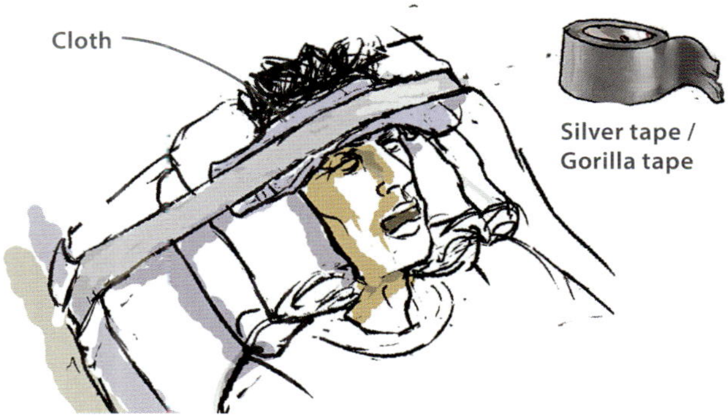

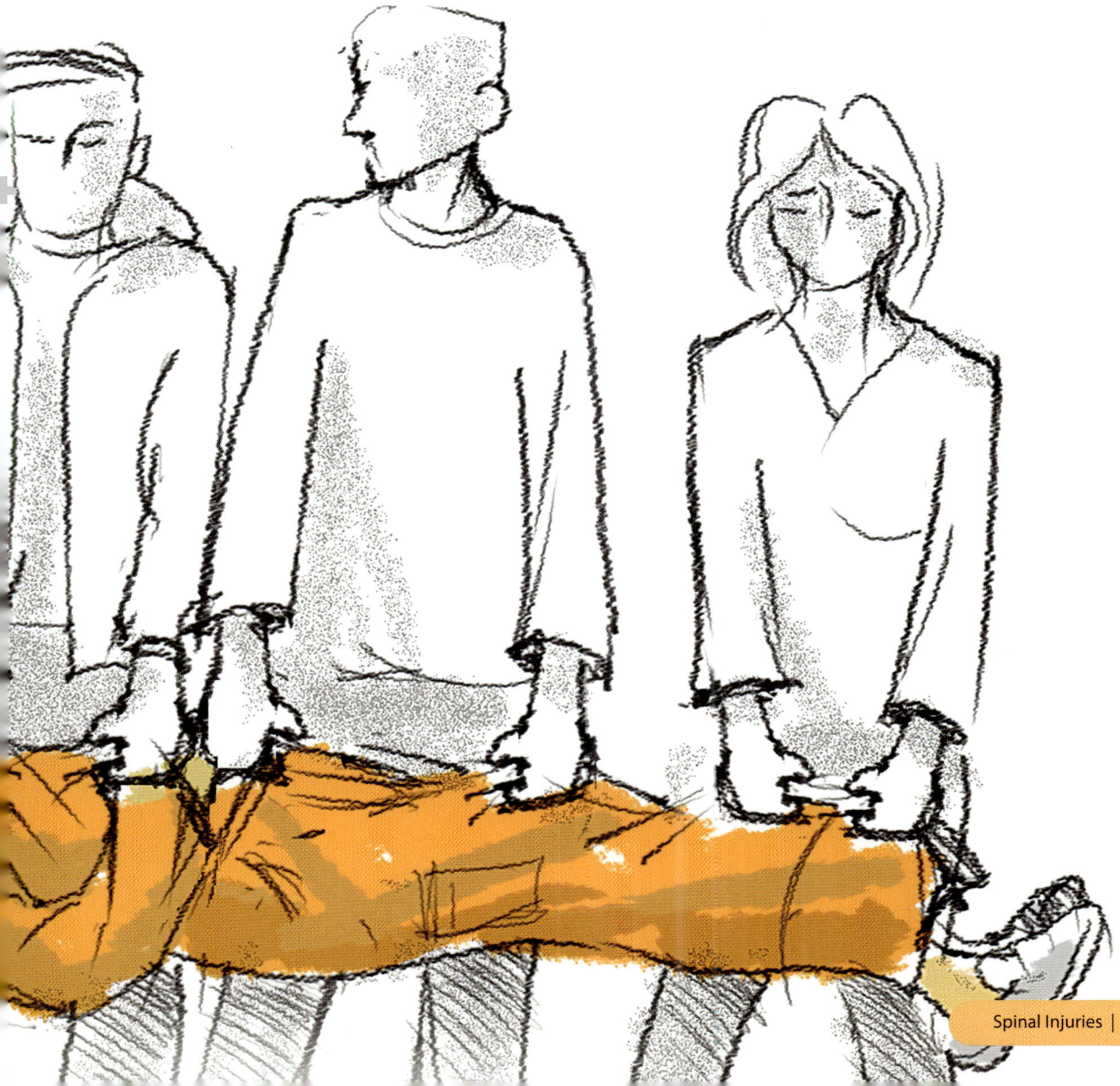

FRACTURES OF THORACIC AND LUMBAR VERTEBRAE

The mechanisms of thoracic and lumbar vertebral fractures are like those of cervical spine injuries, typically occurring in younger, active individuals following collisions or severe falls involving significant force. The severity of these injuries varies greatly, ranging from cases that require only pain relief and exercise to those involving a risk of disabling paralysis due to spinal cord compression. The latter can occur after severe trauma when the vertebral arch is damaged or there is displacement between the vertebrae.

Signs and symptoms

Indicators of a severe injury include:

- intense pain and tenderness over the vertebrae
- tingling or numbness in the hands and/or feet
- loss of sensation
- weakness or difficulty moving the arms and/or legs

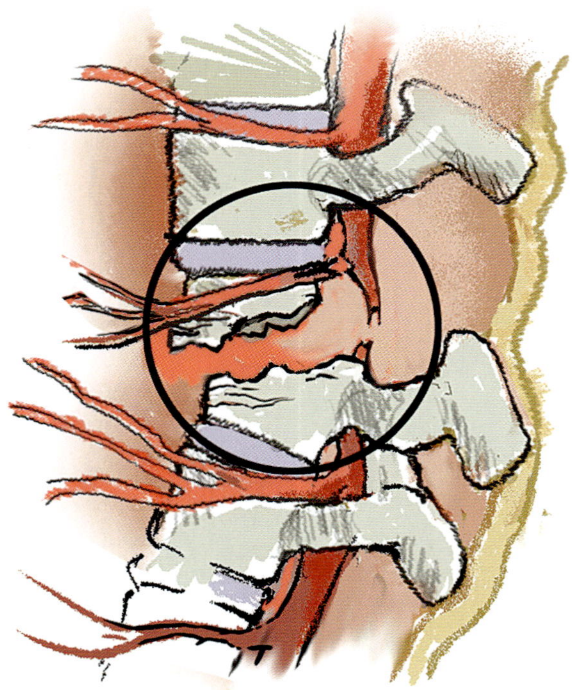

Immediate action / Treatment

A person with such an injury should be treated as if they have a severe spinal cord injury until proven otherwise.

- Conduct a careful examination.
- Avoid any movement of the spine.
- Arrange for transport to a hospital by ambulance for further assessment.
- Wait for assistance from ambulance personnel before attempting to move the person.
- Keep the person warm.
- Stabilise the spine before moving.
- Provide pain relief.

Far from help

If such an injury is suspected in a remote location, contact medical professionals for advice and assistance with planning an evacuation.

Preventing vertebral fractures

- Avoid jolts – adjust speed in rough seas.
- Prevent falls and collisions – anticipate risks.
- Use double safety measures when climbing the mast.
- Do not dive head first.

In cases of falls, such as from a mast, a vertebra may sustain severe damage. The spinal canal can become completely displaced, causing severe nerve damage to the spinal cord.

ACUTE BACK PAIN

Acute back pain is a common reason for seeking medical attention. Causes include muscle strain, wear and tear in vertebral joints, and herniated discs. Boating activities often involve uncomfortable positions, confined spaces, heavy lifting, rope pulling and sudden unplanned movements.

Signs and symptoms

Lumbago (lower back pain): A painful condition in the lumbar region, usually triggered by lifting or overexerting a back muscle. The pain often appears suddenly and can be bothersome. It is typically localised to the lower back.

Sciatica: Compression of a nerve branch, usually the sciatic nerve, causing pain that radiates into the groin or down one leg, sometimes reaching the foot.

Incorrect lifting techniques are a common cause of acute back pain.

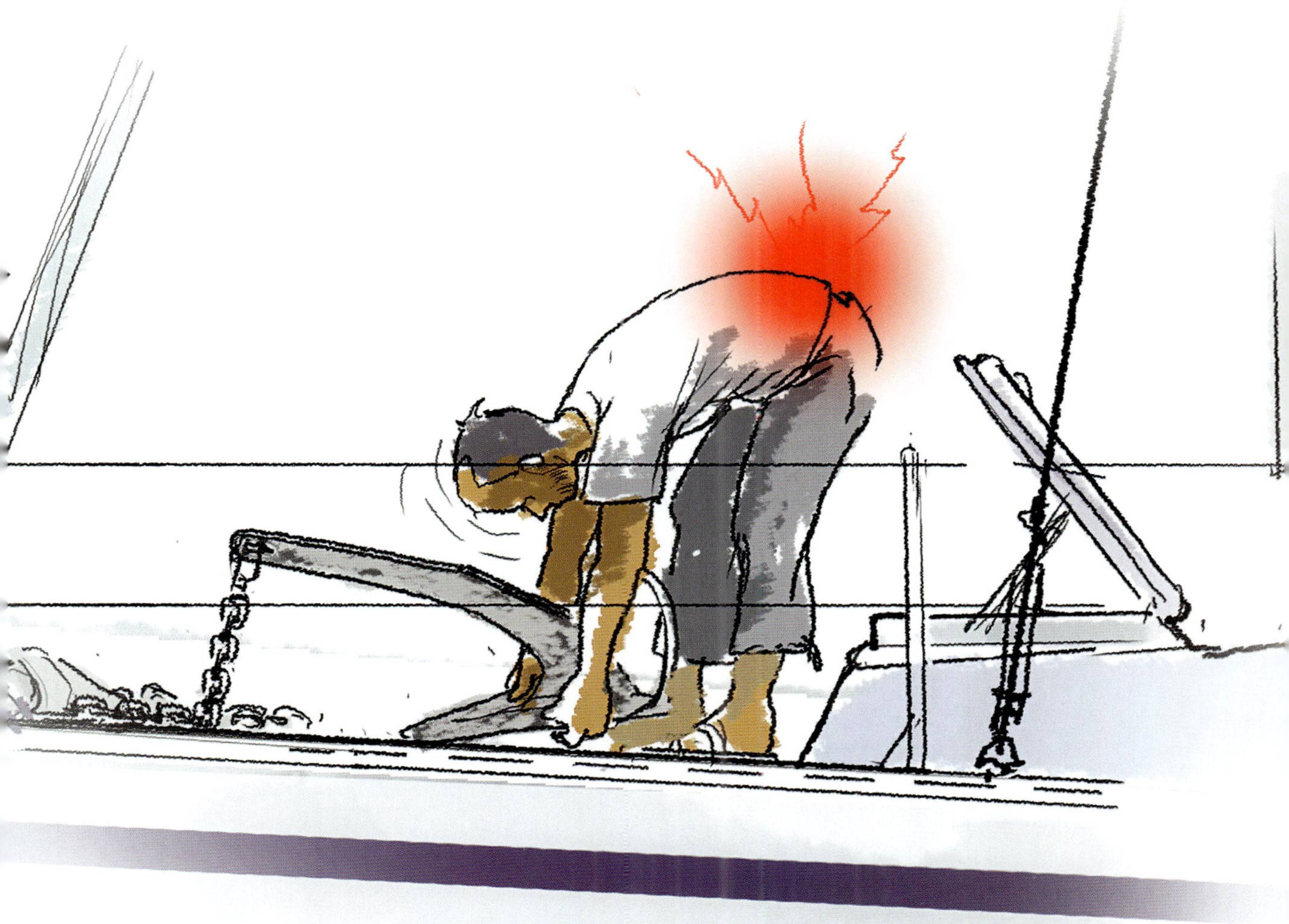

Herniated disc: This condition may start suddenly or develop from acute lower back pain that worsens over several days.

- Severe radiating pain, sometimes extending to the toes. The location of the pain indicates the level at which the herniation compresses the nerve root.
- Numbness in the area supplied by the affected nerve.
- Muscle weakness, such as difficulty walking on the heel or toe, also suggests the level of injury.
- Increased pain in the leg during activities that raise abdominal pressure, such as sneezing or straining during a toilet visit.

How to test nerve involvement? Different ways but this is simple.

SUSPECTED HERNIATED DISC

If the person reports sensory loss around the genital or anal area (often noticed when wiping after using the toilet) or lacks the urge to urinate despite a full bladder, urgent transport to an orthopaedic clinic is necessary. Emergency surgery may be required to prevent lifelong disability, including incontinence.

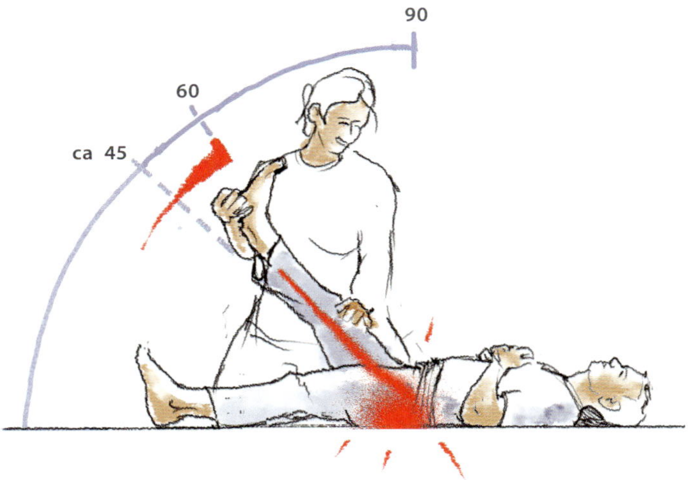

Lasegue's test: Have the person lie flat and relax. If the leg cannot be lifted beyond 45–60 degrees due to pain, it suggests nerve root involvement.

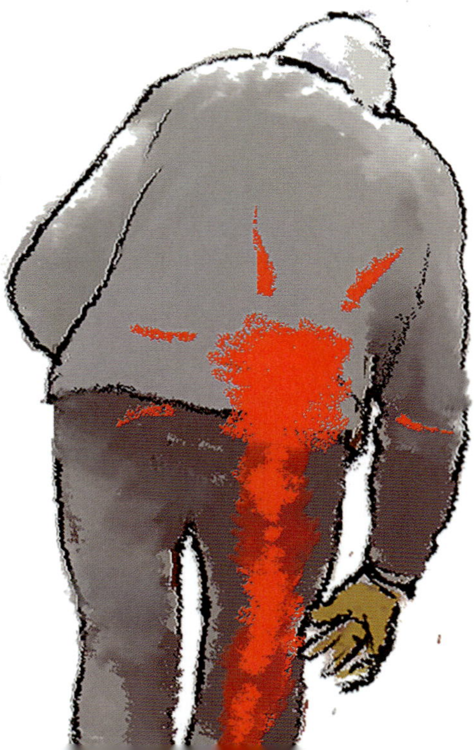

Muscle cramps on one side of the back may cause a stiff and crooked posture (scoliosis).

Immediate action

- Stop all activities.
- Provide pain relief using paracetamol and NSAIDs.

Treatment

Breaking the cycle of pain and muscle spasm is key.

- Provide pain relief and anti-inflammatory medication (NSAIDs).
- Advise gentle exercise and movement; standing and lying down are often more comfortable than sitting.
- Encourage walking to relax back muscles but avoid bending forward or lifting with a twisted back.
- Rest in the psoas position, which maximises relaxation of the back muscles.

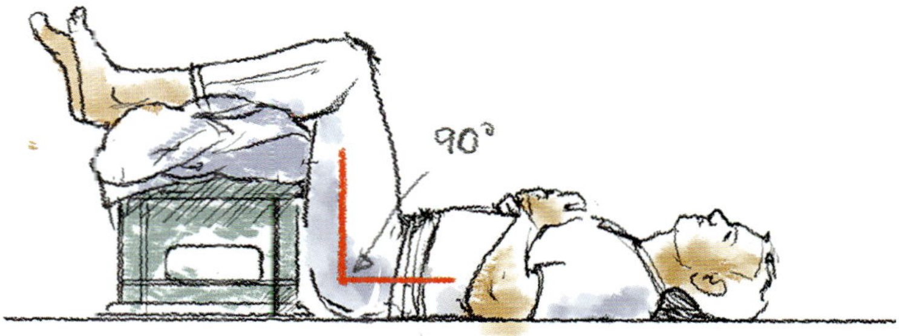

Resting in a supine position with psoas relaxation can help alleviate back muscle tension.

Prevention

- Maintain physical fitness with exercises that strengthen the back muscles.
- Plan physically demanding tasks, such as heavy lifting or pulling mooring lines, to ensure ergonomic techniques are used.

Lift with your legs, not your back. The same technique applies when hauling in a line.

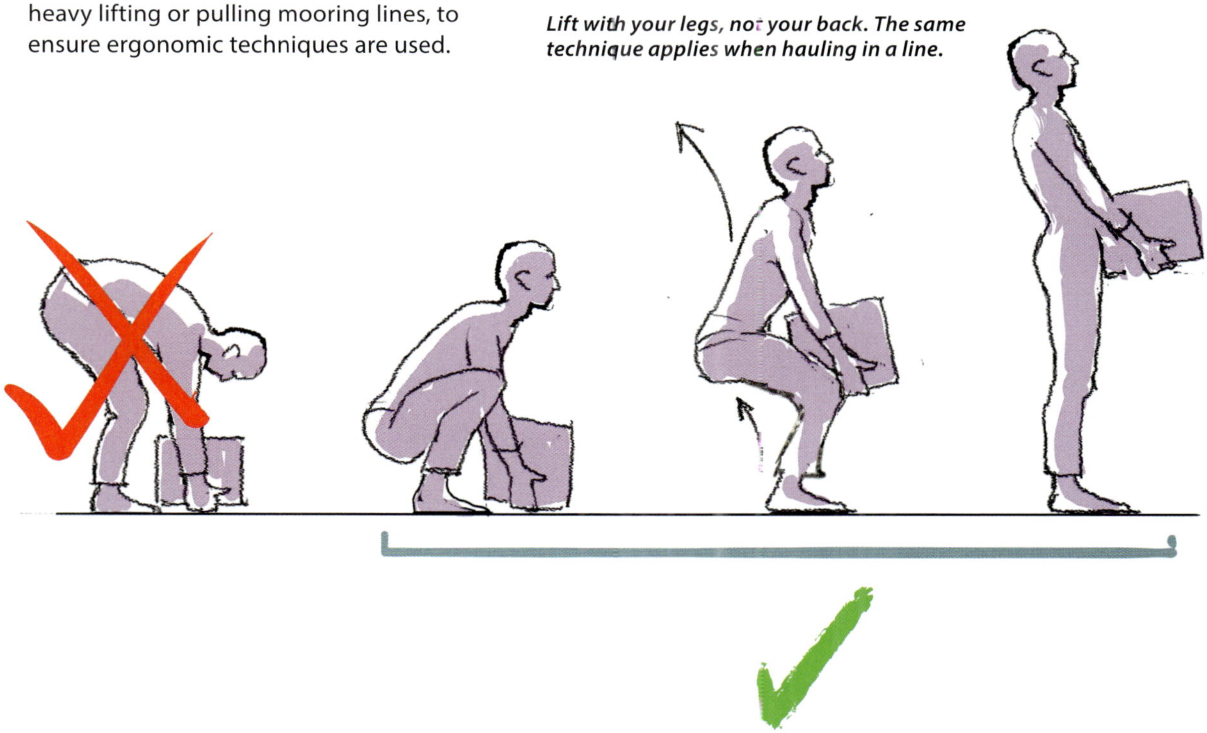

21. SHOULDER AND ARM INJURIES

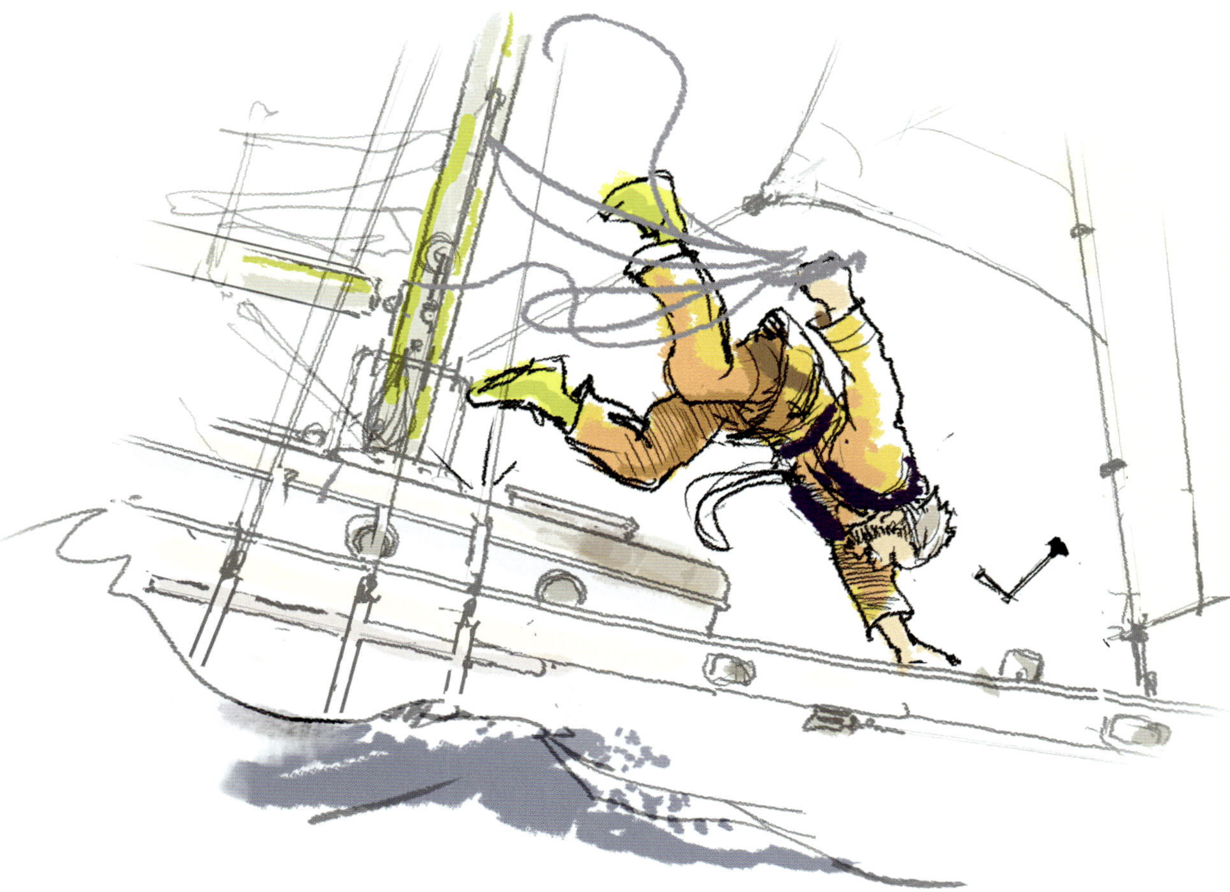

Shoulder injury – fall on an extended arm.

Injuries to the upper extremities, including the shoulder, upper arm, elbow joint, forearm, wrist and hand, are commonly caused by falls or direct trauma. The arm and hand are extensively used, making them susceptible to many accidents and injuries.

Prevention

- Always hold on to something when on board and think carefully before moving around.
- Be cautious when handling winches and ropes.
- Never jump ashore; step ashore carefully.
- On land, be attentive to the terrain, such as rocks, roots and slippery surfaces, and wear shoes with a good grip.
- Be careful with fingers when handling winches or bollards.
- Avoid wearing rings while sailing.
- Never wrap a rope around your hand; fingers can become trapped.
- Never attempt to stop a slipping rope with your hand; release it or use a cleat.
- Be cautious with heavy hatches or objects that may cause crushing injuries.

SHOULDER ANATOMY

The shoulder joint – technically the joint between the upper arm and the shoulder blade – has a relatively small joint surface and is stabilised largely by a complex system of muscles, ligaments and joint capsules. Functionally, the shoulder is our most mobile joint and includes the collarbone and its joints with the shoulder blade and breastbone, as well as the movement of the shoulder blade against the chest wall.

Skeletal anatomy of a shoulder joint.

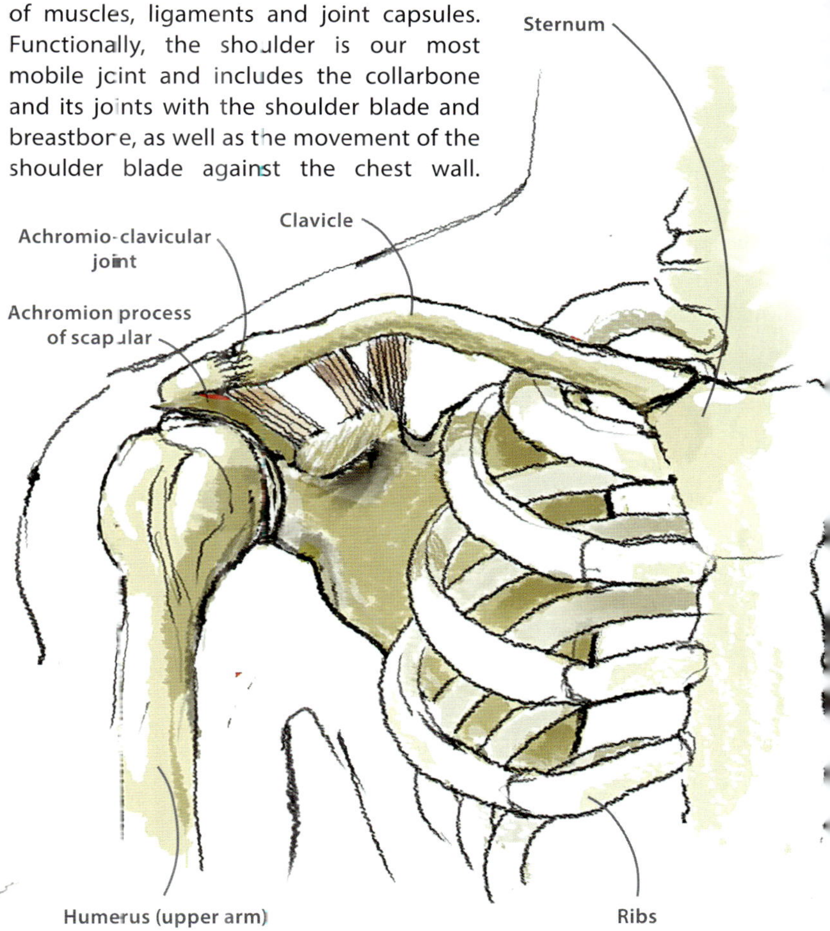

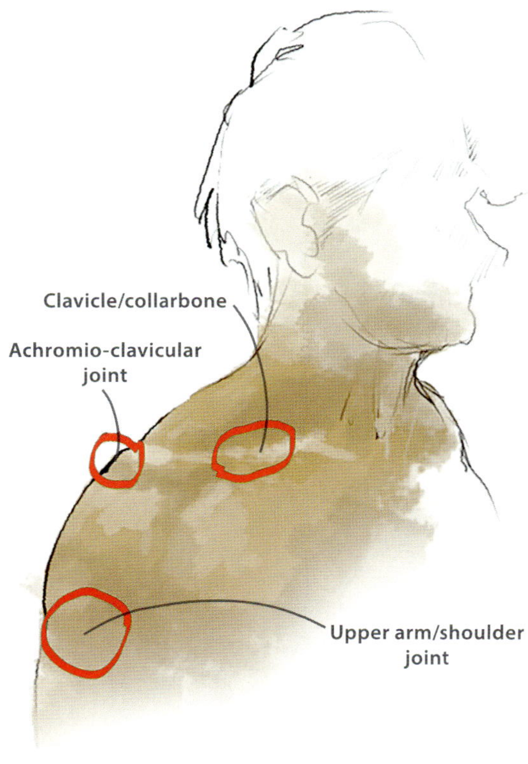

Common shoulder injuries and their exterior anatomical location:

- *sprained outer collarbone joint*
- *collarbone fracture*
- *upper arm fracture near the shoulder*
- *dislocated shoulder*

SPRAIN OF OUTER COLLARBONE JOINT (THE ACROMIO-CLAVICULAR JOINT)

Cause is often a fall on an extended arm.

Signs and symptoms

- Localised swelling and tenderness at the outer collarbone joint
- Painful shoulder movements
- Difficult to distinguish from a collarbone fracture near the joint, but treatment is the same

Immediate action

- Stop activity.
- Check distal status, see page 165.

Treatment

With typical symptoms and findings (see image), this injury can often be managed on board:

- Provide pain relief with paracetamol and ibuprofen.
- Encourage early movement exercises as soon as pain allows.
- If uncertain, seek medical care for possible X-rays to rule out more severe injuries.

Far from help

- Follow the same recommendations as above.
- Early shoulder movement is essential to prevent complications like a frozen shoulder (see below).
- Surgery is rarely required, and evacuation is unnecessary. Seek medical evaluation at the next port.

Sprained acromio-clavicular joint with torn ligaments.

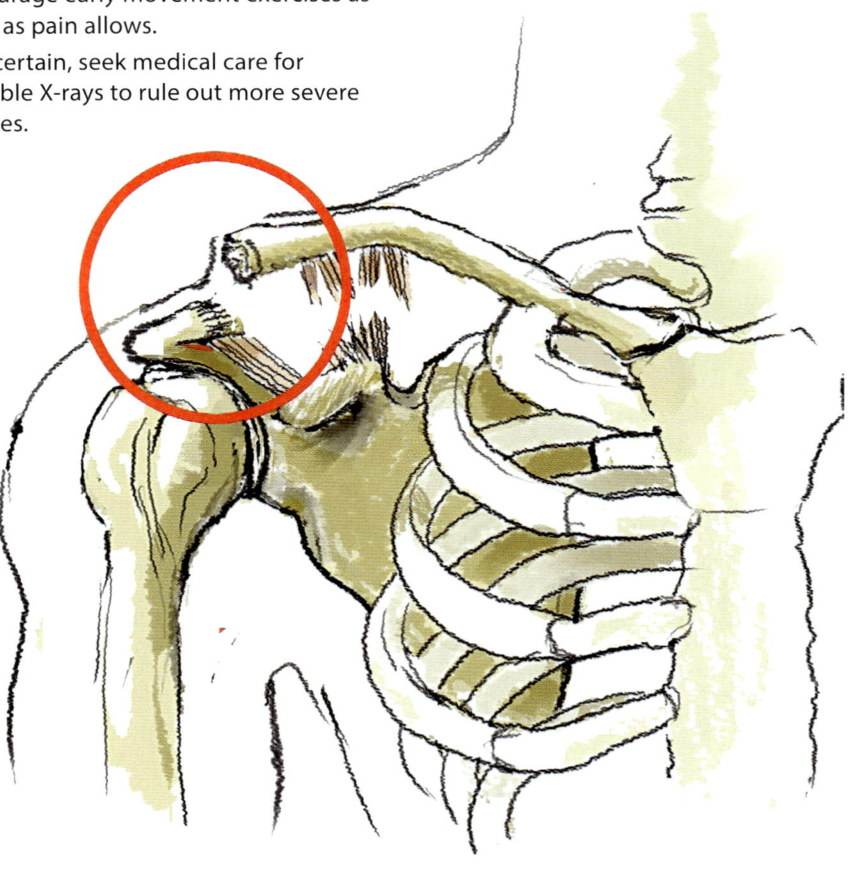

COLLARBONE FRACTURE

Signs and symptoms

- Pain with movement, swelling, and tenderness over the fracture site
- Most common in the middle of the collarbone but can occur along its entire length
- Occasionally, a 'crunch' can be felt at the fracture site

Immediate action

- Stop activity.
- Check distal status, see page 165.

Treatment

- Near the coast: Seek medical attention the same day. Stabilise the arm with a collar and cuff or a sling.

Far from help

If you are far from medical help, the treatment is similar. Give pain relief (see page 248). Evacuation is not necessary, and medical evaluation should be done upon reaching the next port. Start rehabilitation exercises early when pain allows.

The effect of a 'figure-of-eight' bandage has been debated but it might provide some pain relief of value when far from help. Such a bandage often needs to be reapplied because it will stretch.

Typical fracture of the collarbone.

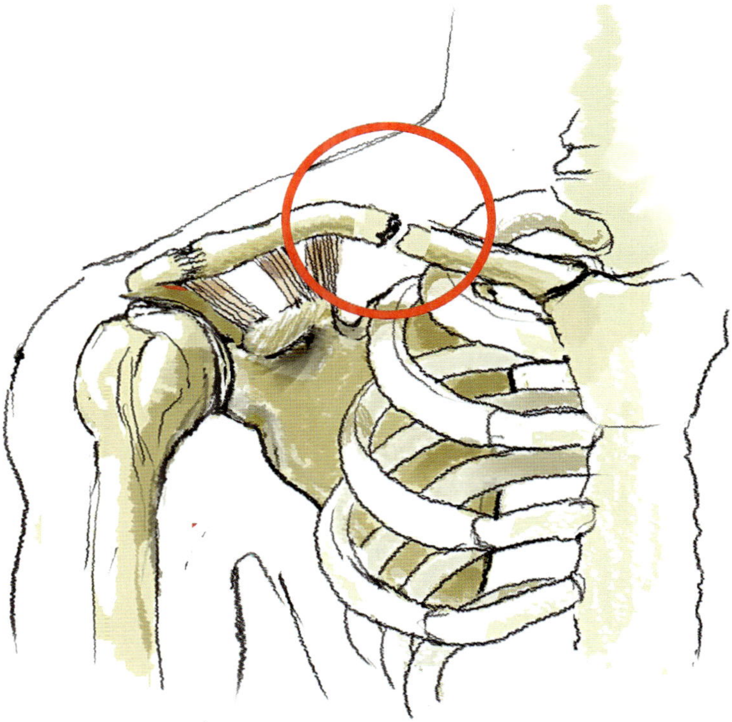

A 'figure-of-eight' bandage applied for a collarbone fracture.

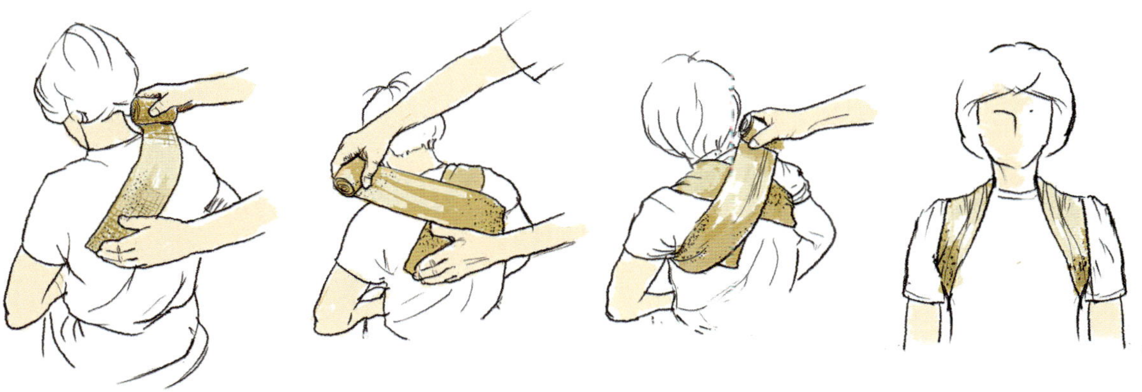

CAUTION – FROZEN SHOULDER!

A significant complication of shoulder injuries is rapid shrinking of the joint capsule, leading to severe and painful restriction of mobility – a 'frozen shoulder'. Early movement exercises are crucial to prevent this condition, which may require extensive physiotherapy.

Shoulder injury rehabilitation

1) Shoulder rolls

- Sit or stand with your arms relaxed by your sides.
- Slowly shrug both shoulders as high as you can towards your ears.
- Pull them back by squeezing your shoulder blades together.
- Relax your shoulders as you go back to the starting position. Repeat 10 times.

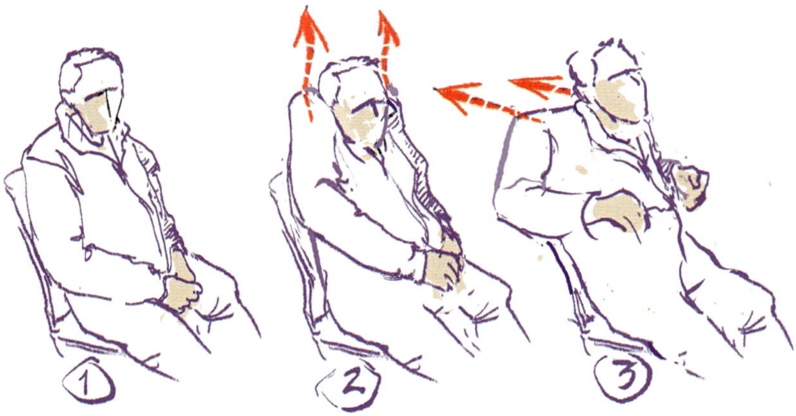

2) Finger walk

- Stand facing a wall, about a foot away.
- Touch the wall at hip level with your fingers, keeping your elbows bent.
- 'Walk' your way up the wall until pain limits movement.
- Steadily 'walk' your way down. Repeat 10 times.

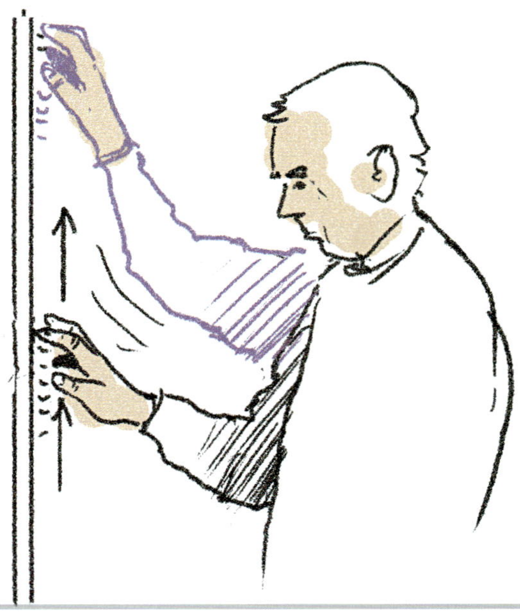

CAUTION – FROZEN SHOULDER!

3) Arm circles

- Sit with your back straight.
- Rest the hand of the affected arm on the shoulder of the same side.
- Slowly draw circles with your elbow, first clockwise, then anticlockwise.
- Repeat 10 times in each direction.

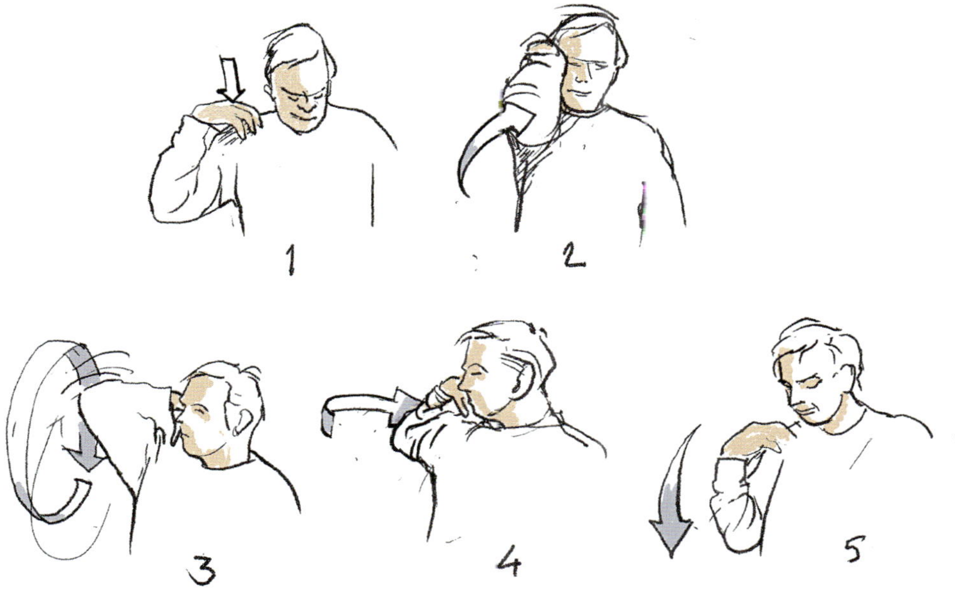

4) Tabletop slides

- Sit at a table with a small towel under your hand.
- Slide your hand forward as far as pain allows, then return.
- Repeat 10 times.

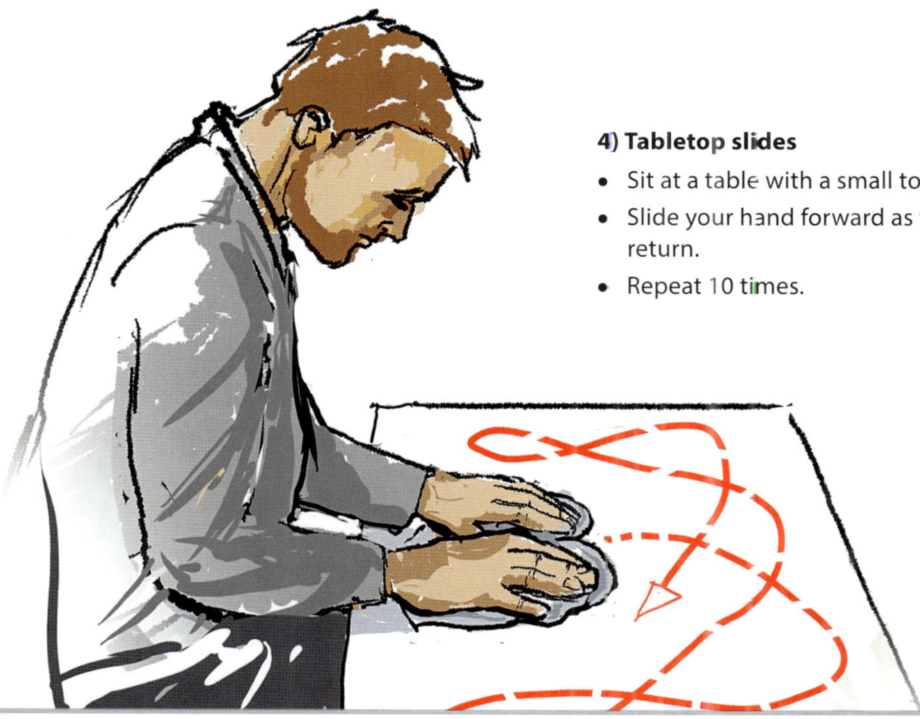

FRACTURE NEAR THE SHOULDER JOINT

Diagnosis is difficult without an X-ray.

Signs and symptoms

- Tenderness and swelling high on the arm near the shoulder joint
- Pain with movement

Immediate action

- Check distal status (see page 165).
- Immobilise and provide pain relief.

Treatment

- Diagnosis is difficult without X-rays; seek medical attention as soon as possible.
- While awaiting care, stabilise with a collar and cuff or a sling.

Far from help

Give pain relief (see page 248). Immobilise with a collar and cuff or a triangular bandage. Need of evacuation is unlikely. Medical evaluation must be done when reaching the next port. Start rehabilitation exercises early, as soon as pain allows, see above.

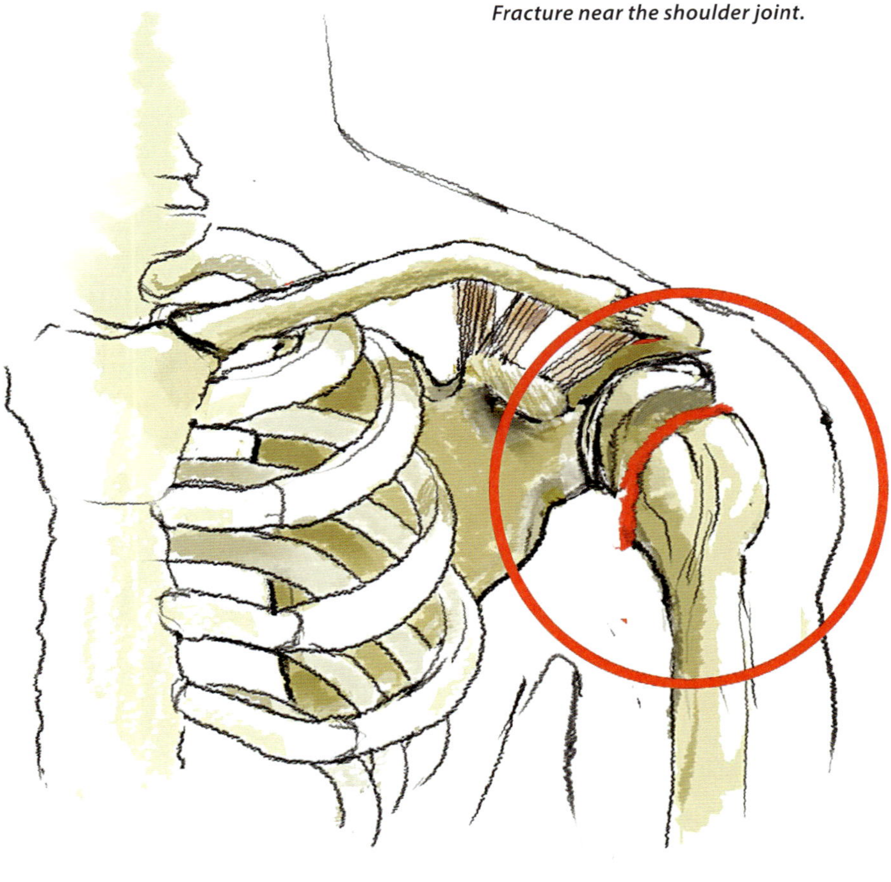

Fracture near the shoulder joint.

FRACTURE OF THE UPPER ARM

Signs and symptoms

Fractures near the middle of the upper arm are common in older individuals. Pain, swelling, tenderness and instability are common signs. Findings can vary depending on whether it is a crack without major misalignment or a severely dislocated fracture. Diagnosis is more obvious if dislocated or open fracture. Otherwise test direct and indirect tenderness (see page 164).

- Pain, swelling, tenderness and instability
- Risk of vascular or nerve injury

Immediate action

- Check distal status (see page 165).
- Control bleeding.
- Immobilise with a collar and cuff or triangular bandage.

Treatment

There is a high risk of vascular or nerve injury with upper arm fractures. If a fracture in the middle of the upper arm is suspected or confirmed, seek medical attention immediately. It is not possible to determine the extent and location of the fracture without an X-ray. Many of these fractures can be treated with the described bandages and movement exercises as the only treatment. However, there are fractures that must be treated surgically, which is why evaluation at a hospital is important.

A collar and cuff allows elevation and free finger movement.

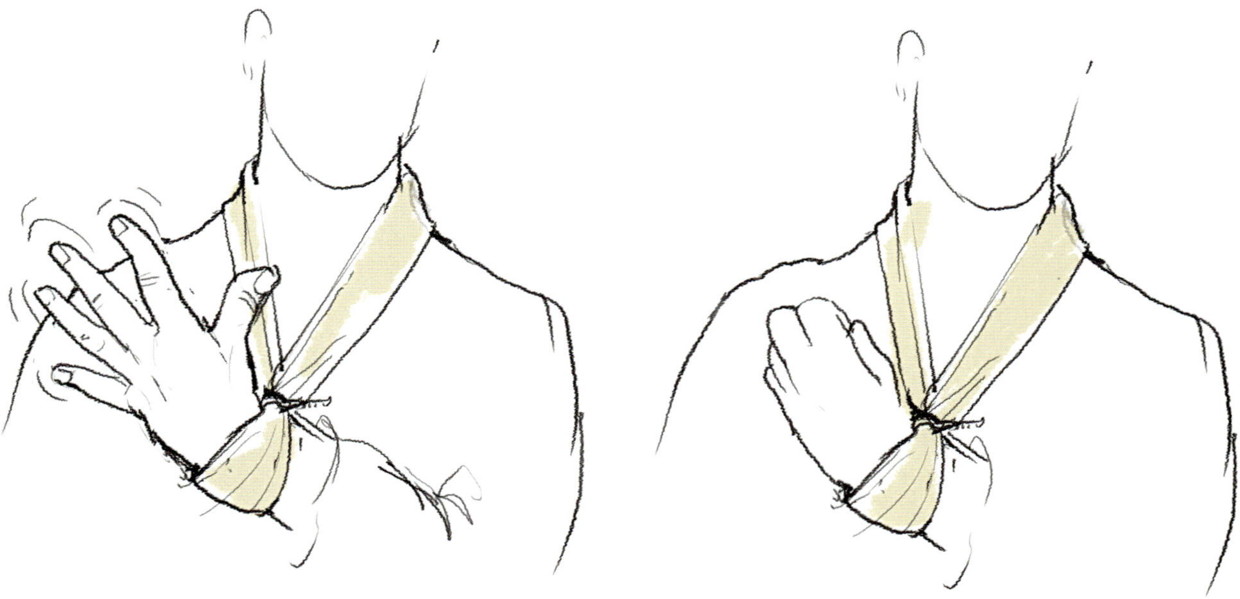

A collar and cuff and the slight pull provided by the arm's weight are often sufficient for stabilisation. A U-shaped cast or aluminium splint can provide acceptable stabilisation of the fracture. A fracture close to the elbow joint needs surgery.

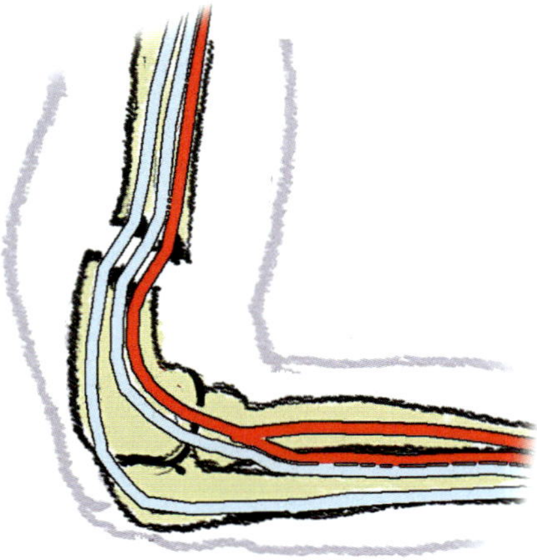

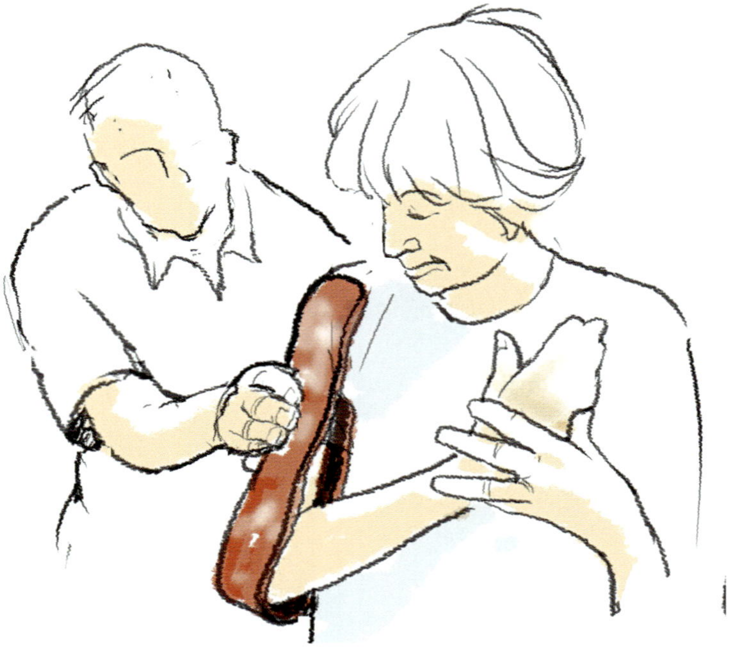

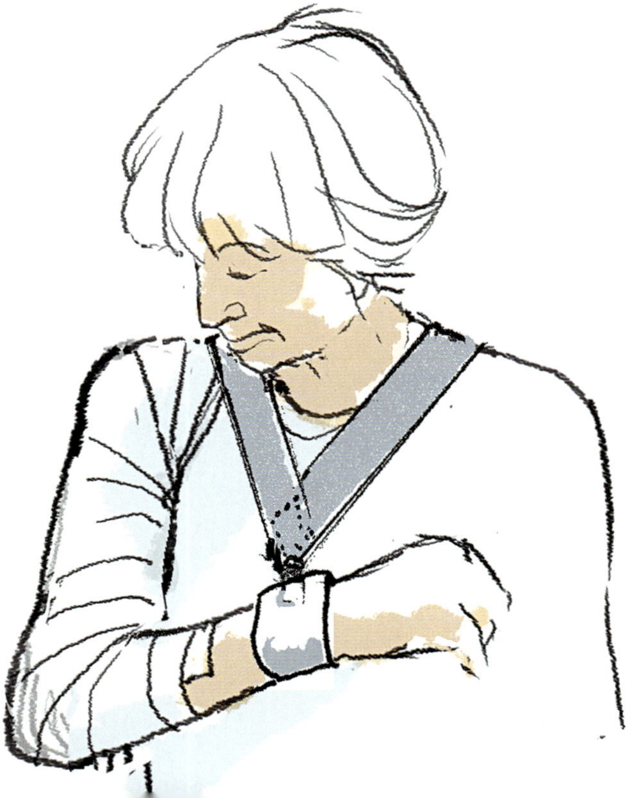

If the fracture is very unstable, additional fixture to the chest may be necessary. Remember to check distal status before and after fixture.

Far from help

- If vascular or nerve injury is suspected, or if the fracture is open, evacuation is essential.
- For uncomplicated fractures, immobilise, try out best stabilisation, provide pain relief and seek evaluation at the next port. Evacuation may be needed.

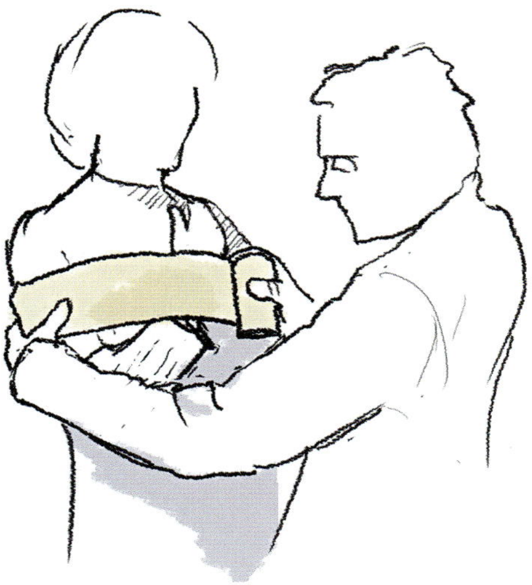

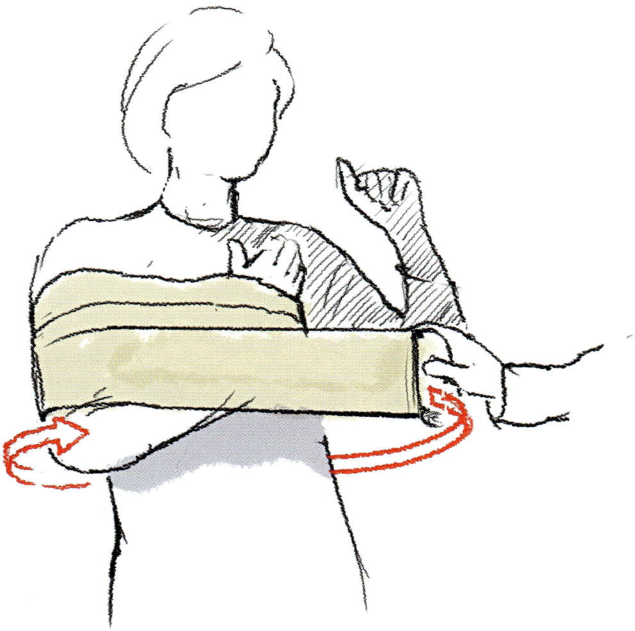

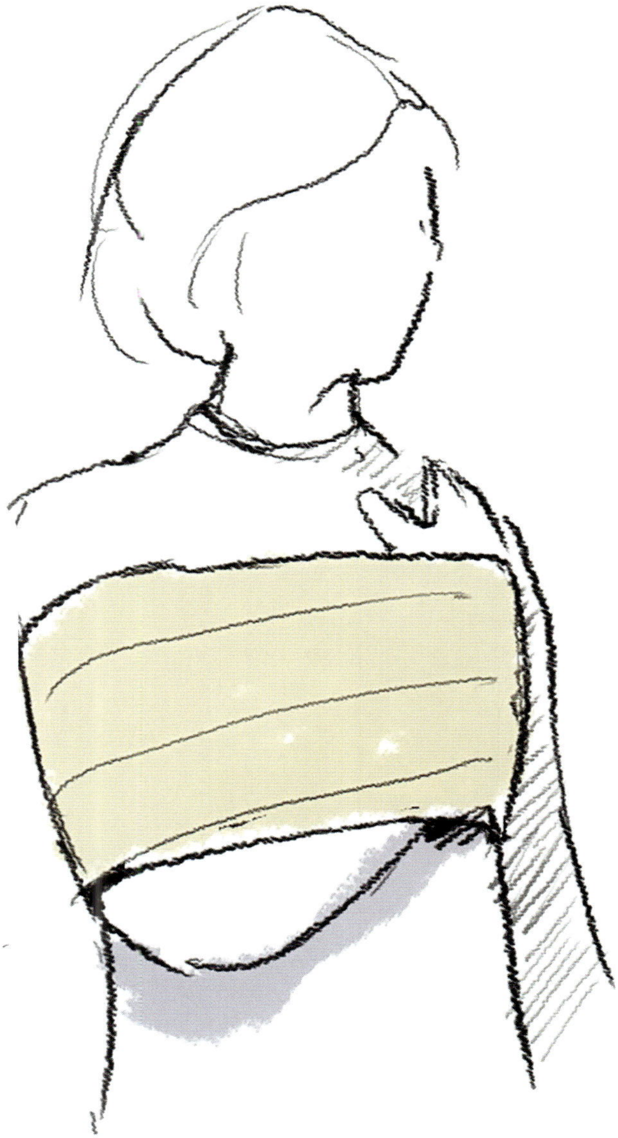

FRACTURES AT THE ELBOW

Signs and symptoms

These fractures result in severe pain, swelling and visible dislocation around the elbow. Elbow fractures pose a high risk to blood vessels and nerves. Check distal status (see page 165)! This type of fracture is also common in children.

Immediate action

- Check distal status.
- Elbow injuries require urgent medical evaluation. If vascular or nerve damage is suspected, immediate transport to hospital is necessary.
- Temporary immobilisation with a collar and cuff or sling is advised prior to transport.

Treatment

Urgent examination and treatment by an orthopaedic specialist. Final treatment is based on individual circumstances.

Far from help

If far from medical assistance, contact emergency services for guidance and potential evacuation. Immobilise the arm using a sling or collar and cuff and a splint until reaching shore or being evacuated. Best position of the elbow is usually a 90-degree angle (see image). Another method of stabilisation is fixture of the entire arm to the chest (see page 193). Managing this injury on board for several days would be highly challenging.

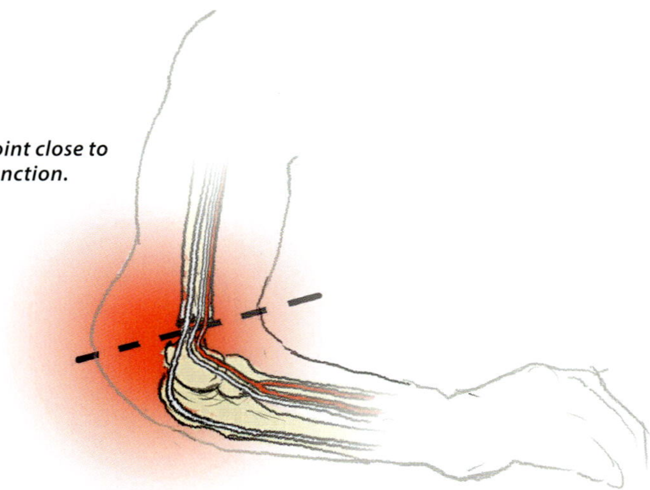

A brachial fracture near the elbow joint close to arteries and nerves critical to arm function.

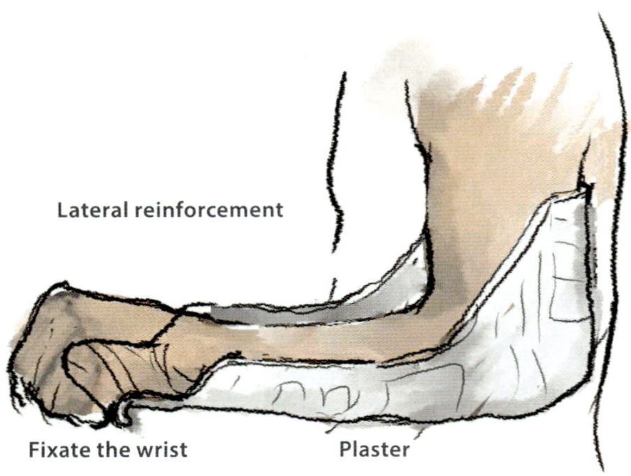

An elbow fracture temporary stabilised with a plaster splint at a 90-degree angle. Secure the splint with elastic bandages. Support with a collar and cuff.

SHOULDER DISLOCATION

Shoulder dislocations are often caused by falls on to an outstretched arm or direct trauma, forcing the humerus to dislocate forward (anterior dislocation). Individuals who have experienced prior dislocations may have weakened joint capsules, resulting in increased instability. Such individuals may sometimes self-reduce their dislocations.

Signs and symptoms

- The humeral head is displaced forward from its normal position
- Comparison with the healthy side may reveal a visible difference in shoulder contour
- Palpation reveals a 'pit' where the humeral head should reside
- The arm is held close to the body, with limited movement, often supported by the other arm

Immediate action

- Check distal status (see pages 165).
- Give an analgesic (for example, paracetamol 1g).

Treatment

- Seek medical evaluation and treatment on the same day.
- If sensation or mobility in the hand is reduced, urgent medical assessment is needed.
- Before transport, immobilise the arm with a collar and cuff or sling. At the hospital, X-rays will confirm the diagnosis and rule out fractures. The shoulder will be relocated under full anaesthesia.

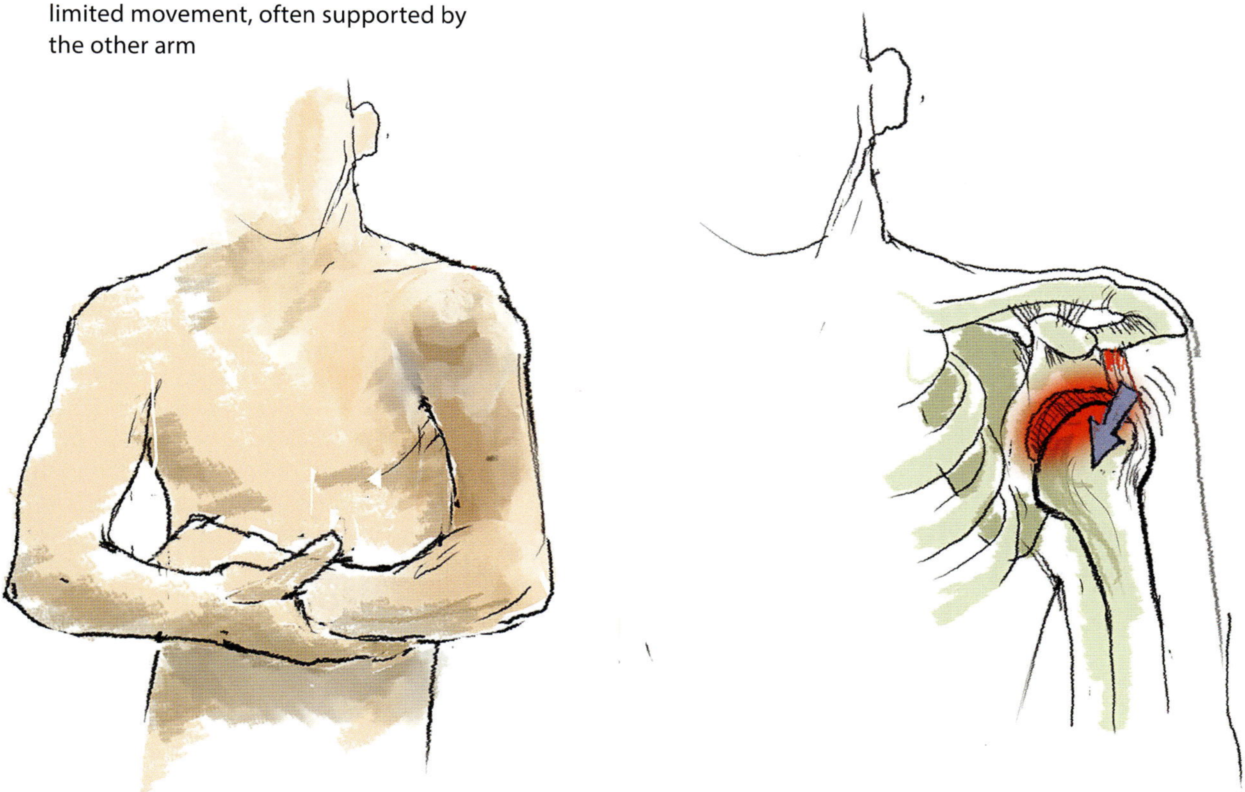

Anterior dislocation of the right shoulder joint: anatomy and typical appearance.

Far from help

The basic principle for a first-time dislocation is evacuation and transport to a hospital for X-ray and treatment. However, evacuation can be challenging if the dislocation occurs in the middle of the sea during a longer voyage. Therefore, seeking medical advice is crucial.

It may be advisable to gently attempt to relocate the shoulder, preferably after consulting medical advice or conducting a risk-benefit analysis. The risks of attempting to reduce the dislocation must be weighed against the risks of leaving it dislocated for several days, or perhaps more than a week. The latter can lead to significantly worse outcomes.

The best chance of successfully relocating a dislocated shoulder is if the procedure is performed soon after the dislocation occurs or on a person with a history of shoulder dislocations.

Provide pain relief and administer sedation, allowing them to take effect for approximately 30 minutes. Morphine preparations may be required, possibly in combination with diazepam or a similar sedative/relaxant.

If the shoulder is successfully relocated, mobility is usually restored immediately. Stabilise the shoulder for a few days using a collar and cuff. Begin rehabilitation exercises as soon as pain allows (see page 188).

How to relocate a dislocated shoulder

There are three different methods that can be used on board. However, these procedures should be performed cautiously and only if you have the necessary knowledge, as complications can arise.

1. Hanging method

Place the injured person face down on a table or a high bunk with the injured arm hanging freely straight down. Ask the person to hold a weight of approximately 2–3kg in their hand or secure the weight to the arm. There is a reasonable chance that the shoulder will pop back into place within 15–20 minutes. If the height is insufficient, be creative: for instance, open a skylight hatch and lay the person on the deck, allowing the arm to hang down through the hatch.

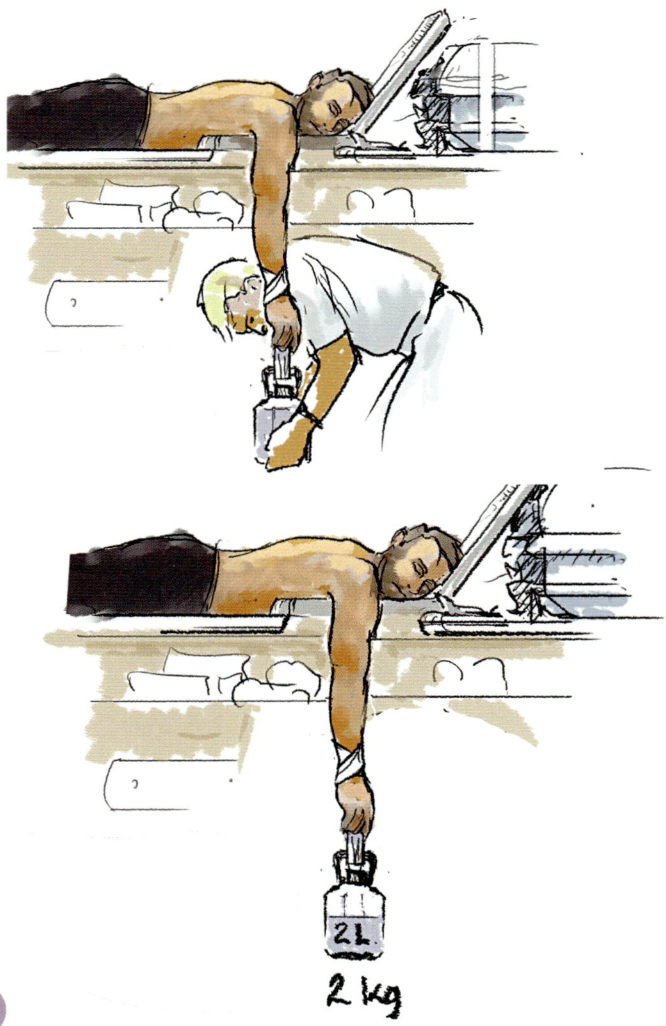

An idea about how to arrange 'hanging reposition' of a dislocated shoulder.

2. Gradual pull method

Alternatively, a crew member can sit comfortably beside the injured person and gradually create increasing tension along the length of the arm. In the final stage, apply gentle forward pressure.

Treat, for example, on a table.

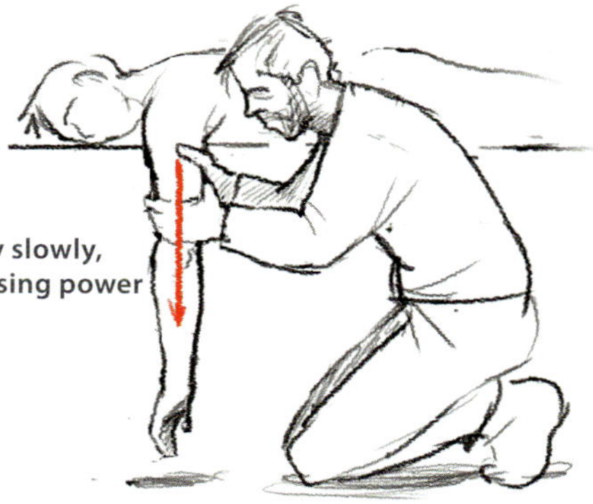

Casualty on bed, face down, arm hanging. Crew member sitting alongside pulls steadily with increasing strength along the upper arm.

3. Kocher method

This is the classic Kocher method for relocation of a shoulder.

1. Place the injured person in a comfortable seated or lying position. Perform all movements slowly and carefully.
2. Keep the injured arm alongside the body and bend the elbow to a 90-degree angle.
3. Rotate the forearm outwards as far as possible.
4. With the elbow still bent at 90 degrees, bring it across the chest until it stops.
5. Finally, lay the hand on the collarbone on the opposite side.

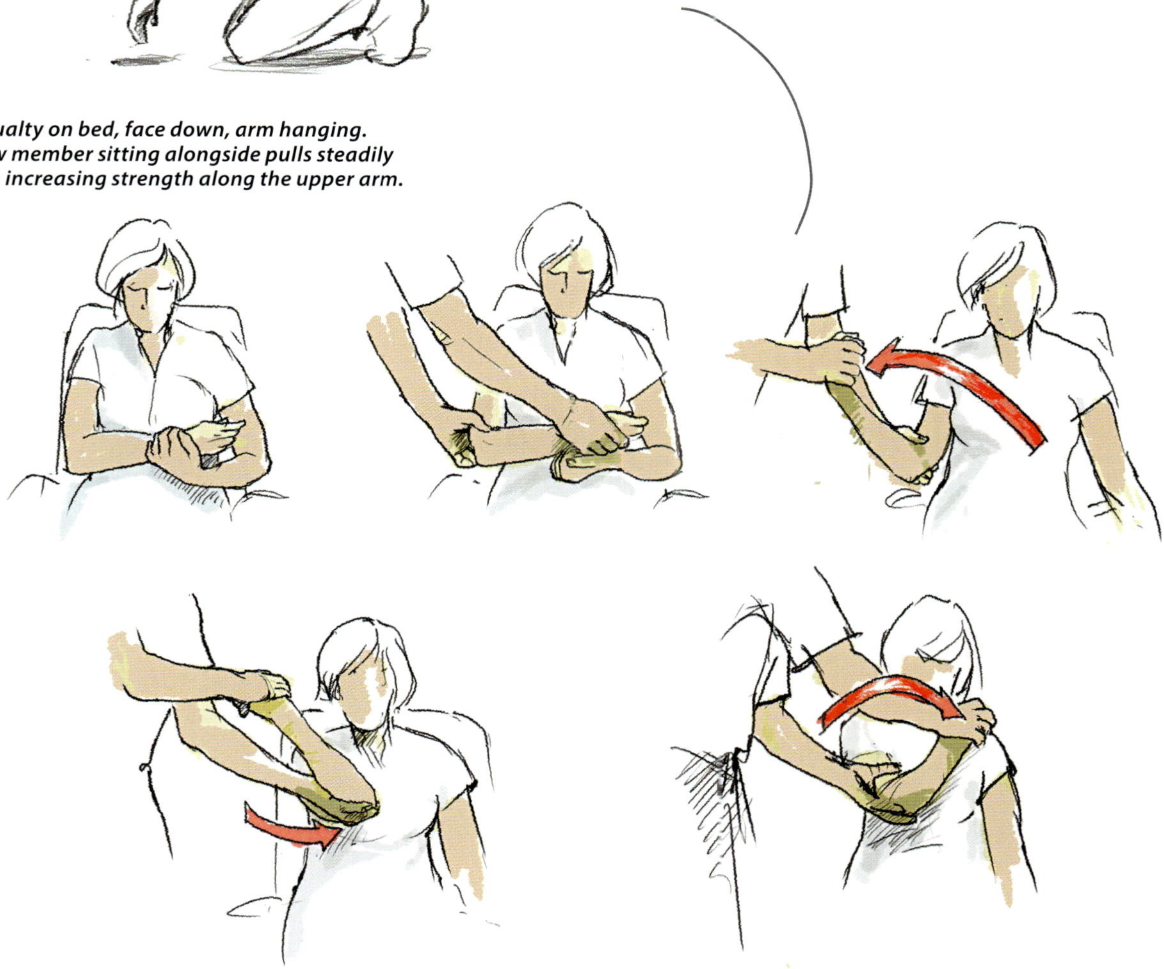

FOREARM FRACTURE

Forearm fractures typically result from falls or direct blows to the forearm. These injuries may affect both bones in the forearm (the radius and ulna) or just one.

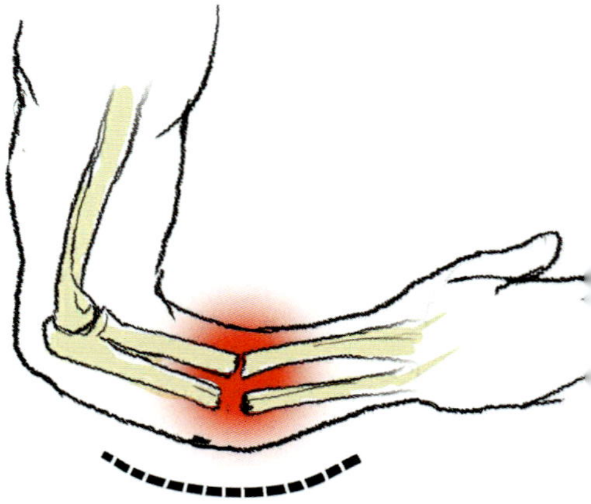

Signs and symptoms

Signs and symptoms vary depending on whether one or both bones in the forearm are affected. When both bones are broken, there is typically a noticeable deformity and instability in the middle of the forearm. Injuries to a single bone often result in localised pain and swelling, making it challenging to determine the extent of the injury without an X-ray. Test for direct versus indirect tenderness.

Immediate action

- Check distal status (see page 165).
- Pain relief and immobilisation with a sling (see page 168) are the primary treatments for forearm fractures awaiting examination by a doctor.

Above: Classic dislocation if both bones are fractured. Left: Only one of the bones is fractured, no dislocation despite a fracture. No indirect tenderness, only direct tenderness.

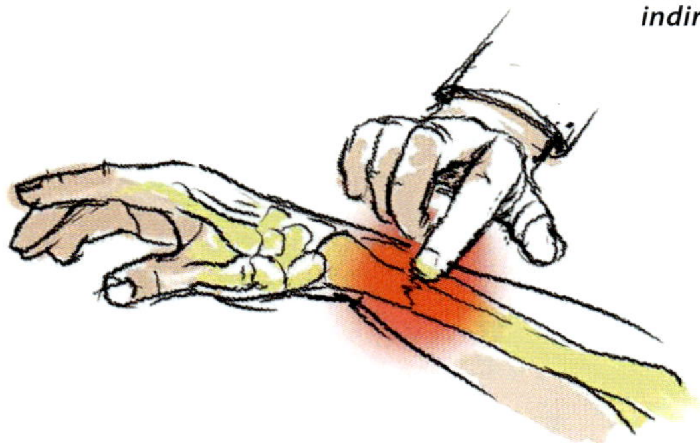

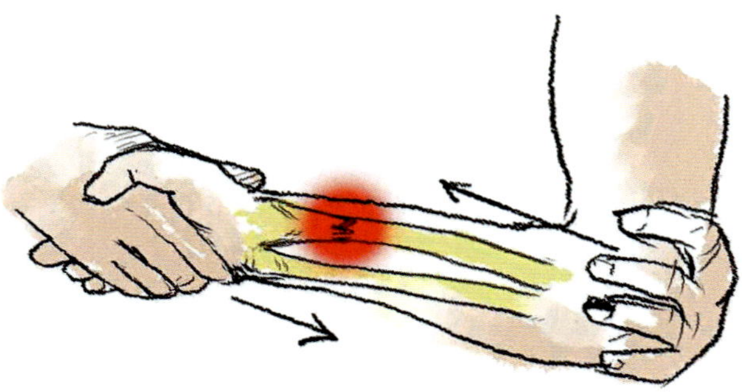

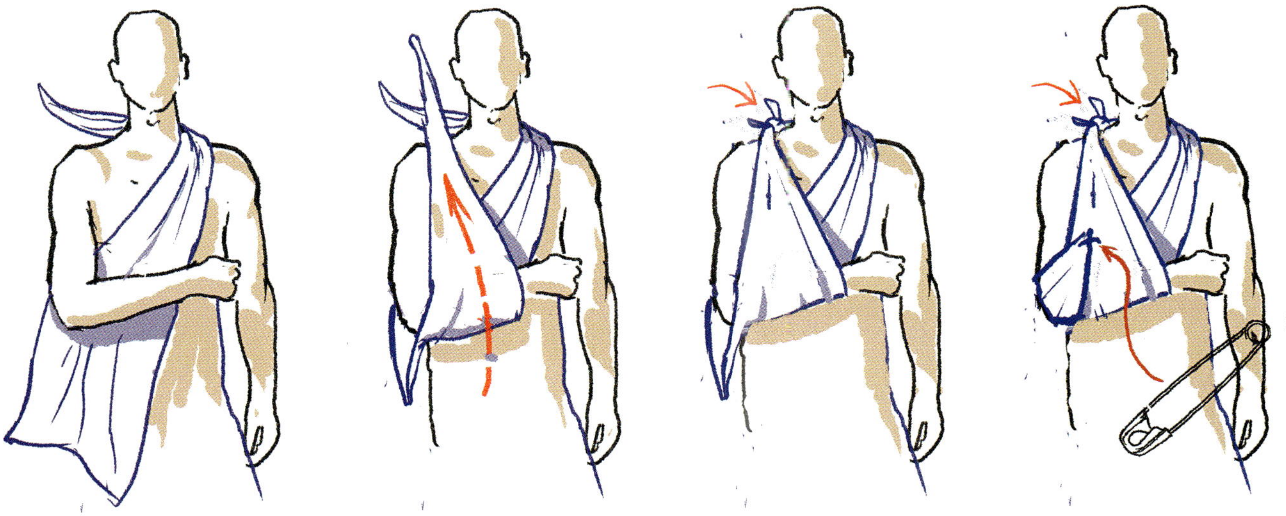

Triangular bandage. For more unstable fractures, additional stabilisation with a U-shaped cast or an aluminium splint may be required.

Treatment

A same-day medical examination is preferable. If there are signs of vascular or nerve injuries, arrange for urgent transport to a hospital. Immobilise and stabilise the fracture with a triangular bandage and/or an aluminium splint.

Far from help

Evacuation may be necessary, depending on the circumstances. If far from medical assistance and the fracture is uncomplicated, it can potentially be managed with immobilisation, a sling or a splint (see page 168) and pain relief until reaching a port. Always check distal status to assess vascular and nerve function.

For severe instability, open fractures or signs of vascular or nerve damage, contact emergency services for evacuation, as urgent medical care may be required. Pain relief is crucial, and evacuation may need to be discussed based on location and the severity of the injury. However, many forearm fractures can be managed without evacuation if the arm is effectively immobilised.

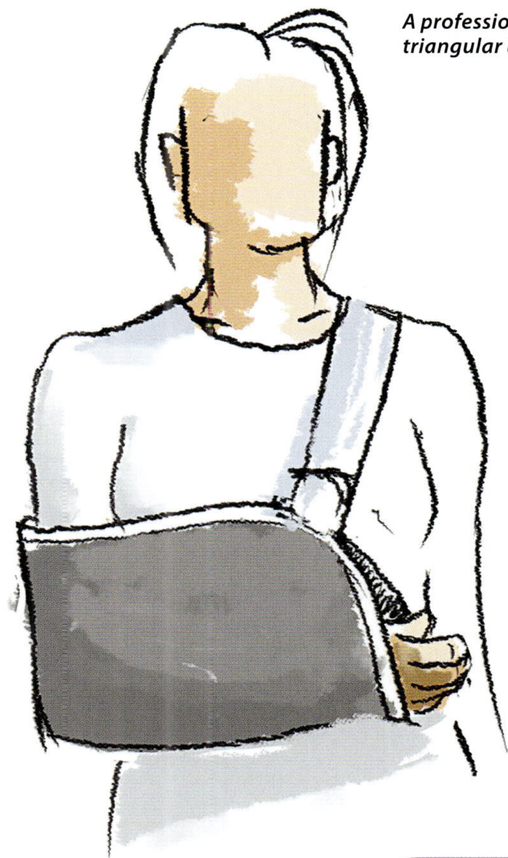

A professional premade triangular bandage.

WRIST INJURIES

Sprains or fractures of the bones in the wrist are common. These injuries often result from falls on to an outstretched hand and can be managed with supportive bandaging or splinting until reaching a port. Fracture of the radial bone is the most common wrist injury.

Signs and symptoms

Symptoms include pain during movement, swelling, and tenderness over the injured ligament or bone. When there is deformity, a fracture is relatively easy to diagnose.

Immediate action

- Immobilise.
- Elevate.
- Give pain relief.

Treatment

- Arrange for a medical examination on the same day. Many fractures may require realignment, and some may need surgery.
- Apply a stretch compression bandage in figure-eight loops, starting from the hand and including the wrist.
- Immobilise the arm in a sling (see page 168) for elevation until a medical evaluation is carried out.
- Regular movement of all fingers is essential to avoid swelling and maintain mobility.

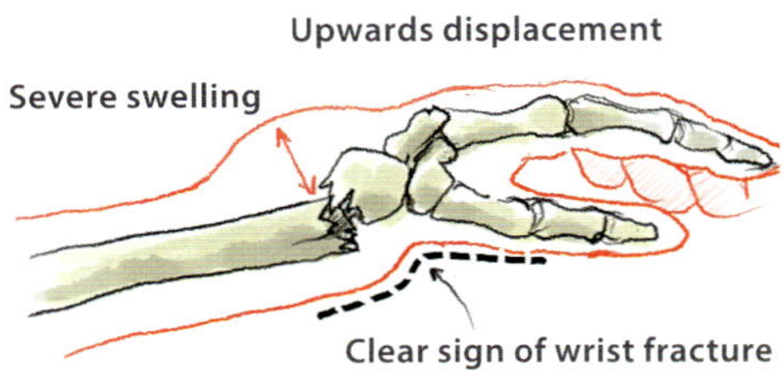

Typical location and misalignment in fracture of the radial bone at the wrist.

Supportive wrist bandage. Start distally on the hand. Add a triangular bandage to elevate the hand.

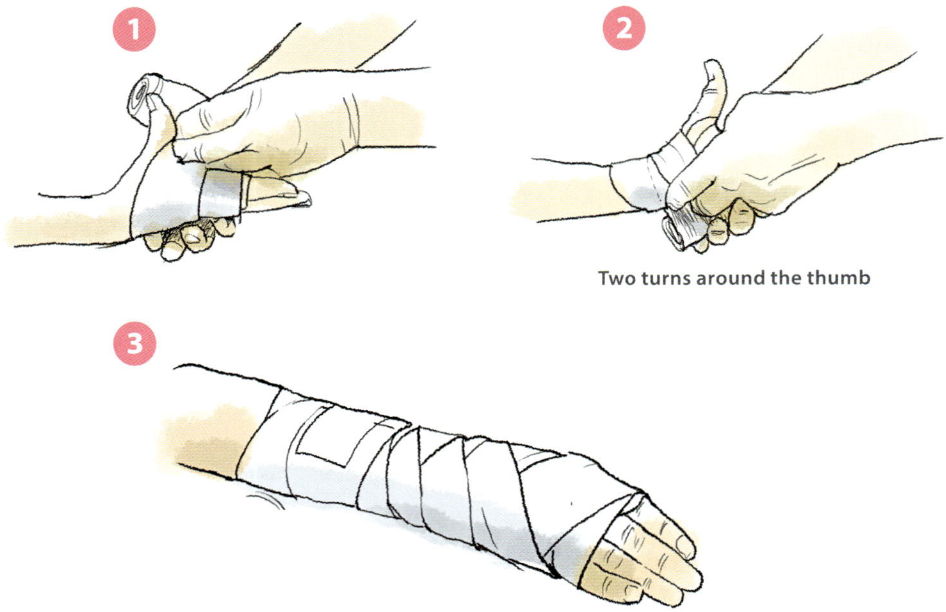

Far from help

If far from medical help, the injury can normally be managed on board. Examination and treatment can wait for several days without serious consequences. Immobilise the wrist with a splint. Pain relief is essential. Evacuation is unlikely but may be discussed depending on location and the severity of the injury.

Choice of splint

There are two main alternatives as described below. Both require some basic medical equipment.

The aluminium splint has the advantage of being fast to apply and is resistant to water but with less perfect anatomical fit

The plaster splint requires more work but has the advantage of giving a perfect anatomical fit, allowing the extremity to be used in some easier tasks. It is, however, sensitive to getting wet.

1. Pre-made padded aluminium splint

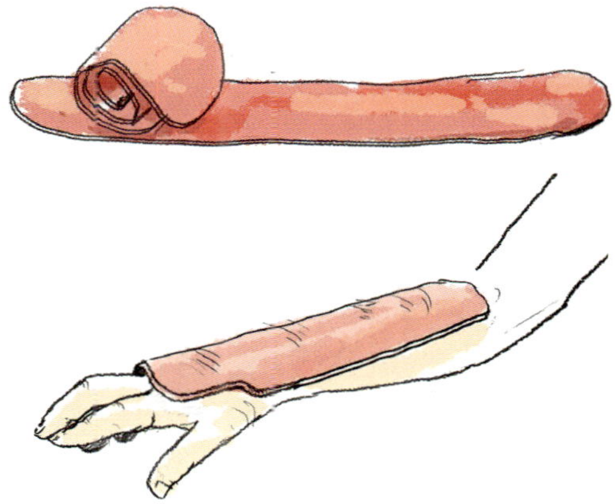

A padded aluminium splint, secured with a durable bandage, is a simple and effective option. Ensure a layer of padding or fabric is placed next to the skin.

2. Plaster splint

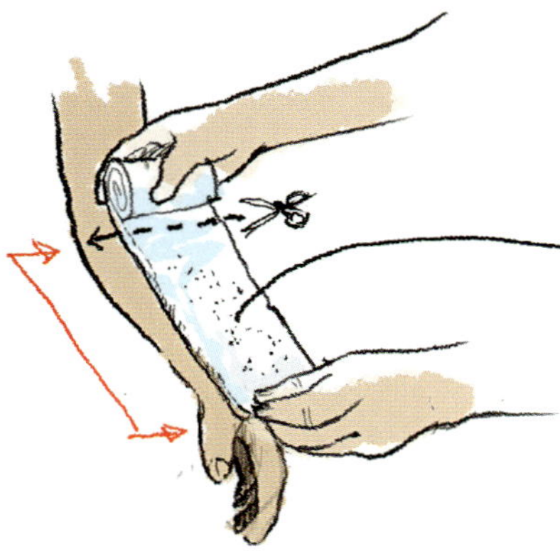

Measure the wadding.

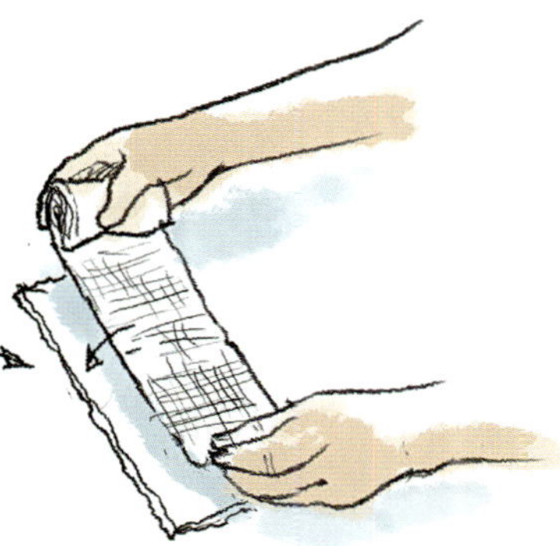

Lay out the plaster fabric.

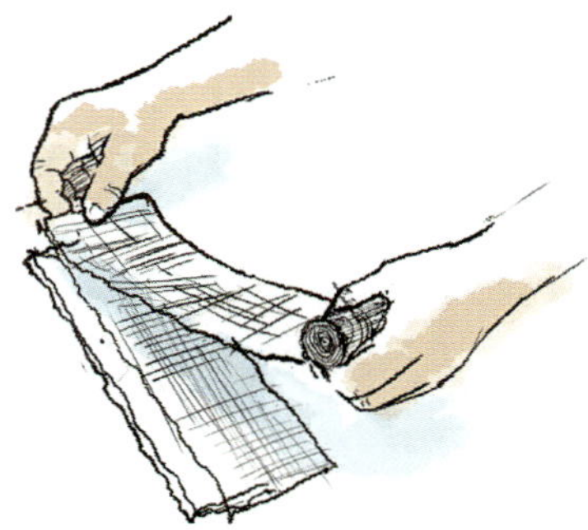

Lay out 9–10 layers.

Making a simple plaster cast: Measure the length of the padding and plaster bandage to cover the forearm and extend to the fingers. The padding should exceed the plaster length by a few centimetres. Fold the plaster bandage into 8–10 layers.

Wet the plaster (not the padding) in water and squeeze out excess water. Place the plaster on the padding, ensuring the padding extends slightly beyond the plaster. Apply this to the injured wrist, leaving the fingers free to move.

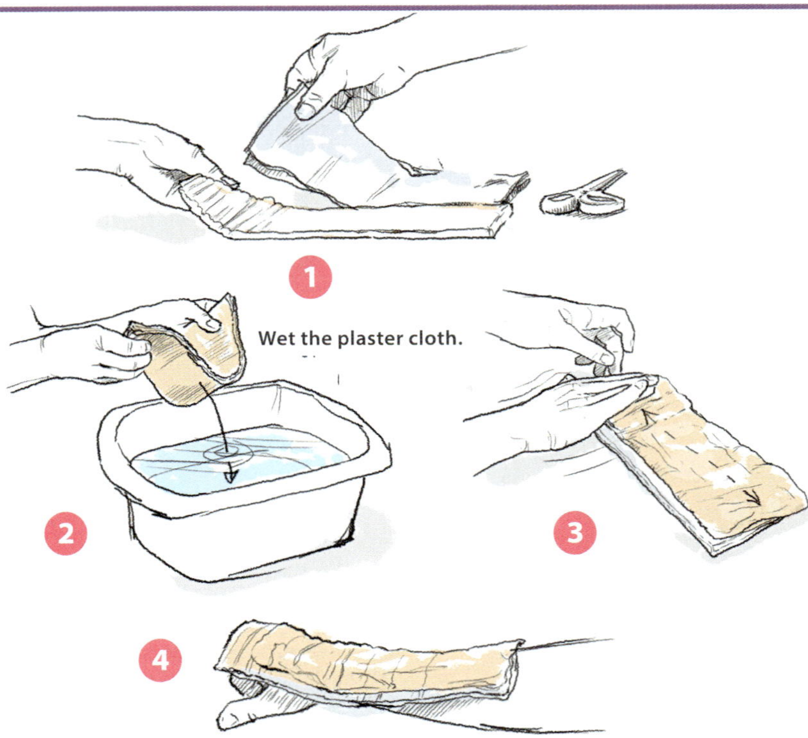

Secure the plaster splint with elastic bandages (8–10cm wide), starting from the outer side of the hand. Hold an object, such as a ball, in the hand to maintain a good joint angle.

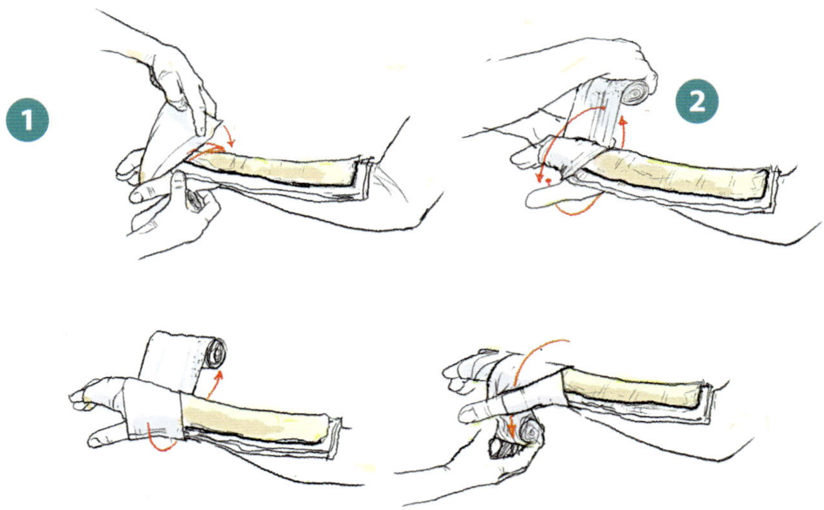

Allow the plaster to set for about 30 minutes before use. Protect the plaster with a plastic bag if showering is necessary.

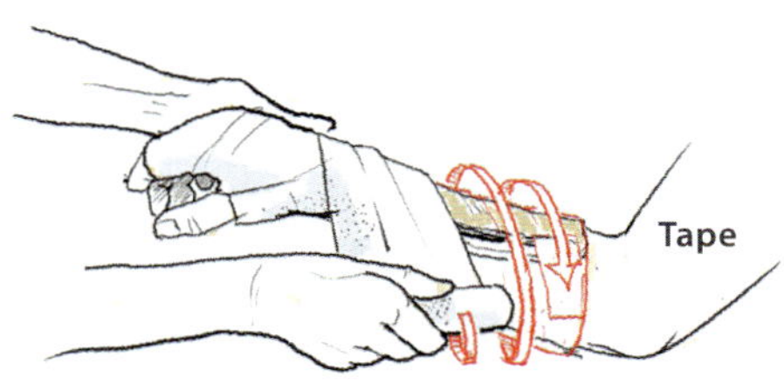

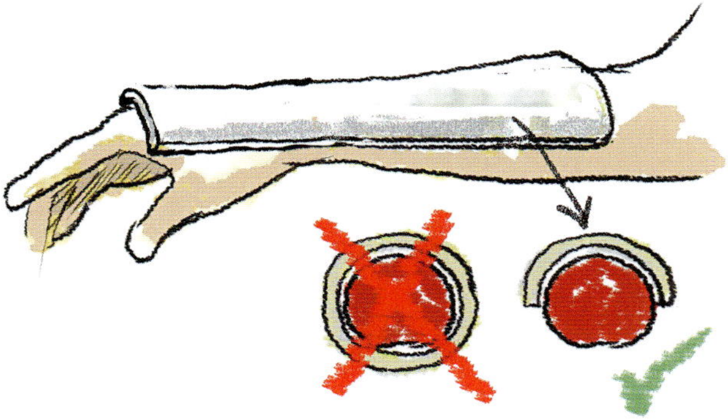

Plastering – never more than half a turn. If the arm is completely enclosed and swells, blood circulation is cut off.

> **CAUTION!**
>
> Never apply a plaster bandage outside of a hospital setting. There is a risk of circulation problems due to swelling. Apply a splint covering at maximum half the circumference.

METACARPAL INJURIES

The metacarpal bones consist of eight small bones that can be sprained, fractured or cracked if you fall on your hand. One of these bones, the scaphoid bone, often called the 'boat bone', is particularly notable because a crack may not always be visible on an X-ray immediately, only appearing after several weeks. An untreated crack in the scaphoid bone can lead to ischaemia and permanent damage to one half of the bone.

Signs and symptoms

In cases of wrist injury without signs of a fracture in the wrist bones but with persistent pain and tenderness in the area, a metacarpal bone injury may be present.

Treatment

If close to medical care, seek examination for wrist pain and tenderness in the snuff box if symptoms persist for more than a few days following a fall.

Far from help

Immobilise the wrist with a splint (see above) until a medical assessment can be arranged.

The location of the scaphoid bone (the 'boat bone') in the metacarpal bones. In a scaphoid fracture, maximum tenderness is in the 'snuff box' between the two extensor tendons of the thumb.

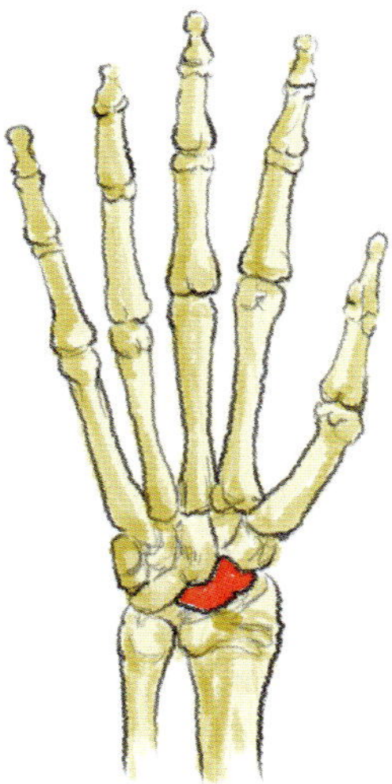

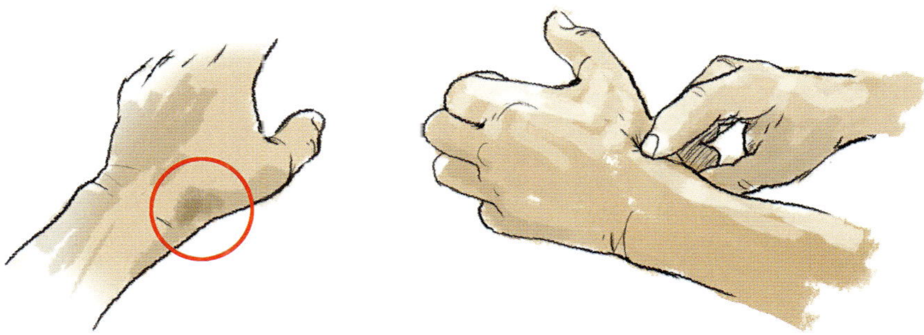

FINGER INJURIES

Finger injuries are common during sailing and can result from crushed fingers in winches, belaying line accidents, fractured finger bones, sprains or dislocated joints. Traumatic amputation of fingers during mooring accidents is also a risk. Rings can become stuck, causing severe injuries.

Fractures / sprains

Signs and symptoms

Signs and symptoms of finger injuries include swelling, tenderness and dislocation, similar to other fractures and sprains.

Treatment

A proper assessment requires medical examination and often an X-ray, though it is rarely urgent.

Far from help

Immobilise the finger with a splint or by attaching it to a neighbouring finger using tape or plaster. Have the injury assessed upon reaching port. If dislocation is suspected, you may attempt to reset the joint immediately.

A dislocated finger can sometimes be reset immediately by applying gradually increasing traction in the direction of the finger's length.

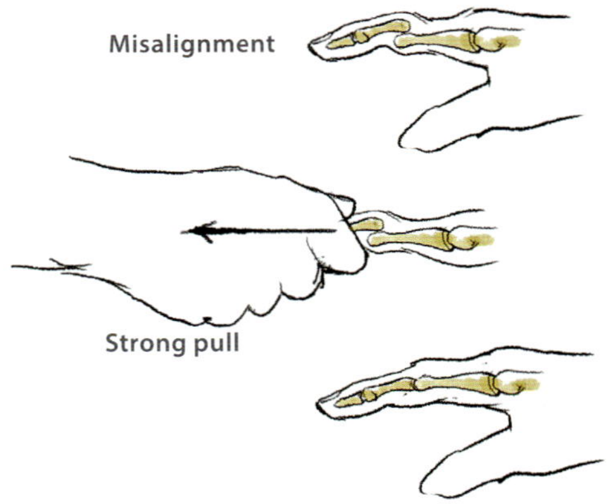

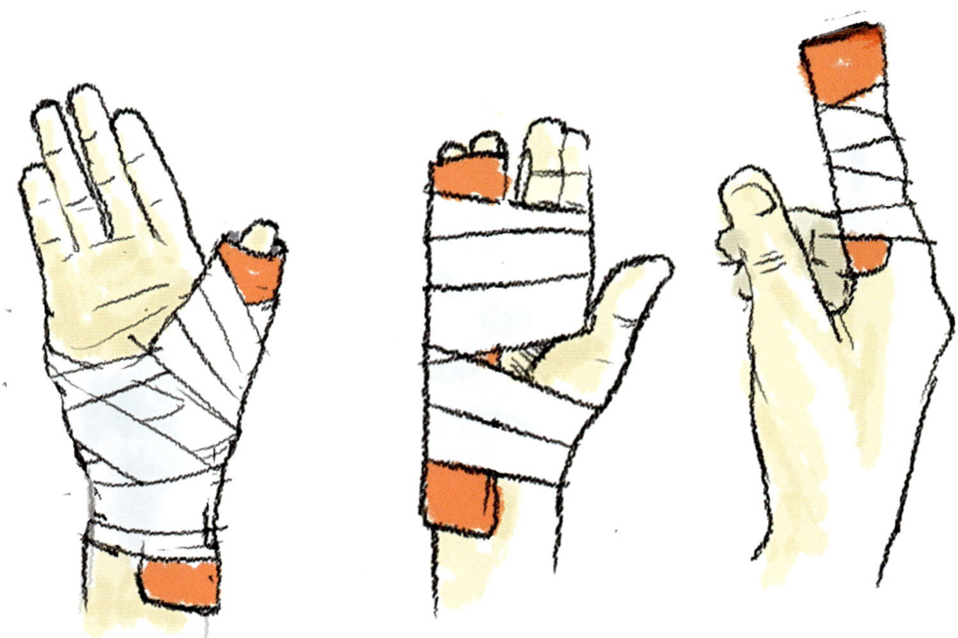

Immobilising fingers with a pre-made aluminium splint. The splint can be shaped with scissors to support the injured finger and a neighbouring one.

Stabilising an injured finger by fixing it to a neighbouring finger is a simple and effective technique. Remember to put padding between the fingers.

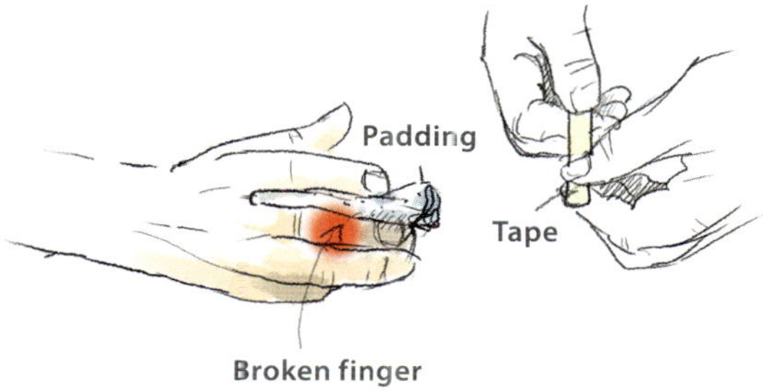

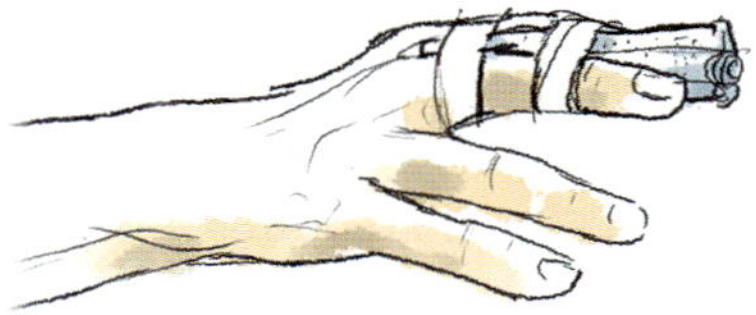

If a plaster splint is needed, adjust its width by cutting it with scissors. The splint should cover the injured finger and a neighbouring one. See above for further instructions.

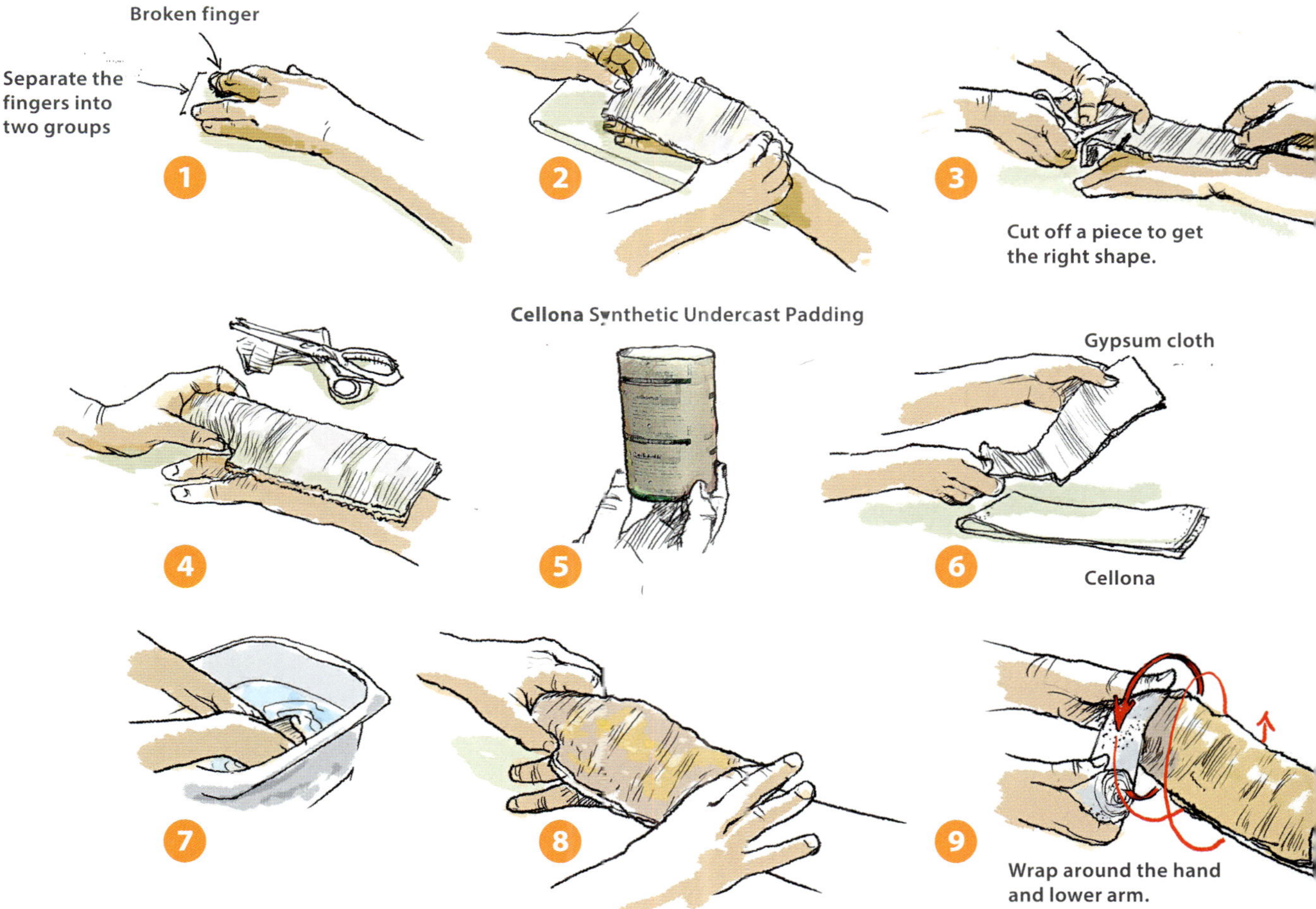

Avoid serious injuries to hands by NEVER wrapping around the fingers. There are sailors with only the thumb left!

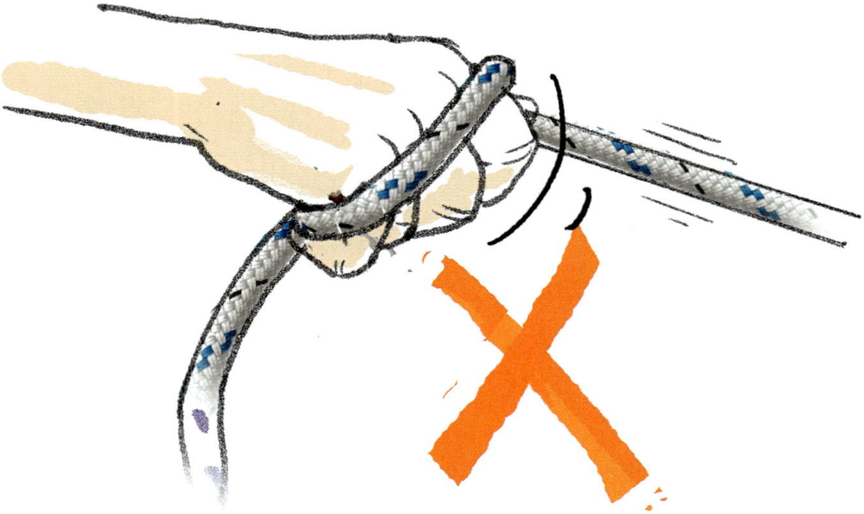

Prevention

A very common type of injury on board is fingers being squeezed by a line, in a winch or by a hatch.

Stuck ring

Hands and fingers are frequently subject to accidents during sailing. Many people keep their rings on, without considering what might happen if they injure a finger.

Immediate action

In all injuries to the arm, hand or fingers, remove rings immediately before swelling makes it impossible. If a ring cannot be removed over the knuckle despite lubrication, try cutting the ring with a saw or wire cutters or use the 'string (dental floss) trick'.

Prevention

Take off all rings and store them in a safe place before leaving the mooring. The ring as well as the fingers will be safer!

CAUTION!

Many fingers are injured during mooring. In one case, all four fingers were traumatically amputated when a rope, looped around the hand, was pulled tight by a cross-wind. Only the thumb remained. Remarkably, there was no immediate pain – just great surprise when the fingers were gone! Never loop a rope around your fingers or hand. If an amputation occurs, bring the fingers to the hospital in a clean plastic bag, preferably with some saline solution, as reattachment may be possible.

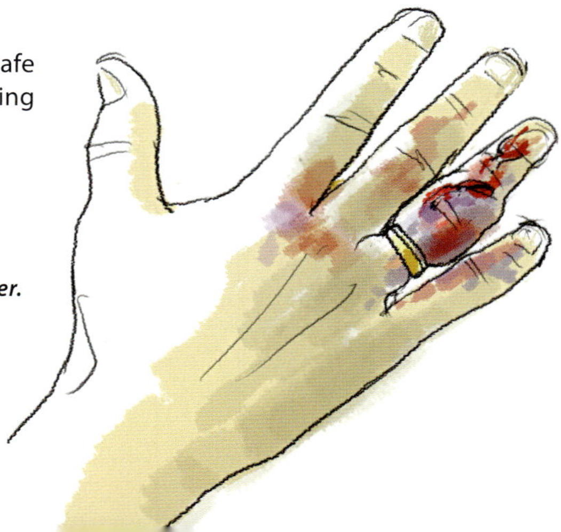

Ring stuck on an injured finger.

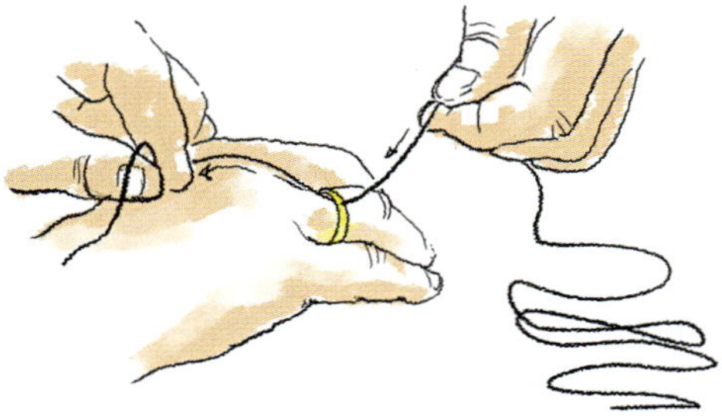

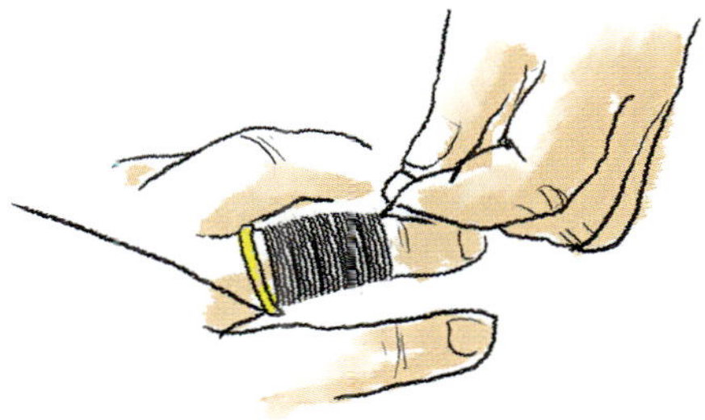

The 'string trick' can remove a stuck ring. Thread dental floss (2mm wide) under the ring. Firmly wind the longer outer end to compress the finger down to the knuckle. Then pull on the inner end, gradually feeding the ring over the knuckle and off the finger.

Wrap tightly!

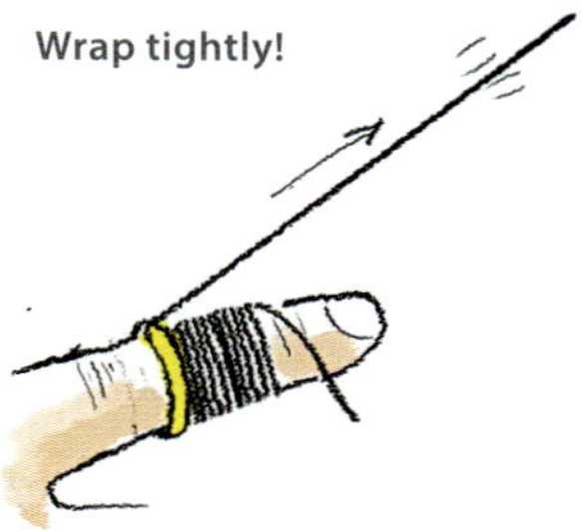

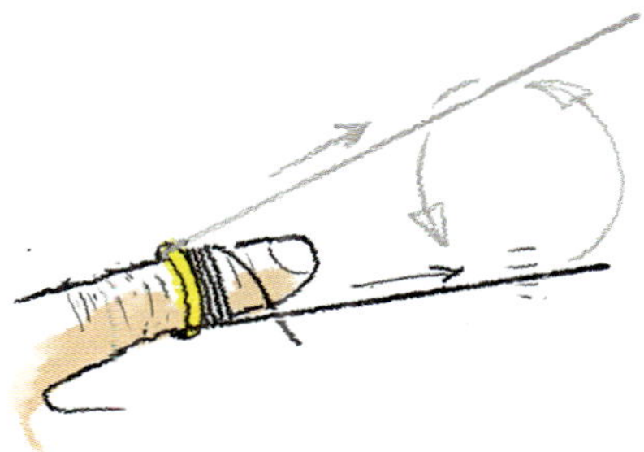

The hard winding reduces the diameter of the finger.

The pull on the thread means that the ring can now crawl forwards and come loose.

'Black nail' – subungual haematoma

A pinching injury to the fingertip may result in a 'black nail', accompanied by throbbing pain. This is caused by blood accumulating under the nail, creating pressure. A simple and effective way to relieve the discomfort is to puncture the nail to release the pressure. Often, these injuries are so severe that the outermost bone in the finger may be fractured or crushed, but this does not typically affect treatment as such fractures do not require special intervention.

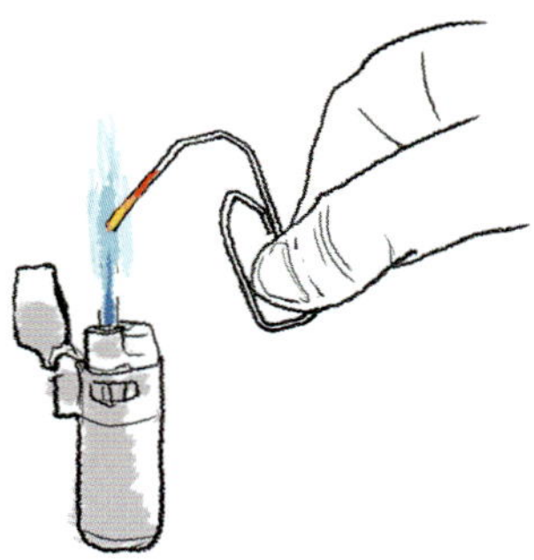

Anneal a paperclip.

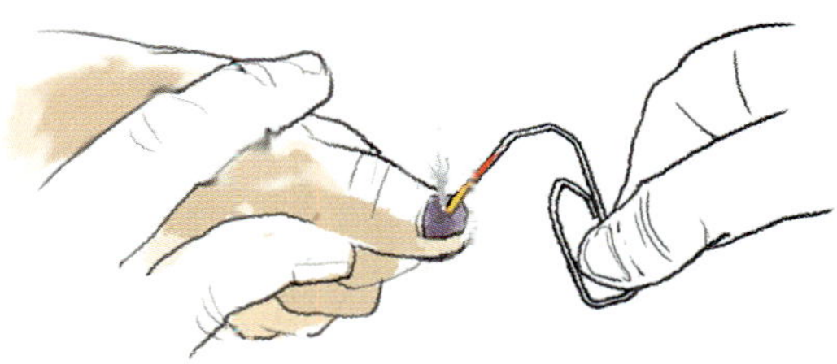

Burn a hole in the nail.

Heat a paper clip until it glows, then press it firmly against the 'black' area of the nail to puncture it. Apply a disinfectant dressing, which should be left in place for one day.

22. LOWER EXTREMITY INJURIES

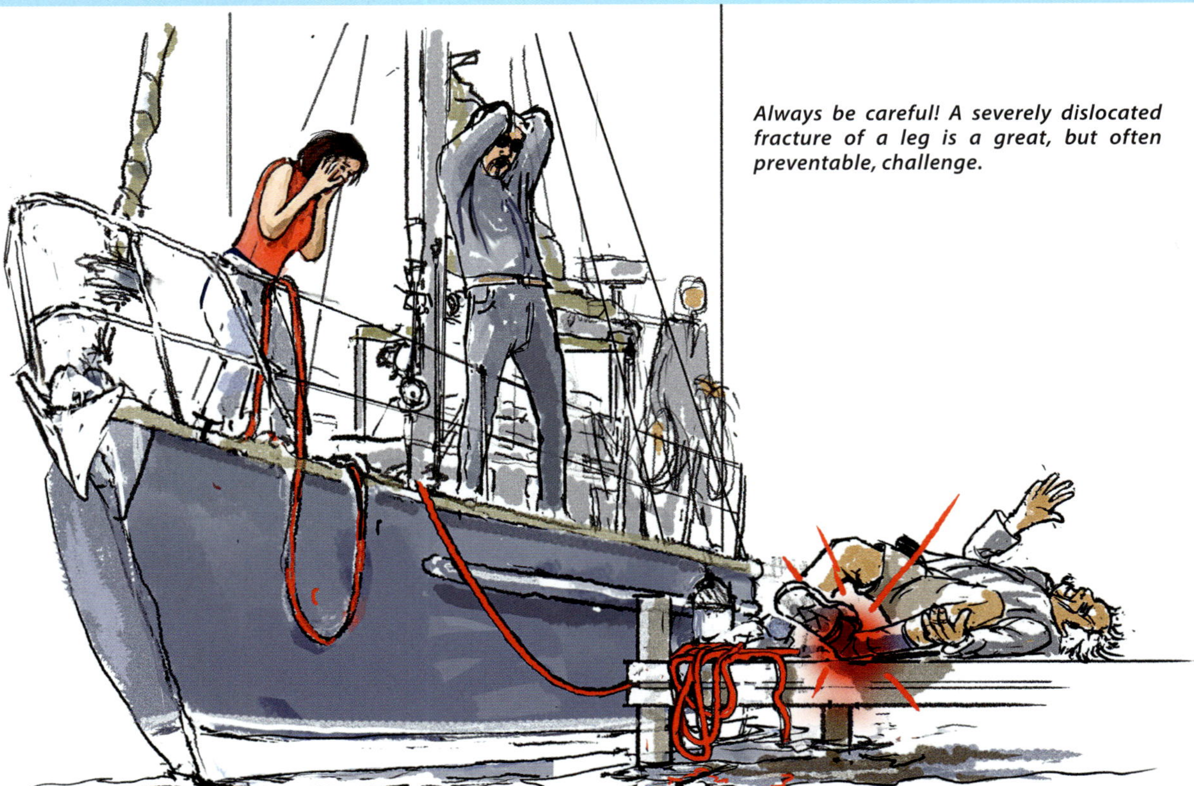

Always be careful! A severely dislocated fracture of a leg is a great, but often preventable, challenge.

This chapter covers the most common injuries of the lower extremities, including the hip, pelvis, femur, knee joint, lower leg, ankle and toes. These injuries are more common after alcohol consumption and in older individuals due to poorer balance and skeletal or muscular issues.

Prevention

General for all parts of the lower extremities:

- Wear sturdy shoes with slip-resistant soles.
- Be cautious on slippery surfaces, rocks and stones.
- Exercise the same care on boats and on land – watch for obstacles like ropes, stones or roots.
- Use support and hold on to something when necessary.
- Avoid alcohol, or exercise extra caution if consumed.
- Think before you act.

PELVIC FRACTURE – UNCOMPLICATED

The pelvis consists of two pelvic wings, the sacrum and the pubic bone, forming a stable skeletal structure known as the pelvic ring. The most common pelvic injury is a mild fracture in older individuals following a minor fall, often resulting in a crack in the pubic bone that does not affect pelvic ring stability.

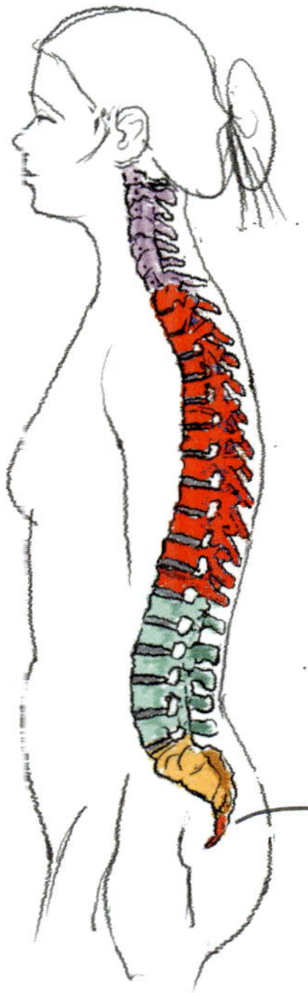

Signs and symptoms

- Localised pain
- Difficulty sitting; walking is usually possible with support
- Tenderness around the injury site

Immediate action

Examine the casualty and make a preliminary diagnosis of pubic or tail-bone fracture.

Treatment

- Administer pain relief.
- If close to home, seek emergency medical assessment.

Far from help

- Manage on board with painkillers and gentle exercise.
- Use a soft pillow or cushions for sitting.
- Diagnosis without an X-ray can be challenging, but differentiating from a severe pelvic fracture is often obvious (see page 210).

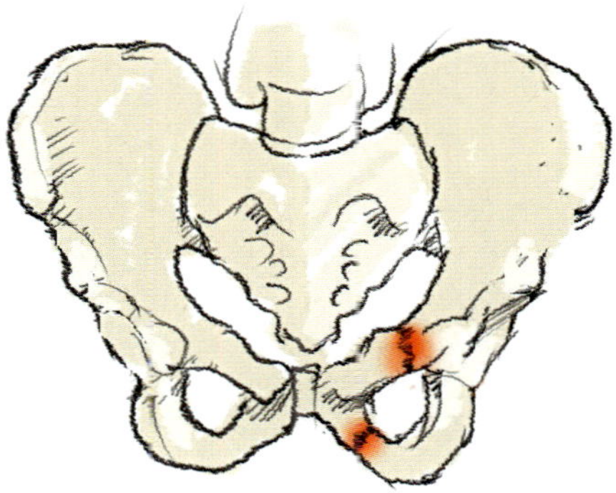

Crack or fracture in the pubic, sitting or tail bone. A common and harmless type of pelvic injury that does not affect the stability of the pelvic ring.

COMPLICATED PELVIC FRACTURE

Severe, unstable pelvic fractures occur after high-energy trauma, such as falls from a height, and traffic or speed boat accidents.. These injuries carry a high risk of internal bleeding, which can cause shock and become life-threatening.

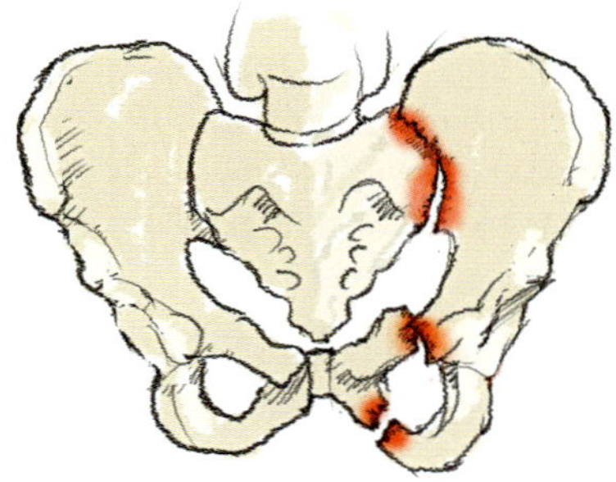

Severe pelvic fracture with an unstable, dislocated pelvic ring. One pelvic half is displaced due to multiple fractures, risking profuse bleeding from large blood vessels inside the pelvis.

Signs and symptoms

- Extreme pain
- Symmetric or asymmetric pelvis
- Signs of impending shock
- Bleeding from the urethra, vagina or anus
- Often associated with high-speed or high-sea boating accidents

Immediate action / Treatment

- Follow DRABC (see page 12), keep the person warm.
- Call for an urgent ambulance transport.
- Examine the pelvic bone (see image right).
- Stabilise the pelvis (see image below).
- Administer pain relief.

Far from help

Same as above under 'Treatment'. Establish contact with medical care for advice and evacuation. Monitor circulation and respiration. Keep the person warm. The situation can become difficult if the wait is prolonged.

As a layperson, you can contribute to a reduced risk of bleeding by bringing the legs together and gently compressing the pelvis with a makeshift belt made of cushions, a wide strap, elastic bandages or a sheet (see below).

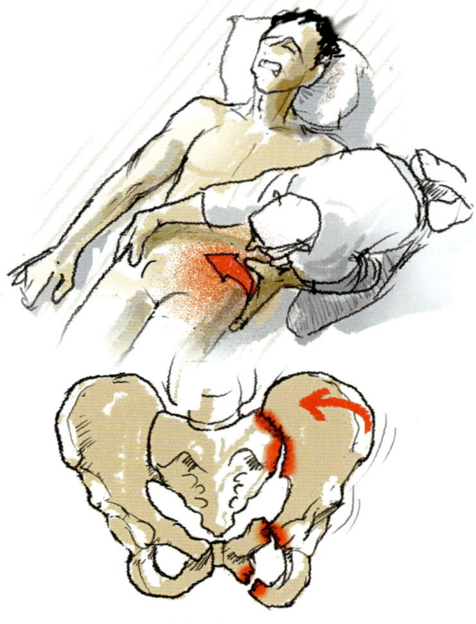

Examination of the pelvic bone. Check for symmetry by placing a hand on each pelvic wing and gently pressing together. Asymmetry, pain or instability indicates a serious injury.

Compression of a fractured pelvis.

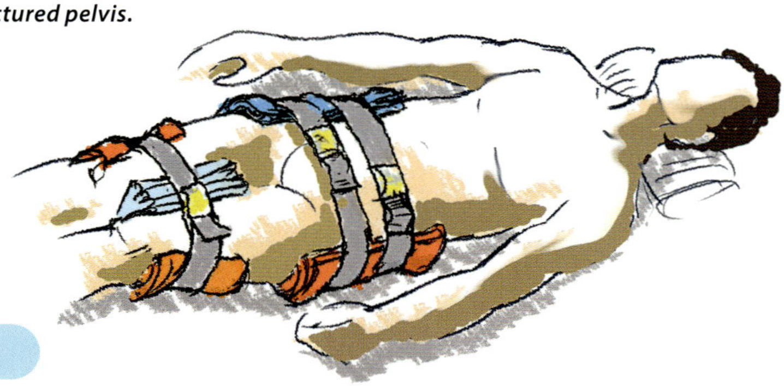

FRACTURE OF THE FEMORAL NECK

This common injury typically occurs after a fall on the hip and is more frequent among older women. However, it can affect younger individuals following significant trauma.

Signs and symptoms

- Pain in the groin or hip area
- Difficulty bearing weight on the leg
- Tenderness over the hip
- Outward rotation and shortening of the leg (in cases of complete fracture)
- Normal leg positioning if only a fissure is present

If misalignment is absent, examine for indirect tenderness:

- Gently tap the sole of the foot with a clenched fist.
- Rotate the foot back and forth.
- Pain in the groin or hip suggests a fracture or fissure.

Fracture of the femoral neck. The fracture may be completely displaced or without dislocation.

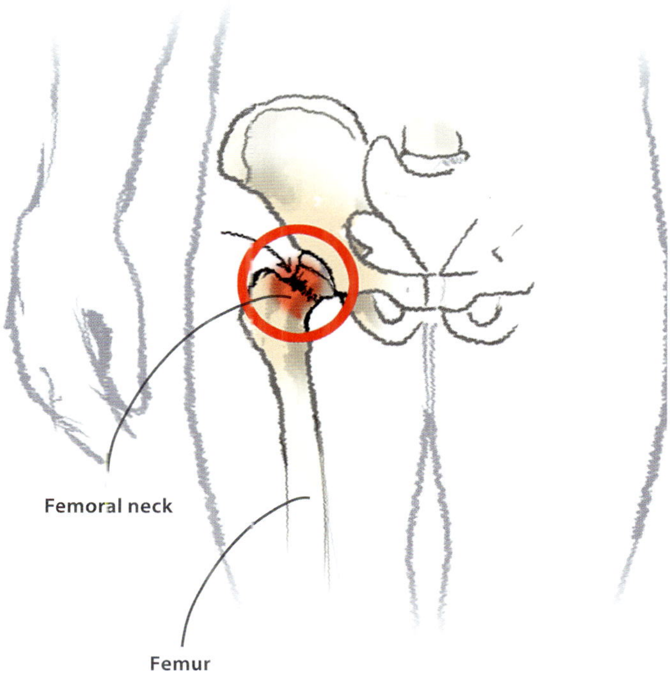

Typical misalignment: the fractured leg is externally rotated and shorter than the healthy leg.

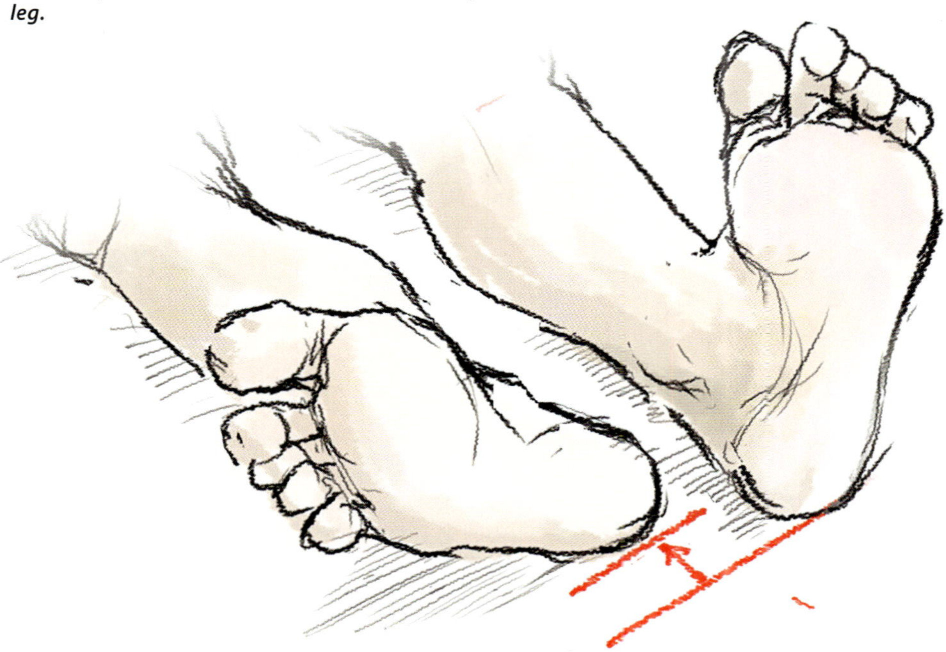

Immediate action

- Follow DRABC (see page 12).
- Keep the casualty warm.
- Stabilise with cushions or splints (see 'Femoral fracture' on page 214).
- Arrange urgent transport to the hospital for surgery, ideally within 24 hours.
- Administer pain relief.

Treatment

- See above under 'Immediate action'.

Far from help

The severity of the injury and your location will determine the level of difficulty in managing the situation. Evacuate as soon as possible; waiting for more than one to two days can be highly challenging. Seek advice and support. Administer pain relief at a morphine level. Make the injured person as comfortable as possible. Move them to a secure area below deck. Stabilise the injury with cushions and splints. Refer to the section on 'Femoral fracture' below for further details.

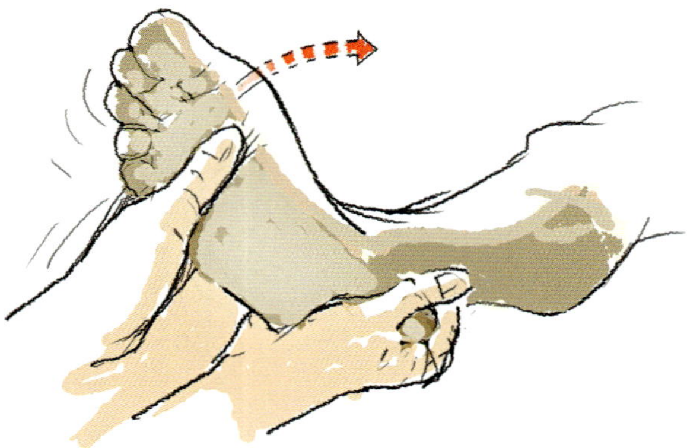

Testing indirect tenderness by carefully rotating the foot and watching pain reaction.

Testing indirect tenderness by applying longitudinal force with a gentle fist tap under the heel.

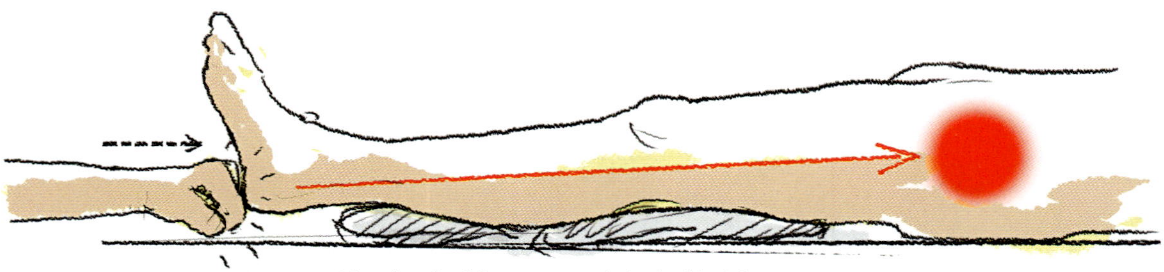

Impact with a clenched fist causes pain in the hip joint.

FRACTURE OF THE MIDDLE FEMUR

A fracture in the middle of the femur usually results from significant force, such as a fall from a height or a collision.

Signs and symptoms

The diagnosis is often clear due to several direct signs of a fracture, including shortening, outward rotation and angular deformity. The injured leg appears markedly different and abnormal compared to the healthy one. The thigh contains a large muscle mass and significant blood vessels, increasing the risk of substantial internal bleeding (1–2 litres), shock, and the development of significant swelling or a haematoma.

- Obvious fracture with deformity
- Shortened, outwardly rotated leg
- Angular deformity and swelling due to internal bleeding (up to 1–2 litres)

Immediate action / Treatment

- Follow DRABC (see page 12), keep warm.
- Check distal status! See page 165.
- Cut open clothing, if necessary, to inspect the entire leg and check for any wounds.
- Administer pain relief.
- Call for urgent transport to hospital.
- Immobilise with cushions or splinting, as described below.

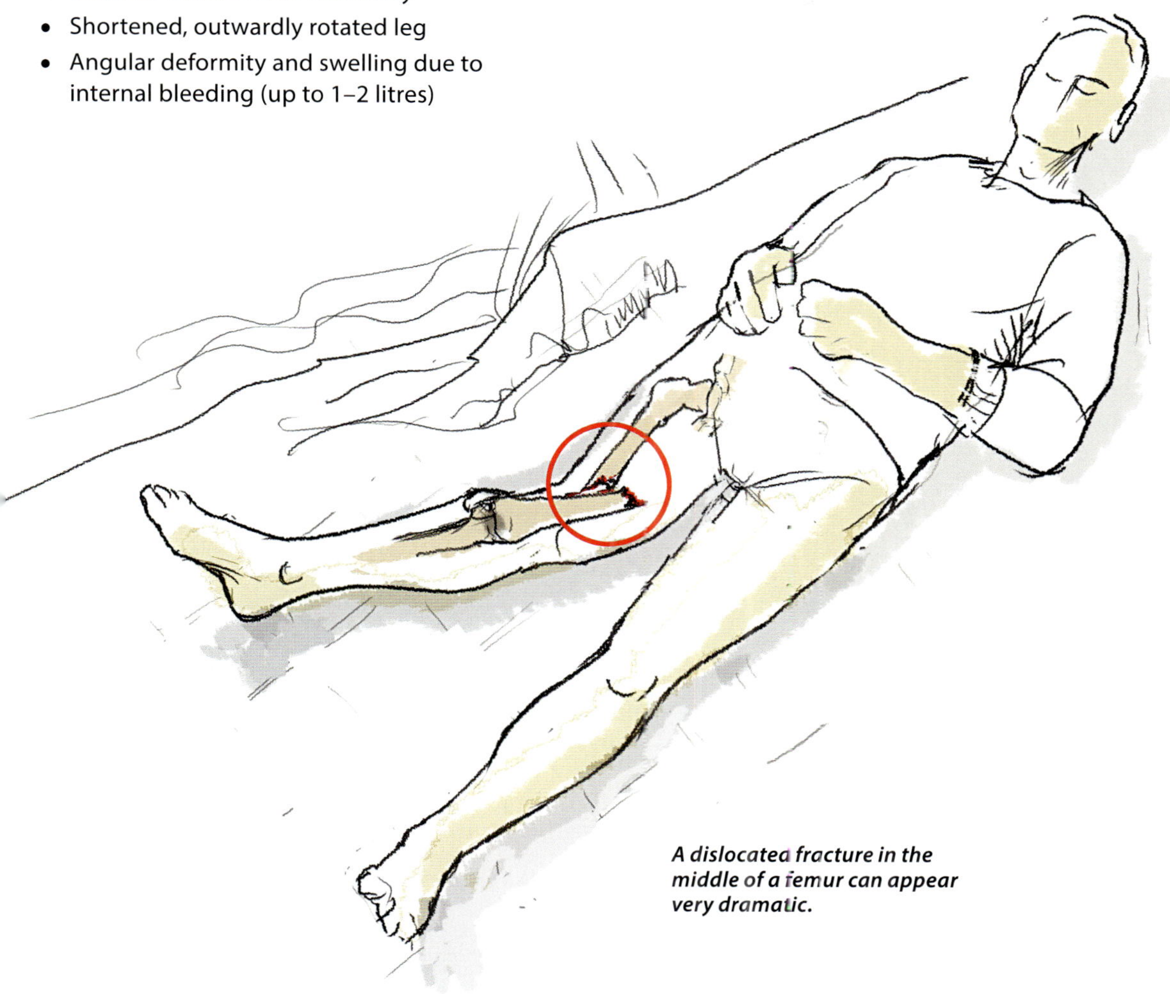

A dislocated fracture in the middle of a femur can appear very dramatic.

Far from help

In cases of significant deformity, consider attempting immediate repositioning (refer to 'Orthopaedics – General' on page 170 for detailed guidance).

Prompt repositioning requires focus and decisive action, despite the stressful nature of the situation.

1. *Grasp the foot and apply steady traction, not a sudden forceful pull, along the length of the leg. Pull to release muscle spasm and straighten or reduce the angulation.*
2. *Rotate the foot to achieve a 'normal' position.*
3. *Stabilise the leg with cushions, splints or other available materials.*

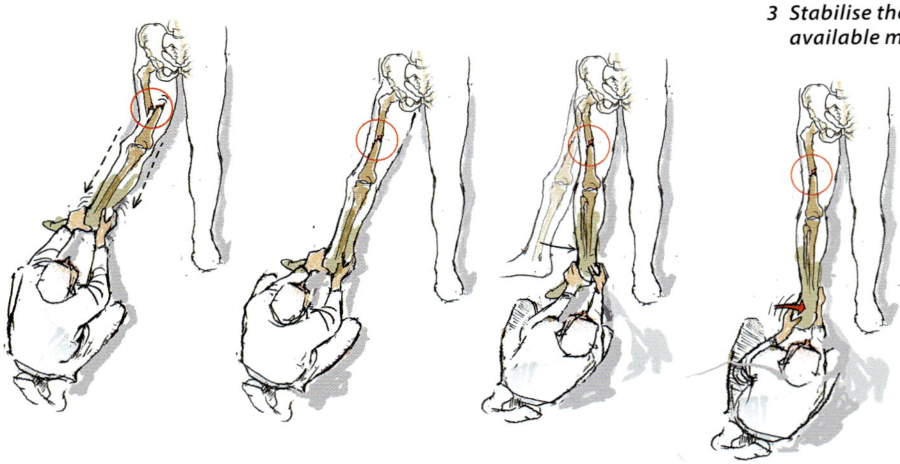

Evacuation must be arranged as quickly as possible. Contact emergency services. Splinting, or makeshift traction, may be necessary to ease the wait for transport. In the worst cases, the wait could extend to several days, depending on the location. Pain relief at a morphine level will likely be needed.

When a hip or femur fracture is suspected, splinting should include the pelvis and hip joint down to below the knee. Use available items such as oars, a boat hook or boards, ensuring a soft padding is placed closest to the body.

Makeshift stabilisation of a femoral fracture.

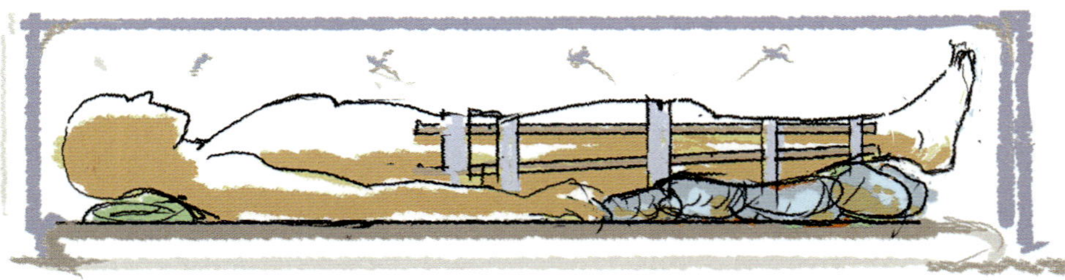

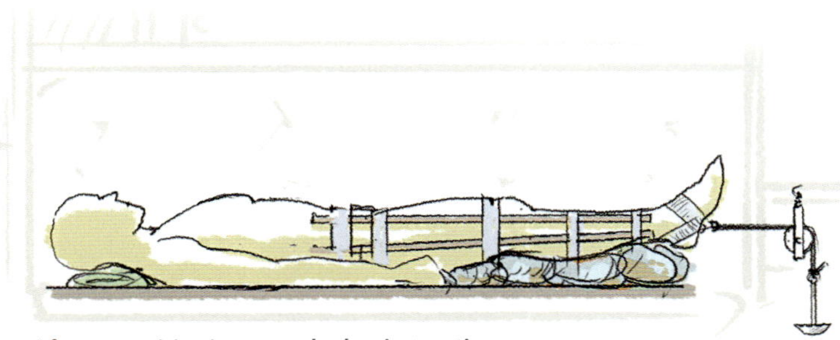

After repositioning, put the leg in traction.

If evacuation delays are prolonged, potentially lasting days, improvised traction can help make the injured person more comfortable. Suggested method: position the person comfortably on a stretcher or bunk. Attach a thin rope with Gorilla/gaffer/duct tape around the shoe, running it through a block at the stretcher's edge. Add weights (approximately 3–4kg, depending on the person's muscle mass). Use in combination with cushions and splints.

KNEE INJURIES

The knee joint is stabilised by a joint capsule, an outer and inner collateral ligament, as well as an anterior and posterior cruciate ligament. There are cartilage discs, called menisci, which act as cushions between the joint surfaces. Knee joints are subjected to heavy weight-bearing, bending and twisting forces, making ligament and joint injuries the most common.

Valgus force injuries

The most common mechanism of injury occurs when the knee is rotated outwards and simultaneously loaded or bent while being pushed inwards. The inner ligament, the inner meniscus, and often the anterior cruciate ligament can be injured – sometimes individually, but combined injuries are also possible. The degree of injury can range from ligament stretching to complete tearing.

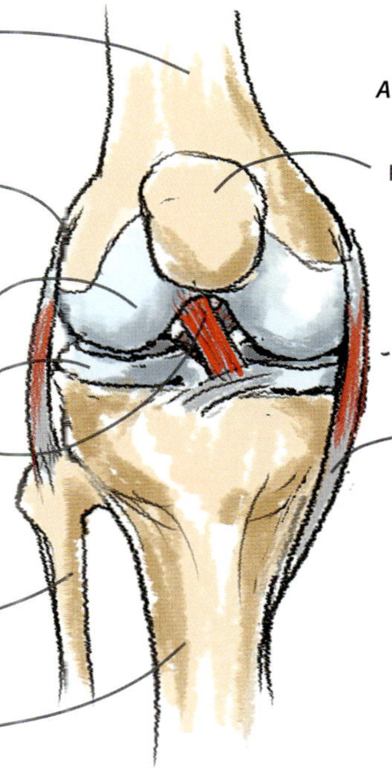

Anatomy of the knee.

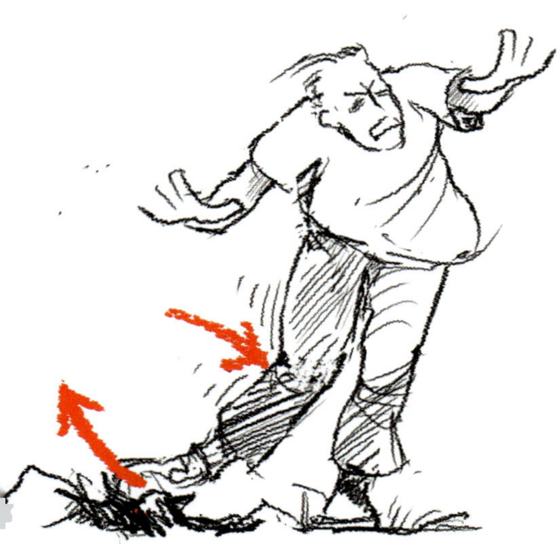

Typical combination of outward rotation and inward angulation (valgus) force.

Signs and symptoms

- Inner ligament injury: Symptoms include tenderness over the inner ligament and a swollen knee.
- Cruciate ligament injury: Of the two cruciate ligaments, the anterior is most commonly injured. This typically leads to bleeding within the knee joint, causing significant swelling and a feeling of instability.
- Meniscus injury: There are two menisci, one on the inside and one on the outside of the joint. The inner meniscus is most frequently injured, often causing swelling due to blood or fluid accumulation. A common symptom is painful mechanical locking of the knee, where the joint gets 'stuck'. Tenderness is typically found along the joint line on the inside of the knee.

Immediate action

- Stop activity.
- No weight-bearing.
- Assess signs and symptoms (see above).

Treatment

In the case of an acute knee injury, it is recommended to seek medical evaluation if possible. The person can usually walk and bear weight with caution. These types of injuries rarely, if ever, require urgent surgery or immediate treatment beyond rest and supportive bandaging. Therefore, if the accident occurs at sea, waiting until reaching shore for an examination is generally acceptable. Treatment typically includes pain relief and rehabilitation exercises.

Far from help

A knee injury of this type can often be managed during a sailing journey to the next port, even on a long crossing. Use supportive bandaging with a strong elastic bandage or an orthosis, allowing the person to move cautiously.

Important: An injured knee naturally creates some instability, increasing the risk of secondary injuries.

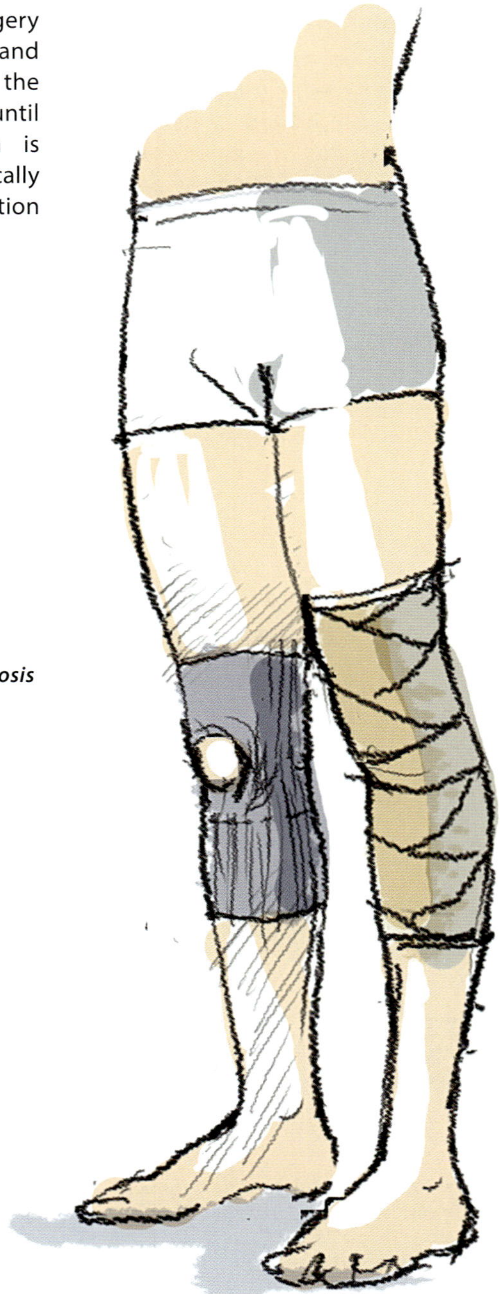

Knee bandages: Right side, a knee joint orthosis – a pre-made stabilising brace. Left side, an ordinary supportive bandage.

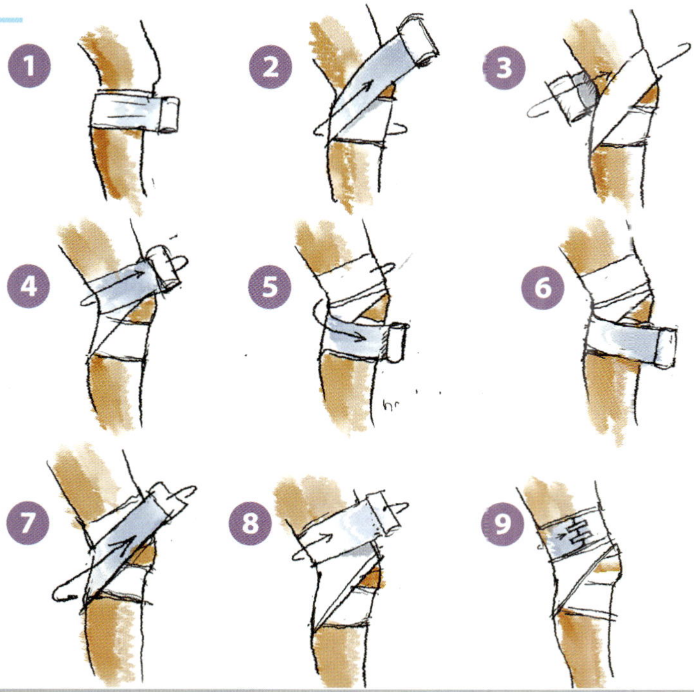

A supportive knee bandage.

REHABILITATION ADVICE

A knee injury can quickly lead to muscle atrophy. Begin rehabilitation exercises immediately, even during extended sailing, without putting weight on the injured knee. The two exercises below will strengthen the thigh muscles, which are crucial for knee stability.

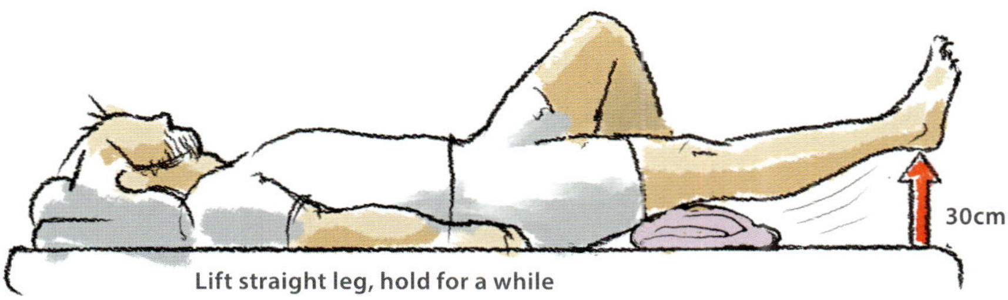

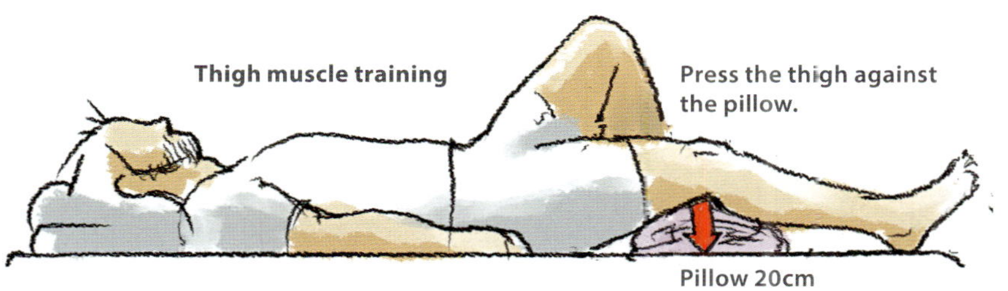

Lie on your back with both legs straight. Lift the injured leg about 30cm above the surface and hold for 15–30 seconds; repeat 10 times. Alternate by placing a pillow under the knee and pressing it by extending the knee joint and holding the position.

LOWER LEG

The lower leg contains two shinbones: the tibia (the larger, weight-bearing bone) and the fibula (the thinner bone). In some cases, only one bone is fractured while the lower leg remains stable, especially if the fibula is the one broken. Lower leg fractures typically occur due to significant collisions or direct trauma.

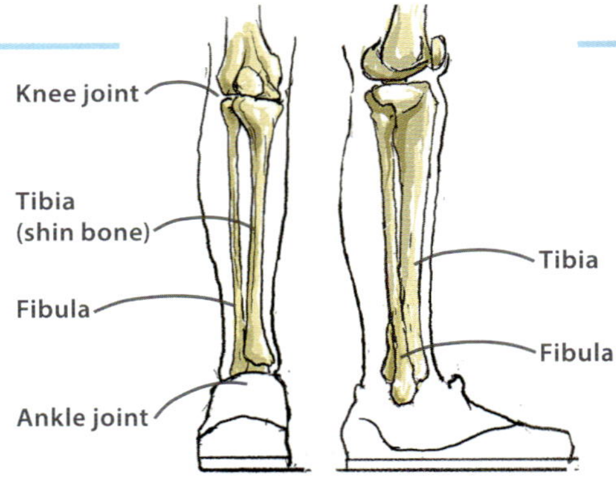

Anatomy of the lower leg.

Signs and symptoms

If both shinbones are fractured, the diagnosis is straightforward due to classic fracture signs – see page 164. There is a risk of sharp bone ends penetrating the skin, resulting in an 'open' fracture with an elevated risk of infection – see page 163. Blood vessels and nerves can also be damaged, potentially causing compartment syndrome – see page 166.

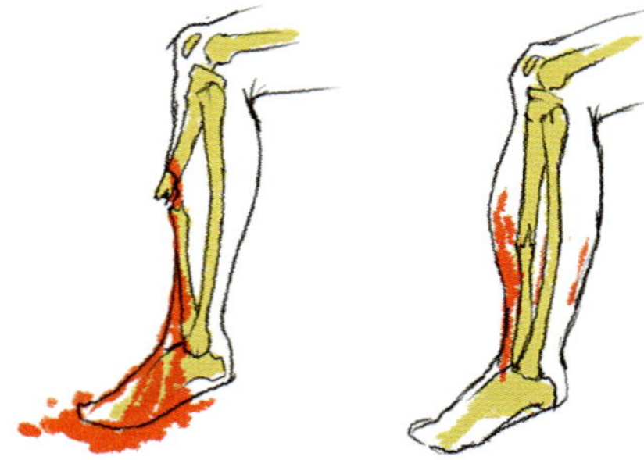

Open and closed fracture of the tibia. The fibula is intact, so there is no obvious dislocation.

Immediate action

- Check distal status (see page 165).
- Check the skin for wounds – is it an open fracture?
- Reduce dislocation if present.
- Immobilise using cushions, splinting, or by bracing against the other leg (see below).
- Keep the patient warm and arrange transport to hospital.

Treatment

Follow the steps outlined under 'Immediate action'. Keep the patient warm and administer pain relief. For an open fracture, start antibiotics such as amoxicillin-clavulanate 875/125mg every 12 hours.

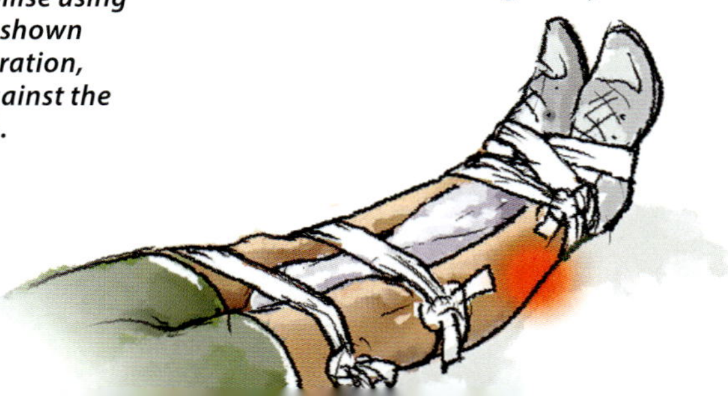

Fractures of the shinbones in the lower leg. Immobilise using a splint, as shown in the illustration, or brace against the healthy leg.

Far from help

Follow the same guidelines as above. Keep the leg elevated and the fracture stabilised until evacuation is possible. Severe swelling can impair circulation and nerve function. Monitor distal status closely to detect the development of compartment syndrome, a potentially life-threatening complication (see page 166).

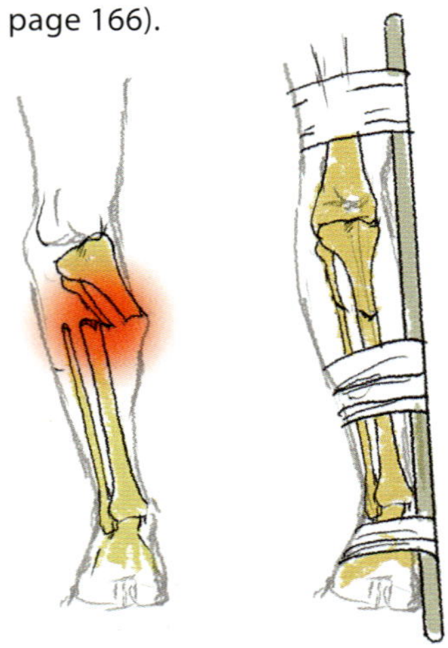

Lower leg fracture

Splinting

ANKLE JOINT – 'CLASSIC' SPRAINS

Ankle injuries, particularly sprains, are common during boating activities. The ankle joint is one of the most frequently injured joints in the body. A 'classic ankle sprain' typically occurs when the foot twists (supinates) and rotates inwards (inversion). This type of injury accounts for approximately 90 per cent of ankle injuries. It is usually benign and easily recognised by laypersons. Other ankle injuries, however, can be more challenging to assess in terms of type and severity. The direction and force applied to the ankle determine the injury's nature and extent.

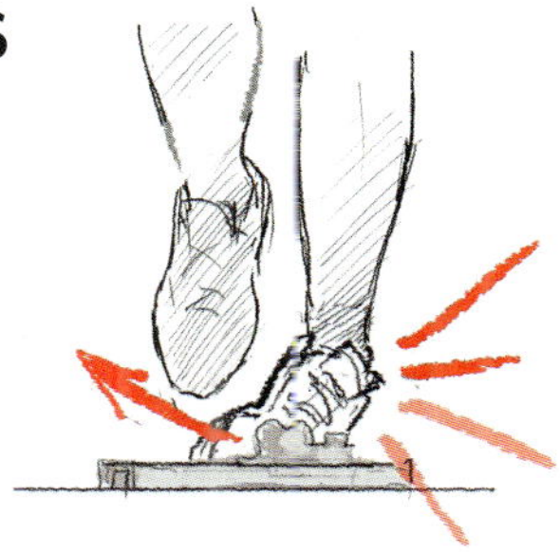

Classic ankle sprain – inversion (inward rotation) is the most common mechanism of injury.

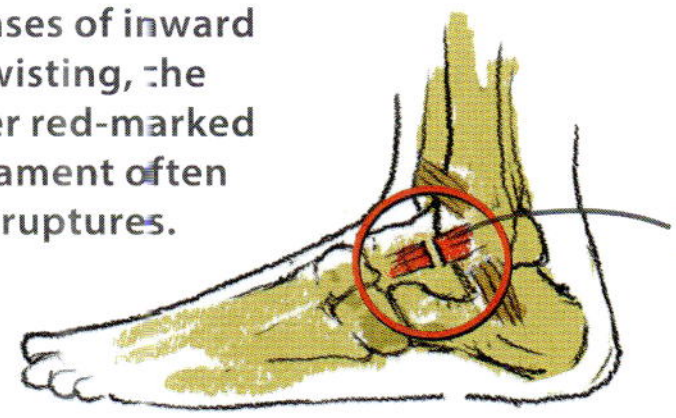

In cases of inward twisting, the outer red-marked ligament often ruptures.

Immediate action

After the injury, follow the PRICE principles.

P – PROTECT	Avoid further injury.
R – REST	Stop activities and rest.
I – ICE	Apply cold therapy primarily for pain relief and to reduce swelling. Do not place ice directly on the skin; use an ice bag for 10–20-minute intervals to prevent frostbite. Note that while ice alleviates pain, it does not reduce bleeding.
C – COMPRESSION	Apply compression with an elastic bandage to counteract bleeding and swelling for 30 minutes to 1 hour. Use a supportive pressure bandage for the next two to three days.
E – ELEVATE	Raise the injured foot to minimise swelling.

Interview the injured person to understand how the injury occurred. Once the worst pain has subsided, remove the elastic bandage and examine the foot.

Signs and symptoms

A classic ankle sprain is likely if the following criteria are met:

- The foot is twisted and rotated inwards.
- Tenderness and swelling are present only on the outside, in front of the outer ankle bone.
- The injured person can walk four steps with gentle support and normal weight-bearing.

Treatment

A classic ankle sprain can generally be managed without professional medical intervention. Treat the injury by elevating the leg as much as possible for one to two days and using a supporting bandage. Begin exercises to restore strength and mobility as soon as possible (see below). However, if in doubt, or if medical care is available, a professional evaluation is recommended.

Far from help

Follow the same guidelines as above.

ANKLE JOINT – ALL OTHER INJURIES

This category includes all sprains, fractures and inversion/eversion injuries that do not meet the criteria of a 'classic' sprain described earlier. If you cannot bear weight, or if there is dislocation, swelling and tenderness around the entire ankle joint, a serious fracture may be present.

Signs and symptoms

Approximately 10 per cent of injuries involve eversion, where the foot twists outwards and the ankle bends in the same direction. This mechanism often causes severe injuries, including tearing of the ligaments on the inside of the ankle and fractures of both malleoli.

If there is tenderness and swelling in one or both of the marked areas (see image below), it is likely not a simple injury. Complex damage, including fractures, may be present. Weight-bearing should be avoided until the injury has been examined at the hospital.

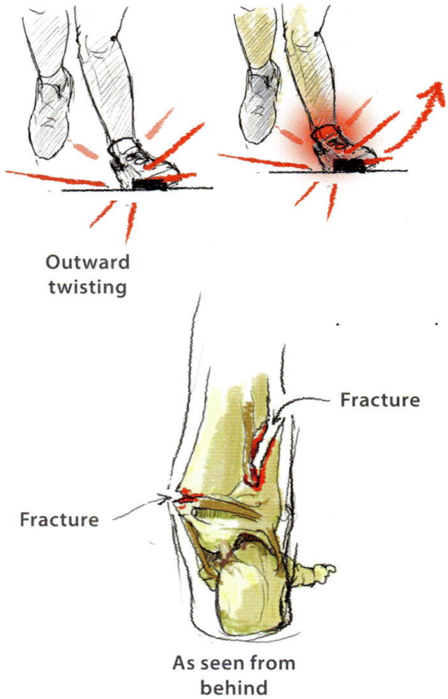

Outward rotation (eversion) leads to more complicated injuries.

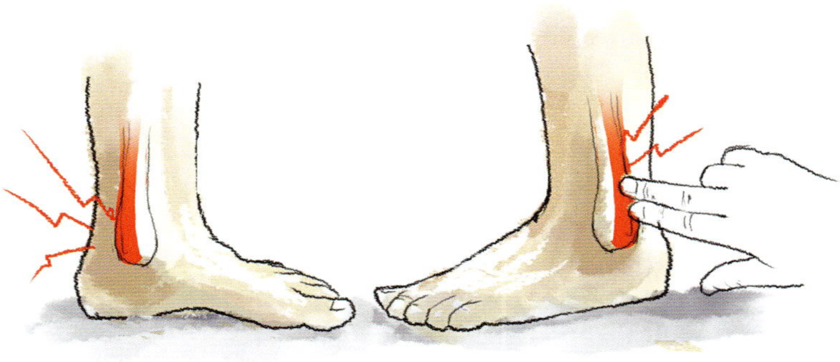

Swelling and localised tenderness from the tips of the lateral and medial anklebones extending 6–7cm upwards along the tibia and/or fibula indicate a possible fracture, necessitating an X-ray.

Immediate action

See earlier section. Follow PRICE principles!

Treatment

- Seek a medical examination as soon as possible.
- Apply a supportive bandage.
- Elevate the leg.
- Avoid weight-bearing until further evaluation. Provide pain relief.

Far from help

Follow the same guidelines as above. In cases of severe fractures with significant misalignment, immediate repositioning may be necessary to avoid skin damage. Overstretched skin over the ankle bones can lose circulation, leading to blisters or ulcers, which complicate healing. To realign, hold the heel and foot with both hands and pull gently in the direction of the leg.

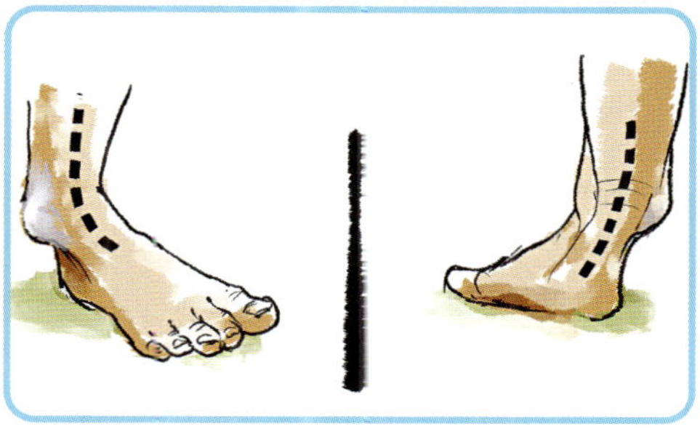

A broken, dislocated ankle with severe misalignment. The overstretched skin over the outer ankle bone shows signs of poor circulation, necessitating repositioning.

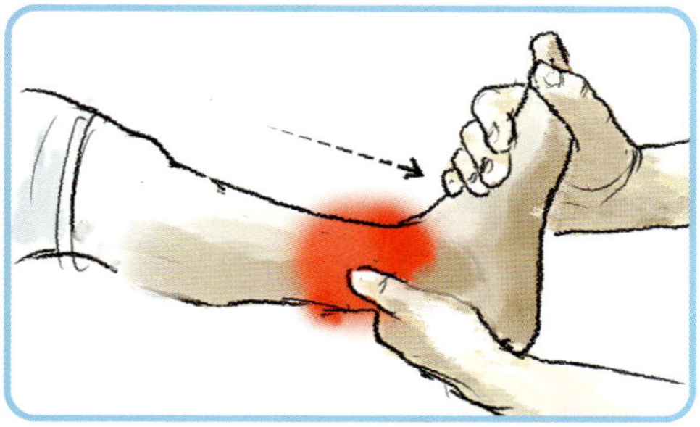

Apply a supportive or fixating elastic bandage (see below). Keep the foot in an elevated position.

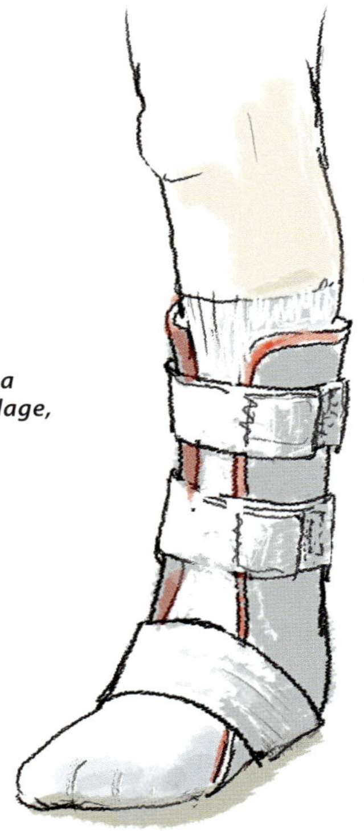

An ankle orthosis is an excellent alternative to a support bandage. It is available in a 'one-size-fits-all' design, provides excellent support, and can be used preventively or effectively for ankle injuries. Consider keeping one on board if ankle sprains are common.

Elastic support bandage: Begin on the outer side of the foot and use figure-eight turns to form a criss-cross pattern at the front. Leave the heel uncovered. A stronger stretch compression bandage, such as a Dauer bandage (10cm wide), may be necessary for larger ankles. Combining with an aluminium splint can improve stability.

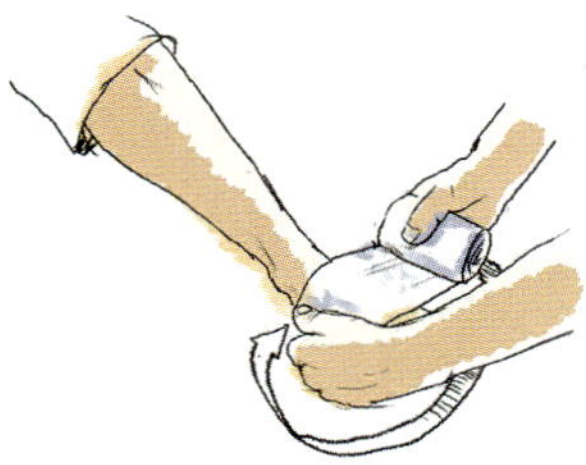

Begin at the heel.

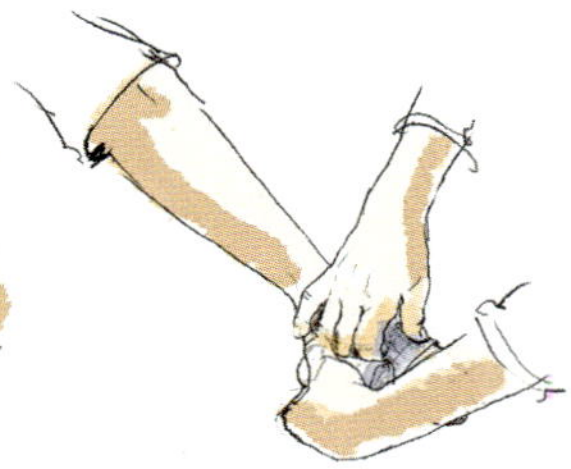

Hold the end.

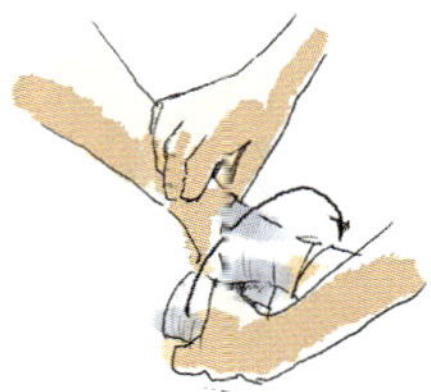

Tuck the end behind the next layer.

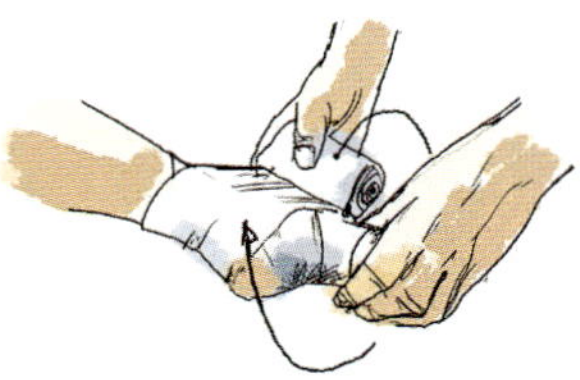

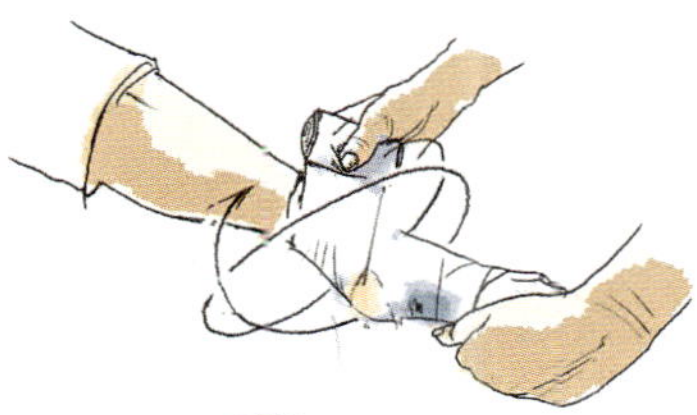

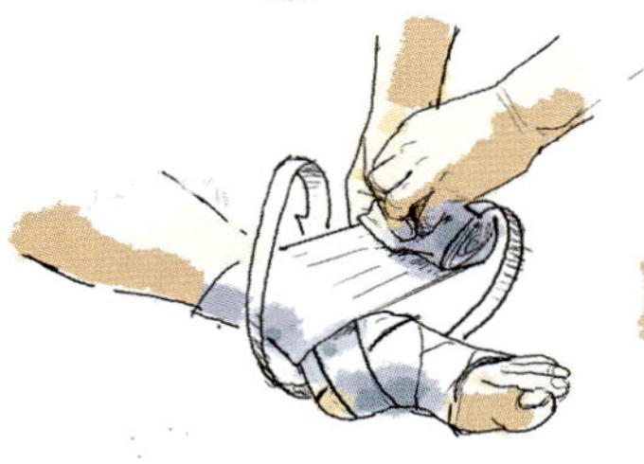

Keep zig-zagging up the leg.

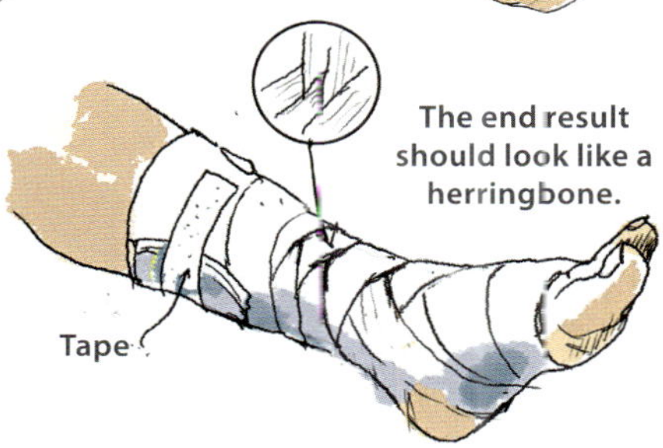

The end result should look like a herringbone.

REHABILITATION OF THE ANKLE

Rehabilitation exercises are essential for ankle sprains to promote faster healing and reduce the risk of recurrence. Begin mobility exercises in all directions immediately, avoiding weight on the ankle. As soon as weight-bearing pain subsides, progress to balance exercises, such as standing on one leg, and strength training with calf raises. Balance board training can be initiated upon returning home.

TARSAL AND METATARSAL INJURIES

Landing on the heel from a height can injure the heel bone, while collisions or crush injuries can break or crush the mid-foot and toe bones. These injuries are very painful but rarely require surgical treatment.

Signs and symptoms

Fractures or sprains typically present with swelling, tenderness, and pain during weight-bearing.

Immediate action

- Stop activity.
- Rest the foot in elevation.
- Provide pain relief.

Treatment

Avoid weight-bearing to minimise pain. Casting or surgery is rarely necessary. Seek evaluation and possibly an X-ray within one to two days if in home waters.

Far from help

A longer passage can continue. Seek medical attention at the next port. There is no need for evacuation. Pain relief, offloading weight, and a stable shoe with a supportive sole can provide relief when walking.

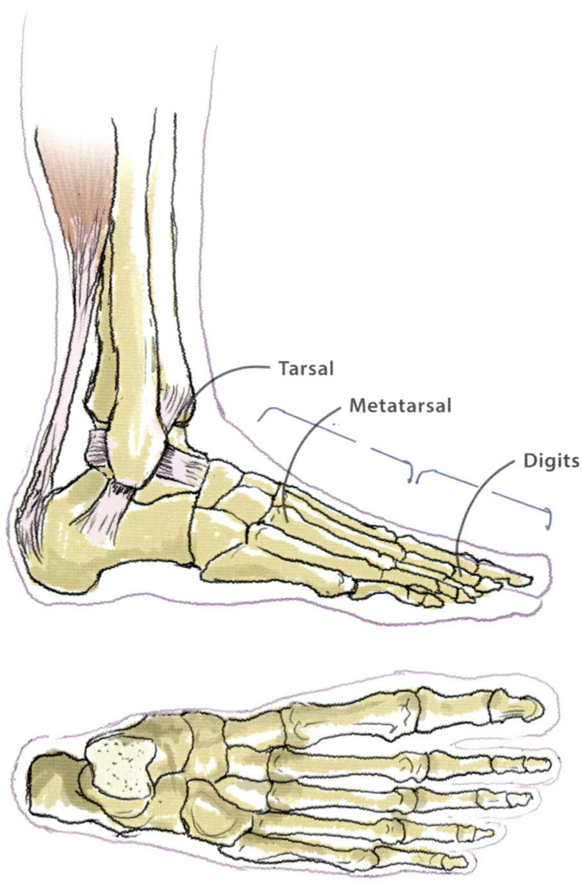

Normal anatomy of an ankle and a foot.

TOE INJURY

Toe injuries often occur on deck when accidentally kicking an object. Severe injuries requiring urgent surgery or X-rays are rare, except in cases of fractures or significant misalignment of the big toe. Open fractures with a wound carry a risk of infection.

Signs and symptoms

Symptoms range from mild swelling and tenderness to severe displacement, wounds or detached nails.

Treatment

- Provide pain relief.
- Apply a temporary bandage (see below).
- Seek evaluation within one to two days.

Far from help

For severe misalignment, attempt to realign the toe. For wounds, refer to the wound care section (pages 26–33). Stabilise the toe by taping it to a neighbouring toe with a soft dressing in between. Use an open-toe shoe or modify an athletic shoe to avoid pressure on the injured toe.

Stabilisation of an injured toe against the neighbouring toe. Remember the padding.

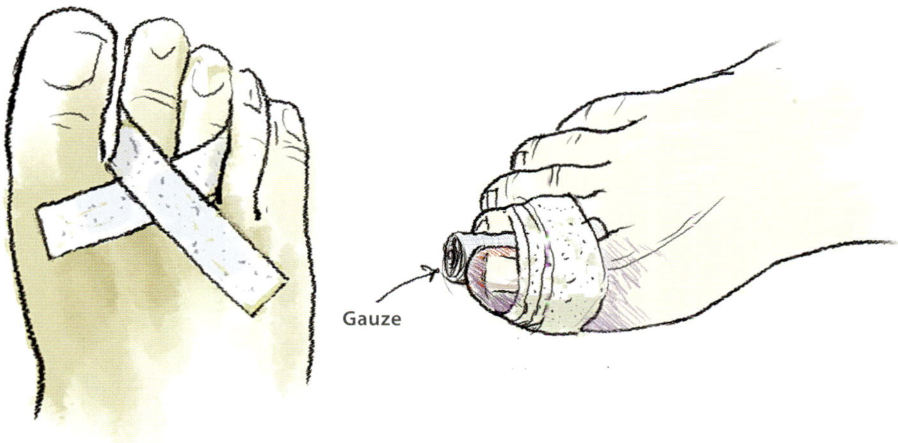

Methods to avoid pressure on an injured toe.

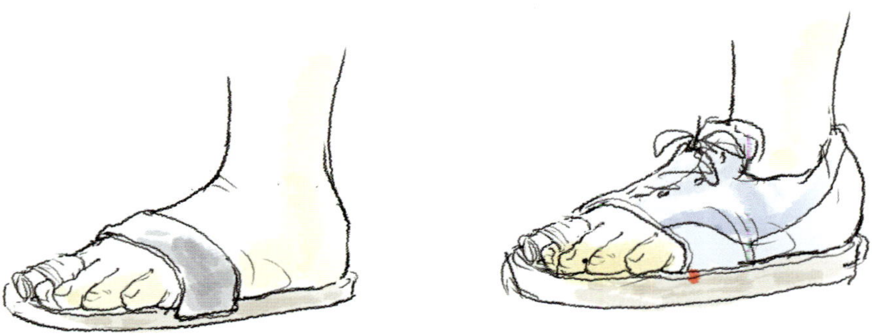

RUPTURE OF THE ACHILLES TENDON

Jumping on to land or a dock can cause the Achilles tendon to stretch suddenly and rupture, either partially or completely. This injury commonly occurs in middle-aged men playing sports without proper warm-up. A snapping sound often accompanies the rupture.

Avoid jumping ashore; step ashore to prevent Achilles tendon injuries.

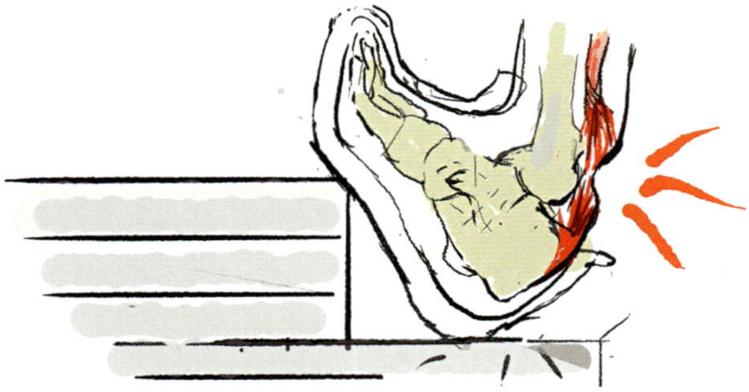

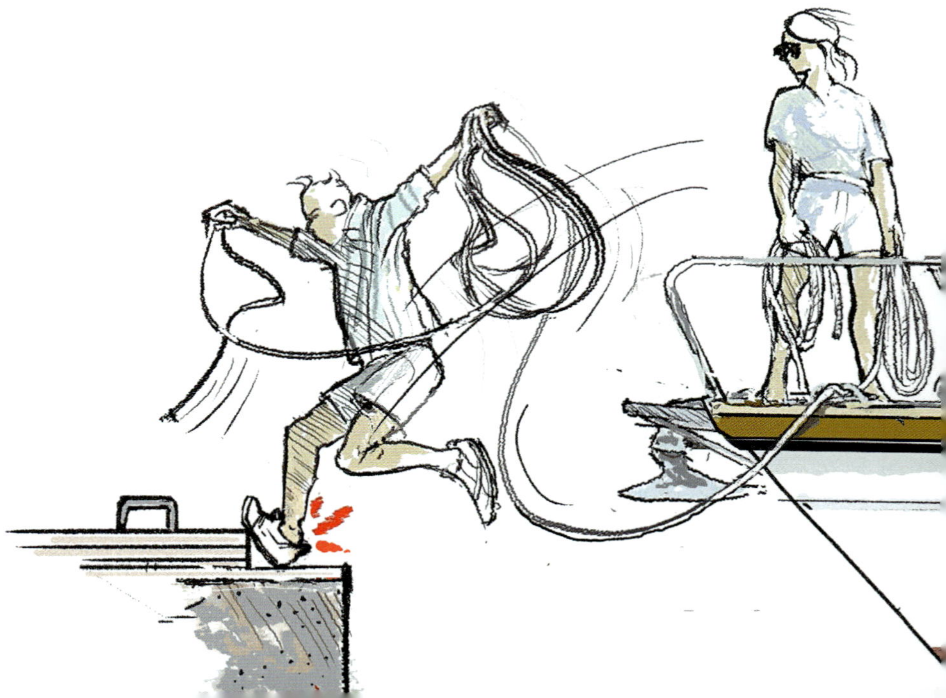

Signs and symptoms

Pain is localised, with difficulty standing on tiptoes, impaired balance, and a detectable 'gap' in the tendon when compared to the unaffected side.

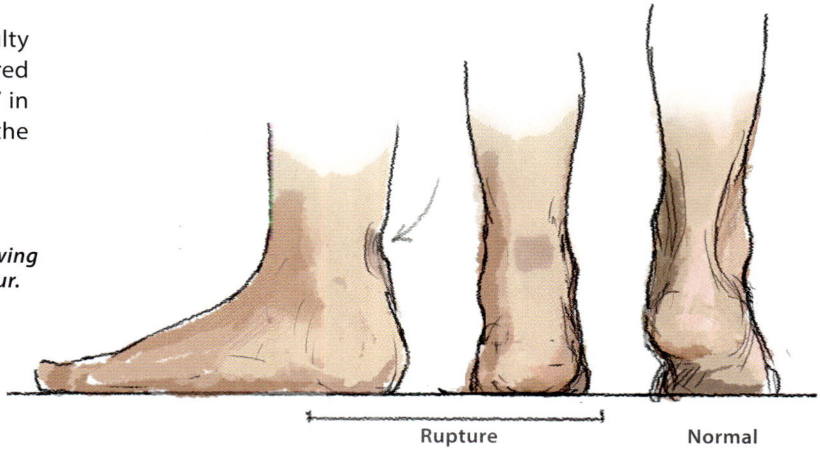

Rupture of the Achilles tendon showing a gap and broadening of the contour.

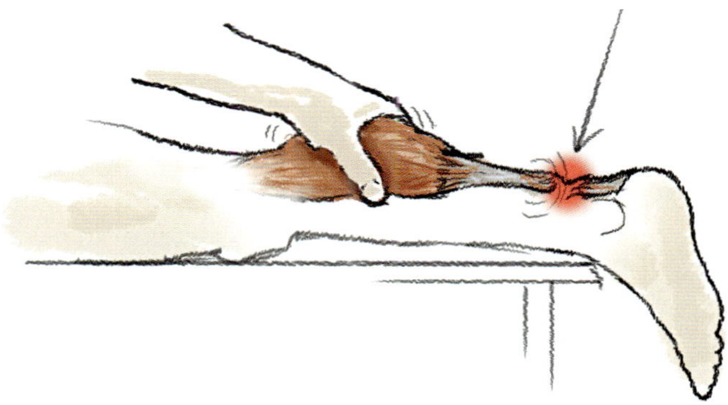

Simple test for Achilles tendon rupture: Have the casualty lie face down and relax. Squeeze the calf muscles and observe foot movement. No movement suggests a total rupture; some movement indicates an intact or partially ruptured tendon.

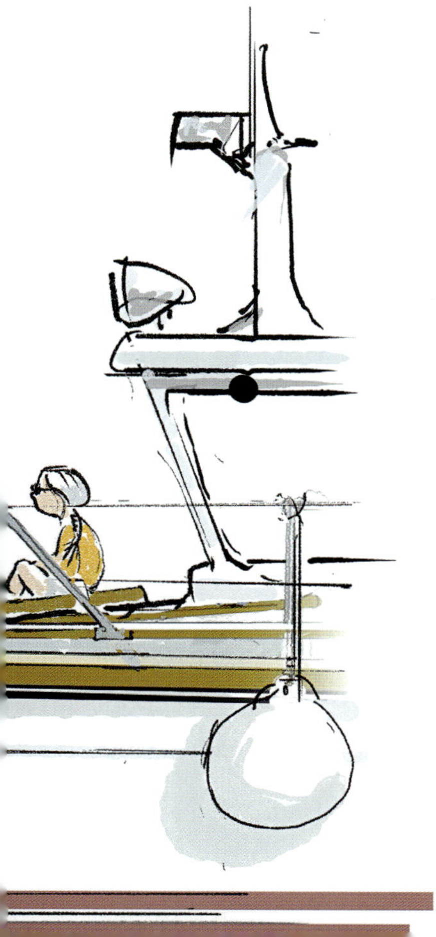

Immediate action

Stop activity and weight-bearing.

Treatment

Use crutches or a cane to offload weight and seek surgical or orthopaedic care promptly. Total ruptures often require surgical repair followed by immobilisation with the ankle extended for four weeks.

Far from help

Follow the same guidelines. Immobilise the ankle to prevent further injury due to impaired mobility. Seek an orthopaedic surgeon upon reaching port. Evacuation is not usually necessary.

23. BITES AND STINGS

Mammals, reptiles, insects, fish and other sea-living organisms can cause bites and stings, some of which are venomous.

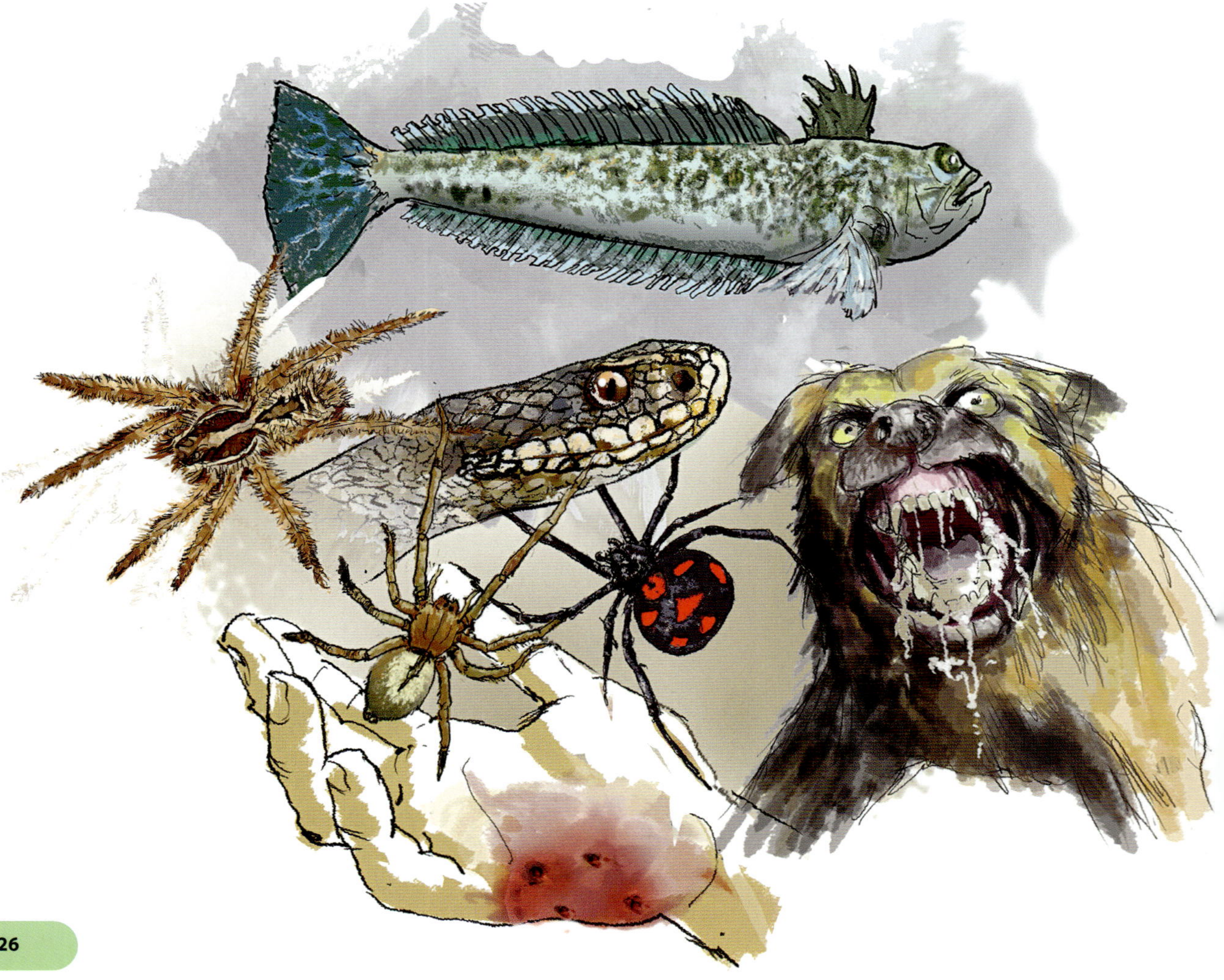

Several animal species are equipped with defence mechanisms that can cause stings, bites or toxic reactions.

ANIMAL BITES

Bites from animals like dogs and cats, or even humans, cause wounds with a substantial risk of infection. This is because teeth often create deep, narrow puncture wounds that are challenging to clean effectively. The bacteria present in the biter's mouth can thrive in these narrow and tight puncture channels. It is essential to have up-to-date tetanus protection.

When on boat trips in other countries, the risk of bites from rodents such as rats and even bats must also be considered. In such cases, there is a different spectrum of diseases to be aware of, including a certain risk of rabies. Consider vaccination against rabies if you want to minimise the risk when interacting with dogs, cats and other animals. Vaccination does not provide complete protection, but it extends the time limit to seek medical care to two days after a bite. The alternative is to seek urgent medical care for serum treatment following a bite.

Signs and symptoms

Inspect and classify the wound regarding the risk of infection and type (for example, puncture or tear injury) and its proximity to joints and tendons.

Immediate action

Stop interaction with the attacking animal. Check and stop any bleeding. Assess distal status (see page 165). Mechanically clean the wound as effectively as possible (see page 30).

Treatment

When at home, visit a doctor to assess the risk of infection and check need of tetanus booster.

Dog bite on hand close to joints and tendons.

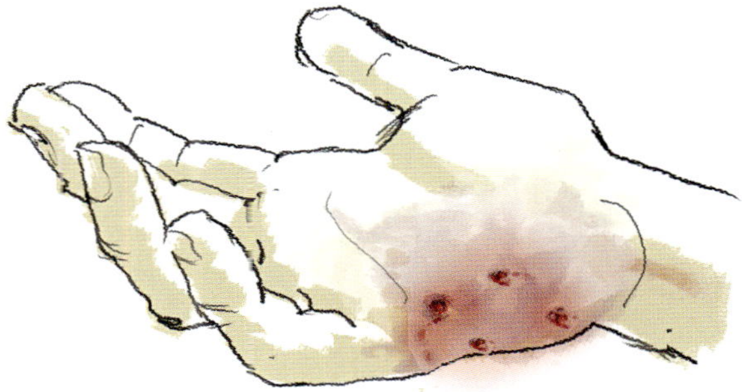

A puncture wound after an animal bite.

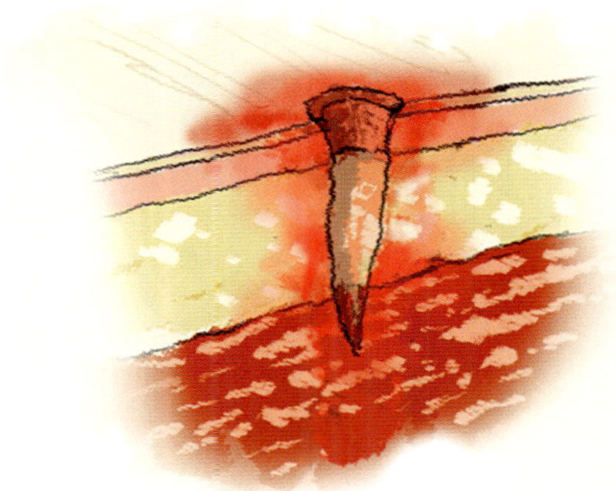

Dogs with rabies can be encountered in many parts of the world.

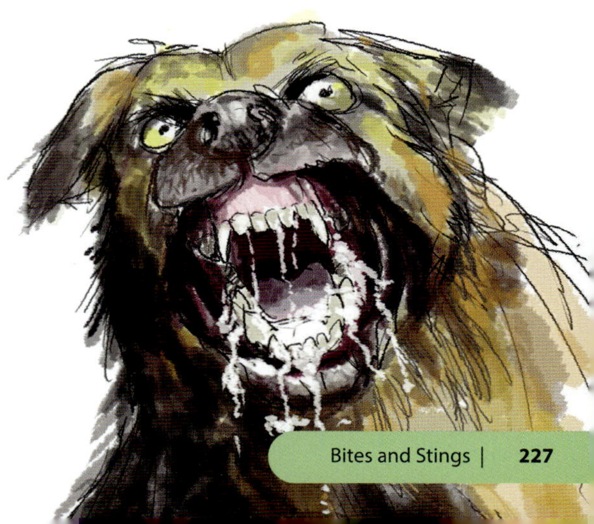

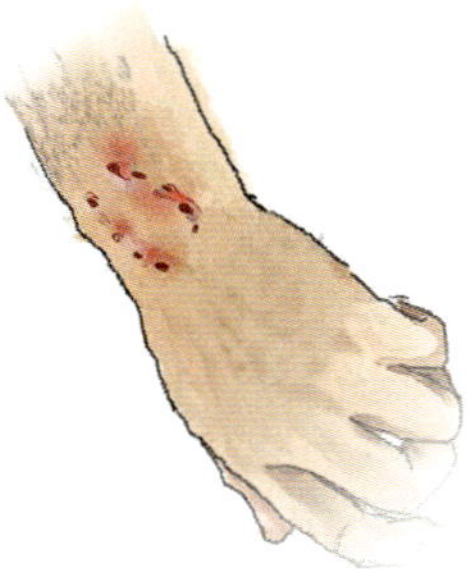

Humans can cause bites with obvious risk for infection.

Far from help

In addition to mechanical cleaning, consider applying a spirit dressing consisting of compresses soaked in alcohol or chlorhexidine solution, secured with a bandage. Be liberal with early antibiotics, especially if the bite is near joints, tendons or the hand (for example, amoxicillin/clavulanic acid). Know when to suspect infection (see page 32). Communicate for advice.

Prevention

- Avoid close contact with unknown dogs and cats.
- Prevent human bites by maintaining kind, respectful interactions.
- Check vaccination status, including tetanus.
- Pack a balanced selection of antibiotics in your ship's dispensary.
- After human bites, most surgeons agree on administering prophylactic antibiotics.

INSECT STINGS AND BITES

To manage stings and bites effectively, it is important to know the local fauna and associated risks. In addition to the risk of infection, some animals are equipped with neurotoxic venoms that can cause acute and sometimes severe reactions. Although fatal reactions are rare, they have been reported.

Signs and symptoms

- Stings from wasps, bees, mosquitoes, horseflies, spiders and scorpions can lead to severe local reactions, including redness, swelling and intense itching.
- Bites from venomous animals, spiders and scorpions can cause severe pain, nausea, anxiety, breathing problems and swelling.
- There is always a risk of insect bites becoming infected, either directly during the sting or due to scratching with dirty fingers. In tropical areas, sailors have reported life-threatening septicaemia following infected bites.
- Mosquitoes in some regions carry serious tropical diseases (see pages 234–40).

There are lots of different venomous biting and stinging insects and spiders, including scorpions, everywhere around the world.

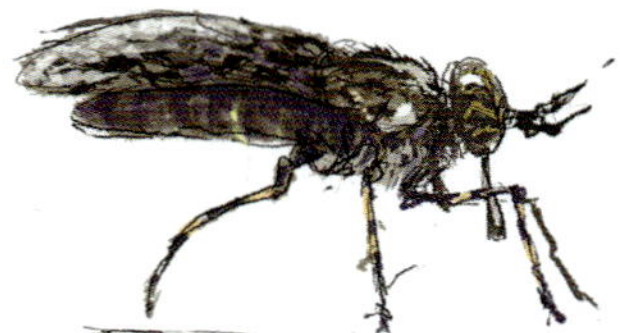

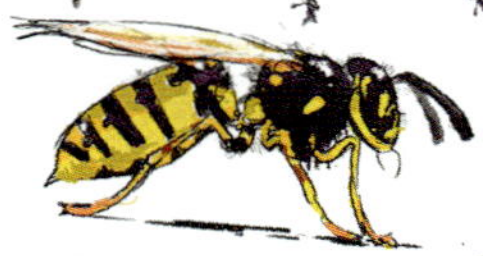

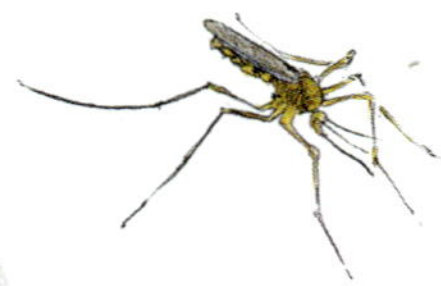

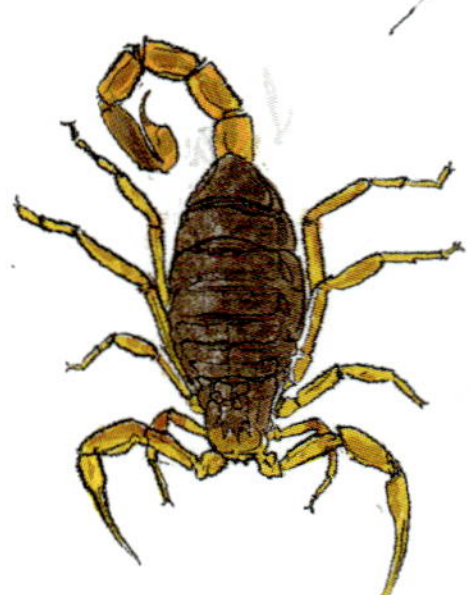

Death Stalker Scorpion

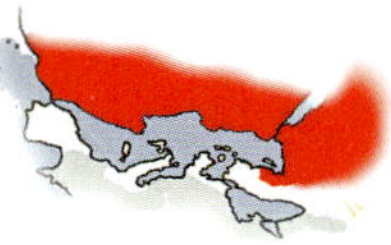

Death Stalker habitat – Mediterranean

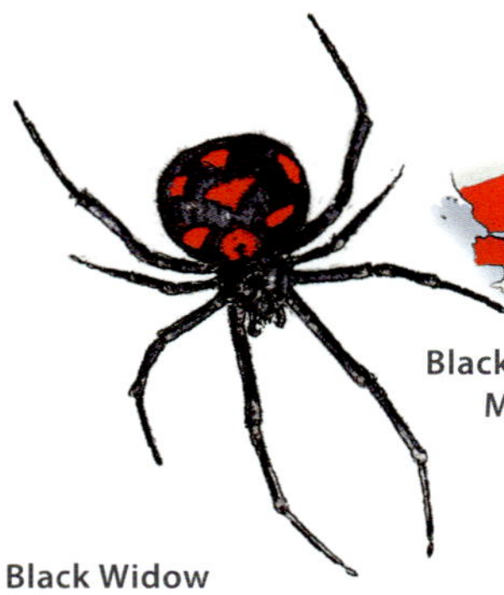

Black Widow

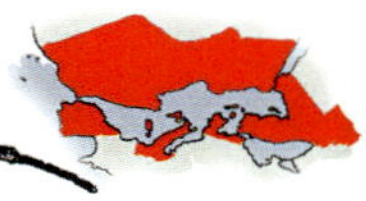

Black Widow habitat – Mediterranean

Immediate action

Move away from attacking insects. Monitor for possible allergic reactions, especially after wasp or bee stings (see page 54). Administer antihistamines if available.

Treatment

- Local reactions: Relieve symptoms with hydrocortisone 1% cream or antihistamine tablets.
- Infections: Treat with antibiotics (for example, phenoxymethylpenicillin).
- Severe bites from venomous animals require medical evaluation and possibly a hospital stay.

Far from help

Monitor for signs of poisoning/allergic reactions (see page 54) and infection (see page 32). Treat symptoms as described above.

Prevention

- Avoid close contact with insects.
- Wear full-cover clothing.
- Stay in breezy areas to avoid mosquitoes.
- Use mosquito nets, especially in malaria-prone regions.
- Avoid scratching itchy bites with dirty fingers.
- Use locally effective insect repellents.
- Check local conditions for specific species, venom risks and prevention techniques.

TICK BITES

Ticks pose specific risks, including tick-borne encephalitis (TBE) and Lyme disease (boreliosis).

Signs and symptoms

- TBE: Severe brain inflammation with no specific treatment. Common in Nordic and eastern European countries.
- Lyme disease: Protozoan infection that can be treated with antibiotics. Symptoms include an expanding red ring (erythema migrans) at the bite site appearing 1–4 weeks after the bite, fatigue, headache, muscle pain and fever.

Immediate action

- Remove the tick as soon as possible to reduce the risk of disease transmission. Use a tick remover to pull it straight out without rotation.
- If the red ring expands to at least 5cm within a week, consider starting a penicillin course.

Prevention

- Wear long trousers and boots.
- Perform a full-body check before bedtime to remove any ticks within 24 hours.

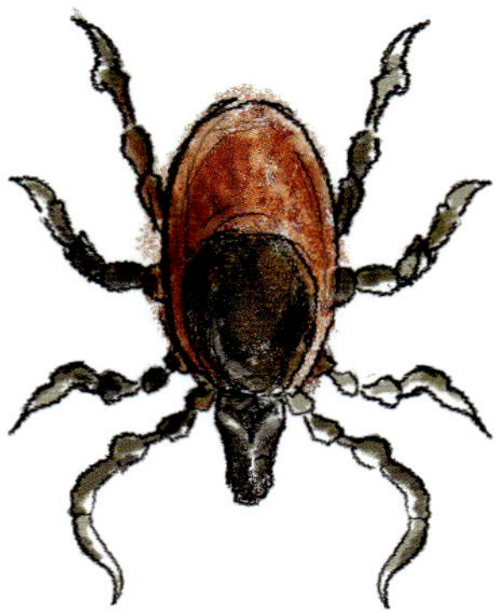

A typical tick, size 2–4mm. Expands after a bite and suction of blood.

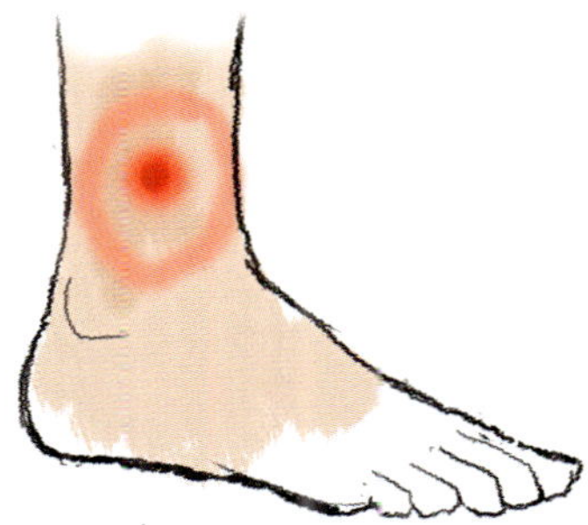

Borrelia infection after a tick bite, with typical ring-formed erythema (erythema migrans). If the red ring expands to at least 5cm in diameter within a week, consider starting a penicillin course for boreliosis (phenoxymethylpenicillin 1g every 6 hours for 10 days).

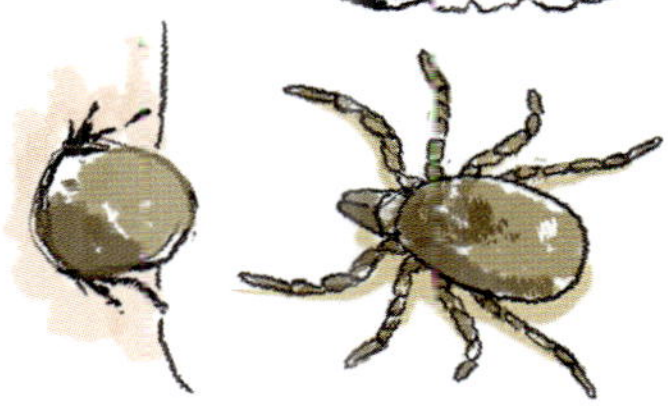

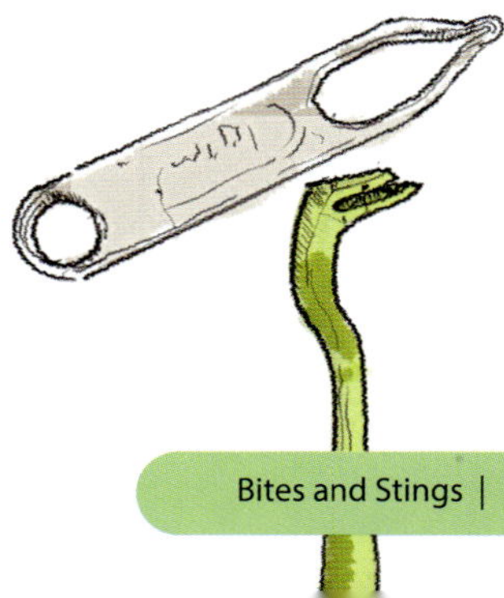

Tick removers.

SNAKE BITES

Signs and symptoms

- Moderate symptoms: Local swelling, pain, discoloration
- Severe symptoms: Nausea, vomiting, allergic reactions, breathing difficulties and signs of shock

Immediate action

- Rest and immobilise the affected limb.
- Seek professional advice and observe the casualty closely.

Treatment

Transport the casualty to a hospital for observation and potential antivenom treatment.

Far from help

See above under 'Immediate action'.

Prevention

- Be aware of local snake populations.
- Wear boots and long trousers in snake-prone areas.

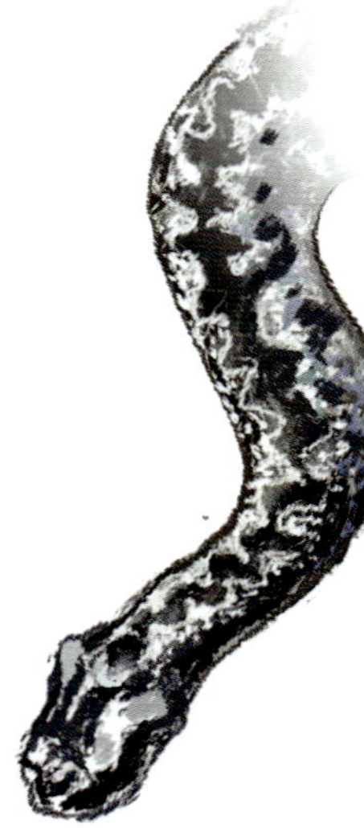

An adder, quite common in all parts of the world, in Europe especially in northern areas.

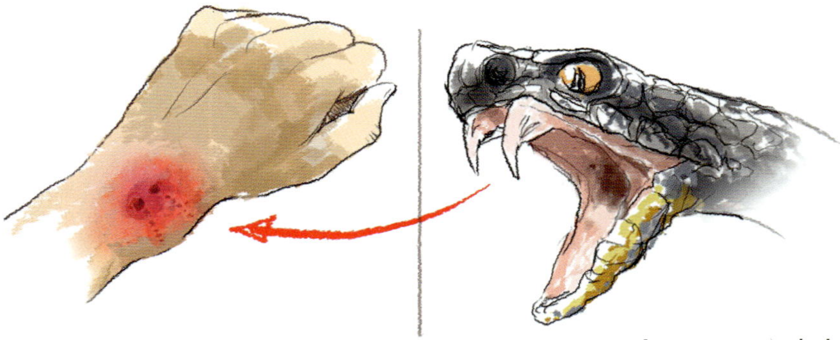

A venomous snake has two venom teeth, leaving a characteristic bite appearance with two skin penetrations 10mm apart. Non-venomous have a different pattern, with several teeth.

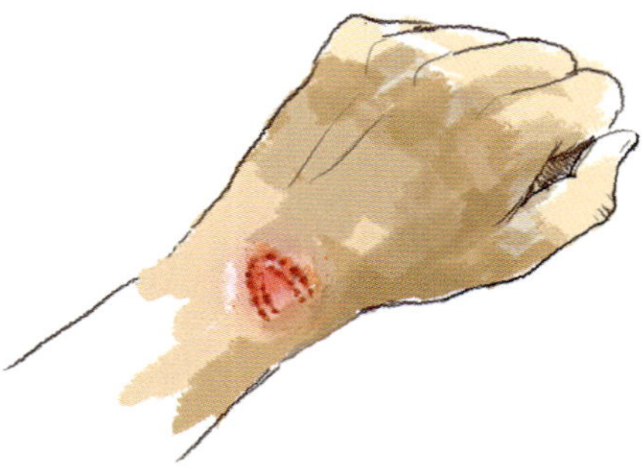

JELLYFISH STINGS

Harmless jellyfish, such as the blue jellyfish, are found all over the world. However, several highly venomous species may be encountered especially in tropical areas like the Caribbean, Australia and the Indian Ocean. The most famous is the Portuguese man o' war, not very large but full of neurotoxins that can severely affect our nervous system. Contact with their tentacles leads to the immediate release of poison, and some of the tentacles may adhere to our skin, continuing to release venom.

Symptoms

- Severe pain, redness and skin burns
- General symptoms like nausea and abdominal pain
- Rare life-threatening reactions with breathing or heart involvement

Typical appearance after contact with a jellyfish.

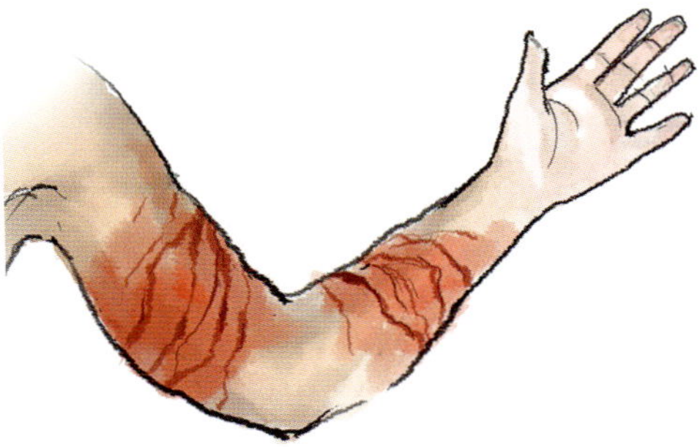

There are several harmless as well as deadly jellyfish existing in our seas.

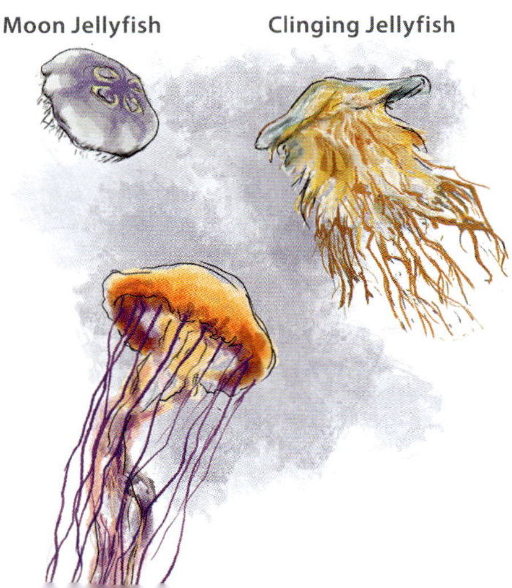

Immediate action

- Move away from the area to avoid further contact.
- Rinse the affected area with sea water and remove tentacles (for example, using a credit card).
- Check the person for possible severe allergic reaction. Seek medical attention.

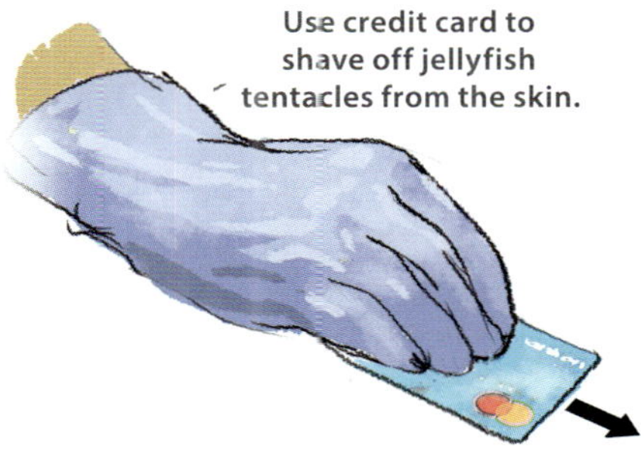

Treatment

- Rinse with sea water or vinegar/acetic acid (12 per cent) for 15–30 minutes.
- Some recommend warm water at 40–45°C.
- Check locally, as different types of jellyfish may require specific treatments.
- Use antihistamines, painkillers or corticosteroids.

Far from help

See above under 'Treatment'.

Prevention

- Be aware of local jellyfish populations.
- Inspect the water surface before swimming.
- Wear a wetsuit.
- Some species gather in large numbers for reproduction, often 8–10 days after the full moon.
- Avoid swimming along leeward coasts.
- Avoid swimming in the dark.

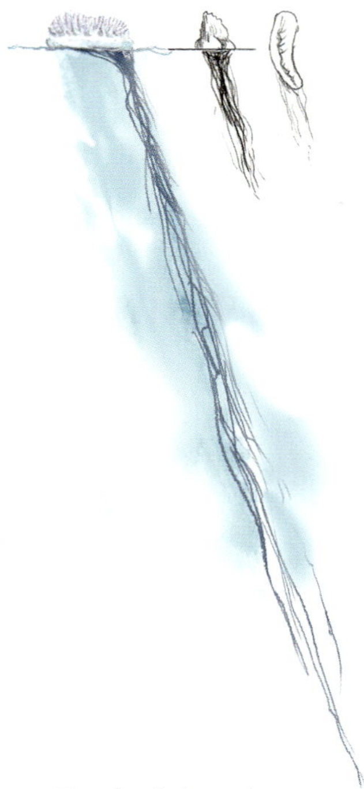

The classic feared jellyfish, Portuguese man o' war. Tentacles up to 8m or more in length. Its shape makes it constantly tack with wind from portside.

WEEVER – 'STING FISH'

These poisonous fish exist mainly in British waters and in the Mediterranean. There are a few different species, but all have venomous fins along the spine as well as on the gill covers. The lesser weever is most venomous. They usually hide in sandy seabeds of shallow waters and are not aggressive unless they are touched or stepped on.

Signs and symptoms

Contact with their fins causes a tremendous pain within a few minutes. Other symptoms are redness, swelling, nausea, breathing problems and anxiety. Symptoms may appear alarming, but fatalities are extremely rare.

Immediate action

Get out of the water as soon as possible. Risk for continued stinging can be dangerous due to pain-related impaired swimming capability.

Treatment

- Apply heat to deactivate the venom.
- Remove any embedded spines.
- Seek medical attention.

Far from help

See above under 'Treatment'. Get medical advice on the phone or radio.

Prevention

Wear protective shoes and possibly also a wetsuit. If you are fishing and get a sting fish on the hook – do not touch it! Cut the fishing line and put the fish somewhere it cannot hurt somebody else.

Weever, with venomous fins.

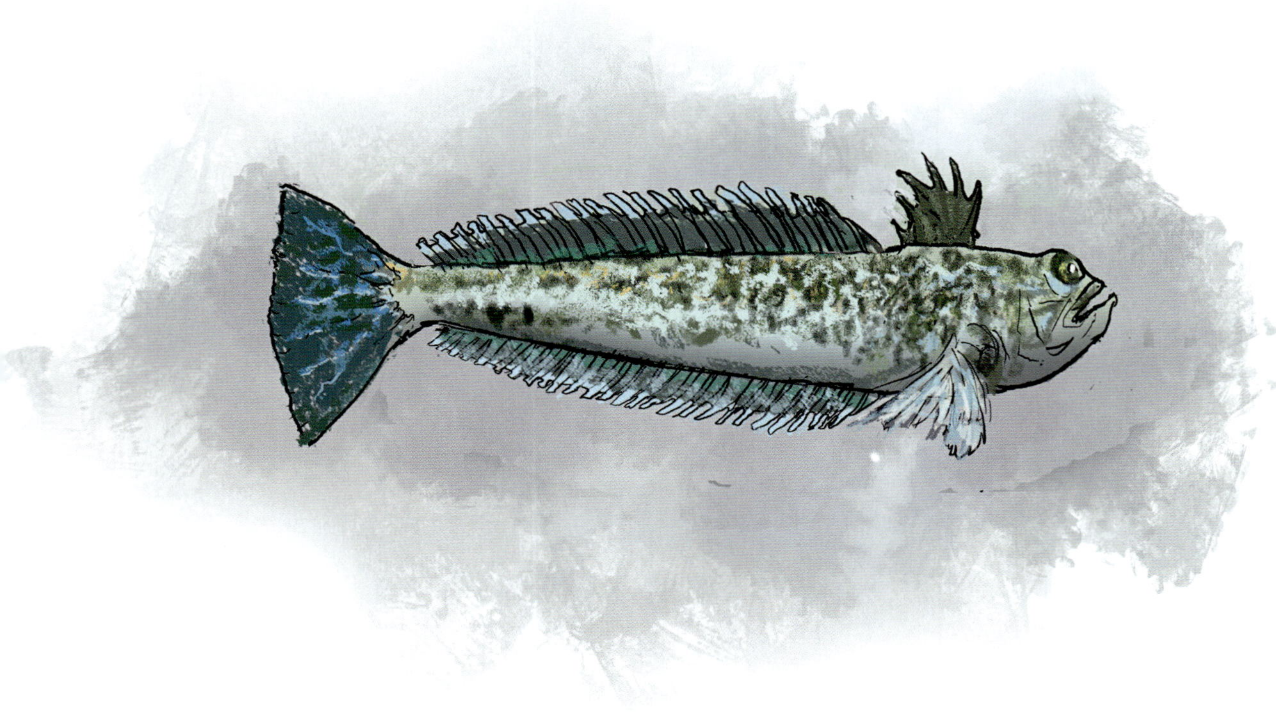

SEA URCHIN

Sea urchin is a common animal in our oceans. There are several hundred different species. They all are venomous but with great variation and mostly causing only local problems and no mortality.

The black needles penetrate the skin and get stuck.

Immediate action / Treatment

- Remove spines with tweezers.
- Apply vinegar or hot water to relieve pain.
- Treat infections with antibiotics if needed.

Prevention

- Avoid stepping or brushing against sea urchins. Wear swim shoes and even a wetsuit if they are abundant.

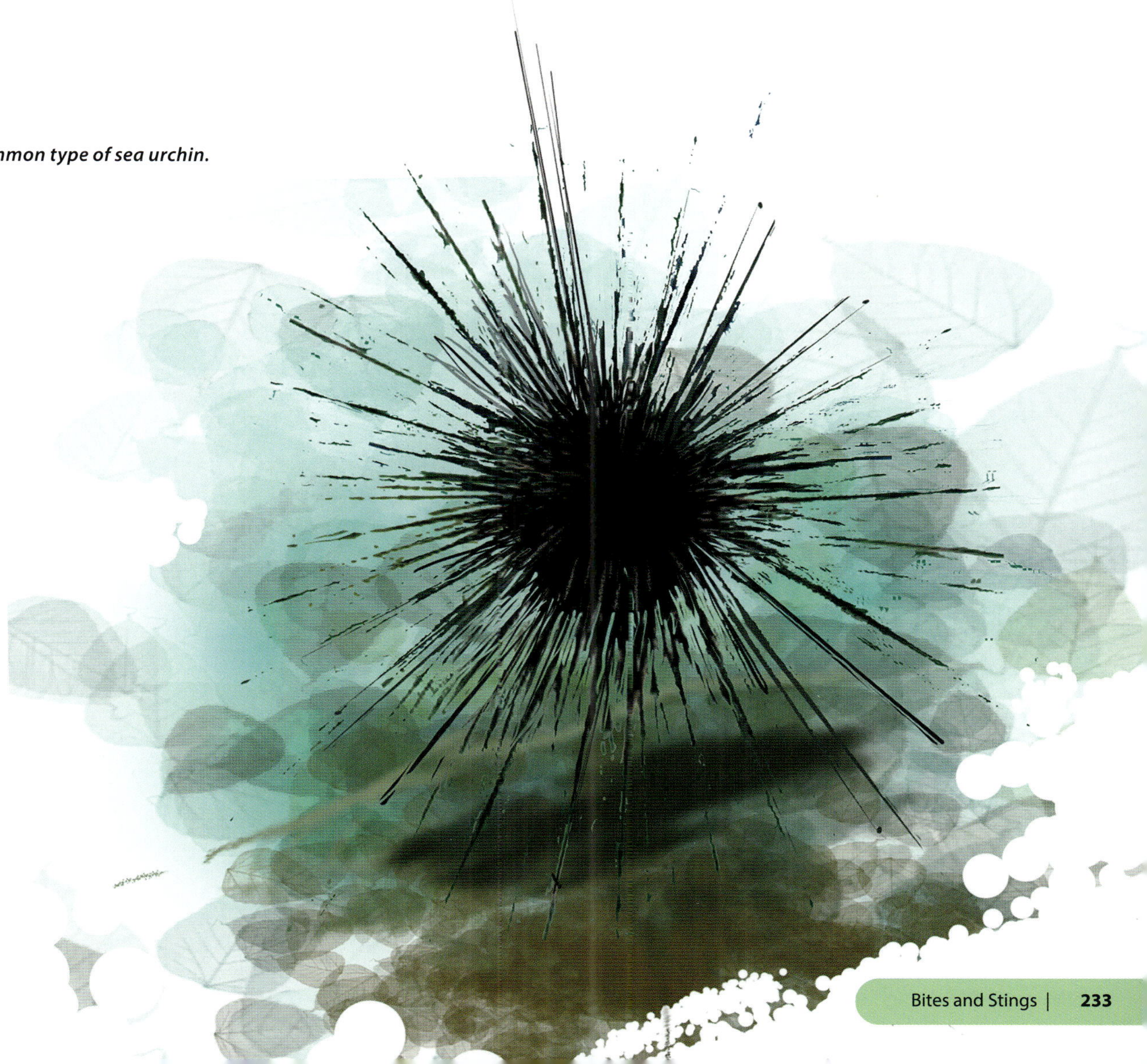

A common type of sea urchin.

24. TROPICAL DISEASES

Protection against mosquitoes is important when in tropical areas.

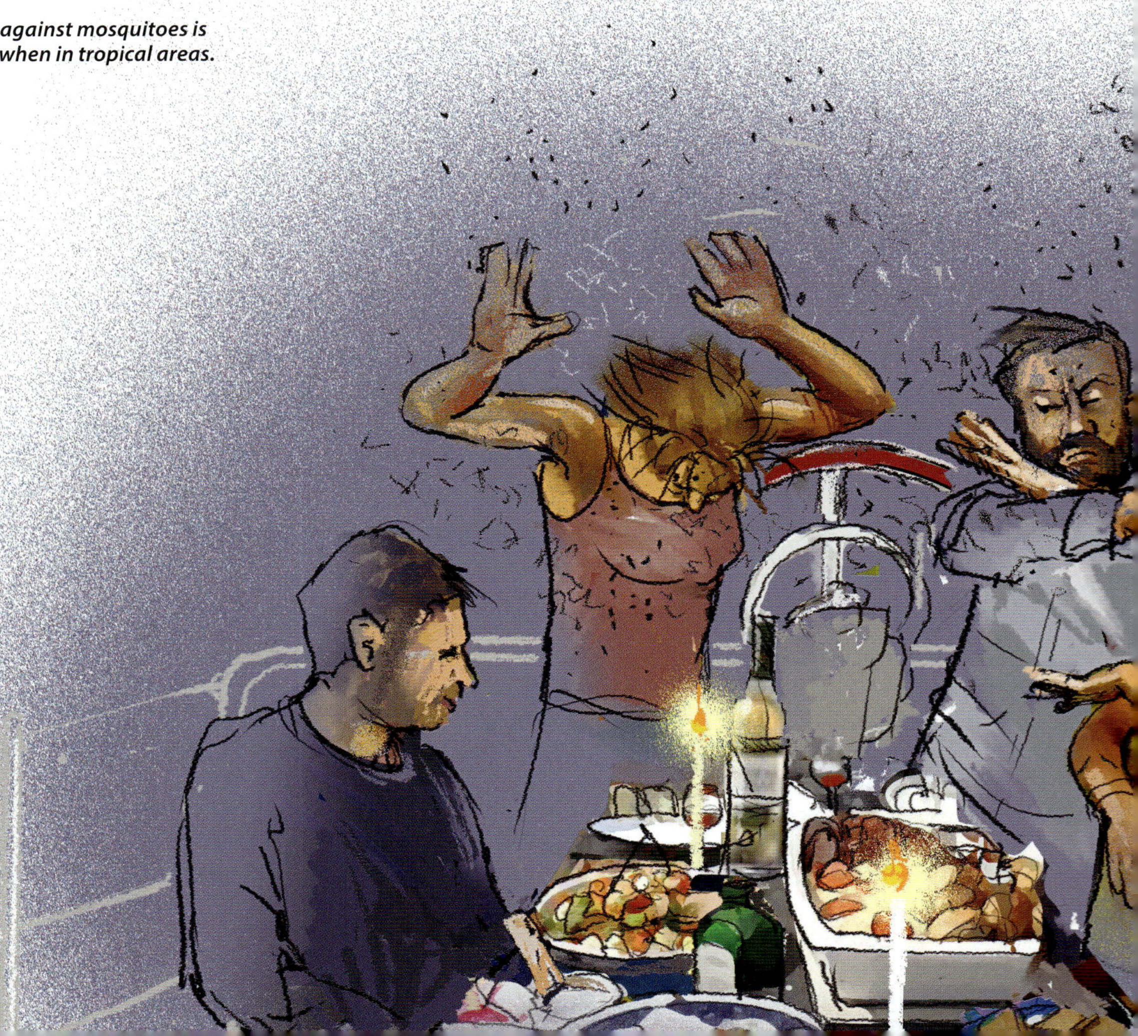

Tropical diseases primarily occur in the tropical and subtropical regions of the world, areas frequently visited by tourists, including those travelling by boat. Specific treatments and vaccines for these diseases are often unavailable, so we can only manage the symptoms. However, we can significantly reduce the risk of contracting these diseases by adopting preventive and thoughtful behaviours.

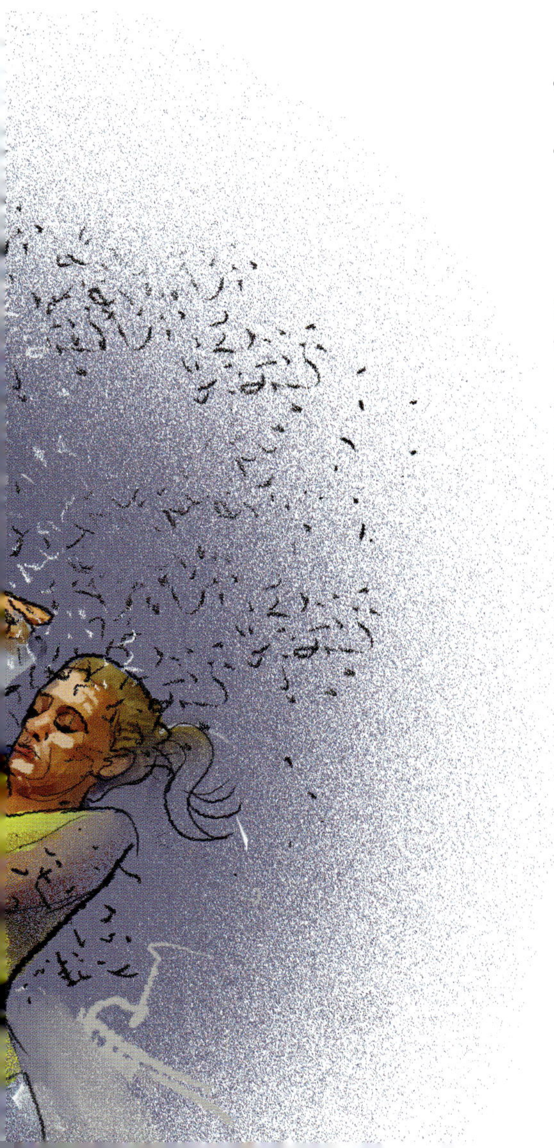

Common routes of infection in tropical diseases:

- Bites of mosquitoes and other insects.
- Contaminated food and water.
- Poor hygiene standards, particularly inadequate hand hygiene.

Prevention

Preventing diseases spread by mosquitoes:

- Use mosquito repellent.
- Sleep under impregnated mosquito nets and install nets on all openings and vents.
- Anchor further out in breezy areas rather than in calm waters near the shore, where mosquitoes are more prevalent.
- Avoid large bodies of fresh water where mosquitoes breed and their eggs hatch.
- Wear full-body clothing, such as long-sleeved shirts and long trousers, even though this may be uncomfortable in the tropical climate.

Diseases transmitted by mosquitoes can occur both day and night (for example, malaria is transmitted at night, while dengue and chikungunya are spread during the day). It's crucial to understand that if someone on board is infected with a mosquito-borne illness like chikungunya, they become a 'host' for the virus. To prevent other crew members from being bitten by mosquitoes that could spread the illness, the infected person should remain surrounded by mosquito nets during their illness.

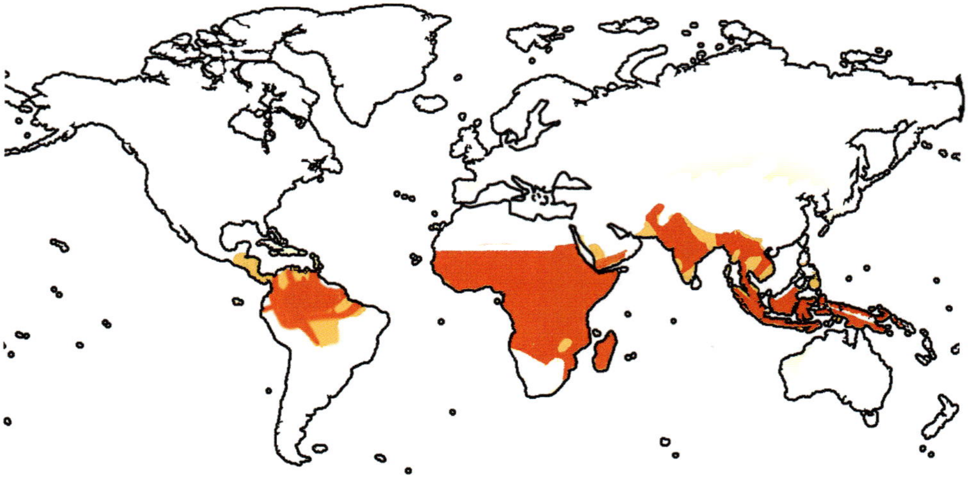

Areas with malaria prevalence.

MALARIA

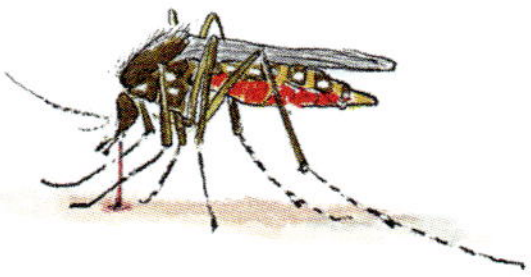

Anopheles – the malaria mosquito.

The most important advice for sailors is always to consult a specialist in infectious disease before sailing or travelling to areas where malaria is prevalent. The spread of malaria varies significantly, and up-to-date information is essential to provide accurate guidance. The risk of infection also depends on factors such as the duration of stay in malaria-prone regions.

Although a malaria vaccine is not yet widely available, protective medication is recommended. Malaria is caused by a protozoan microorganism and is transmitted by the *Anopheles* mosquito, which primarily bites at night. Malaria-carrying mosquitoes are most found in sub-Saharan Africa but are also present in parts of Asia, South America and Oceania.

Despite significant progress in reducing malaria cases over recent decades, more than 200 million people are infected annually, and nearly half a million die from the disease each year. In Europe, 6,000–8,000 cases are reported annually.

The incubation period ranges from one to two weeks, though it can sometimes be longer – rarely exceeding three months.

Signs and symptoms

- Resembles common viral influenza
- High undulating fever (often daily)
- Sweating
- Muscle aches
- Headache
- Nausea
- Diarrhoea
- Dehydration and shock

Immediate action

If any of the symptoms described above develop after visiting a malaria-prone area, seek medical attention immediately, preferably from an infectious disease specialist.

In addition to the preventive measures mentioned earlier, carry malaria prophylaxis in tablet form. Two common types of prophylaxis are available, with slightly different side effects and dosages. Consult a specialist for advice and follow the prescription carefully.

It is important to note that taking preventive medication does not guarantee complete protection. In rare cases, malaria can still occur despite prophylaxis.

CHIKUNGUNYA

Chikungunya, or 'CHIK', is spread by the Aedes mosquito, the same mosquito that transmits dengue fever. It is found in nearly all subtropical and tropical areas worldwide. Reported cases number at least 500,000 annually, with the majority occurring in the Caribbean islands. Hosts include mammals, as well as infected humans and birds carrying the virus. These mosquitoes bite during the day. After feeding on a host, they can transmit the disease to a new host, such as a human, through a subsequent bite. However, CHIK is not transmitted directly from person to person without the involvement of a mosquito.

All Caribbean islands are now affected, and the distribution is very similar to dengue fever. The incubation period following a bite is typically 3–4 days but can range from 1 to 12 days. Symptoms are very similar to those of dengue fever.

Signs and symptoms

- Resembles common influenza
- High fever (> 39°C)
- Severe joint pain and muscle pain
- Headache
- Muscle aches
- Skin rash, often appearing within a day

Joint pain mainly affects the ankles, fingers and wrists (90 per cent), often shifting between joints and leading to acute inflammation, swelling and fluid build-up. Back pain is also common. Symptoms usually resolve within one to three weeks; however, joint problems – and consequently walking difficulties – can persist for several months or even longer. The name 'Chikungunya' translates to 'that which is bent', reflecting the forward-bent, wide-spaced and unsteady gait caused by joint pain.

Other less common symptoms include:

- nausea and vomiting
- diarrhoea
- mouth blisters
- minor bleeding from the nose or mouth mucous membranes

Treatment

There is no specific treatment for chikungunya; the goal is to alleviate symptoms. Treatment typically includes rest, plenty of fluids and fever- and pain-relieving medications. Paracetamol is recommended, and codeine can be added if needed. Medications containing acetylsalicylic acid (for example, aspirin) are less suitable due to the increased risk of bleeding.

Seek medical attention if:

- fever cannot be reduced or lasts more than five days
- pain relief is ineffective
- bleeding occurs
- signs of dehydration appear, such as reduced urine production
- the patient is an infant, elderly, or has underlying medical conditions.

The disease is generally considered benign but rare complications, such as encephalitis or meningitis, have been reported. Deaths directly caused by chikungunya are extremely rare but can occur, especially in the elderly or those with other illnesses.

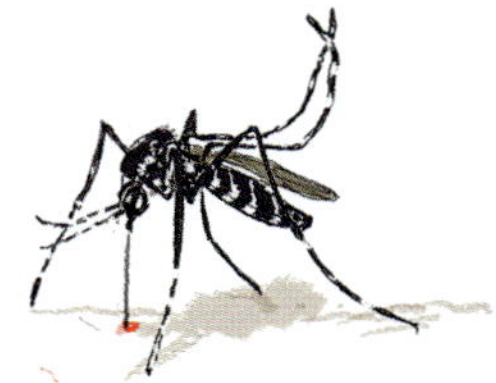

An Aedes mosquito – spreading 'CHIK'.

Areas with risk of Chikungunya.

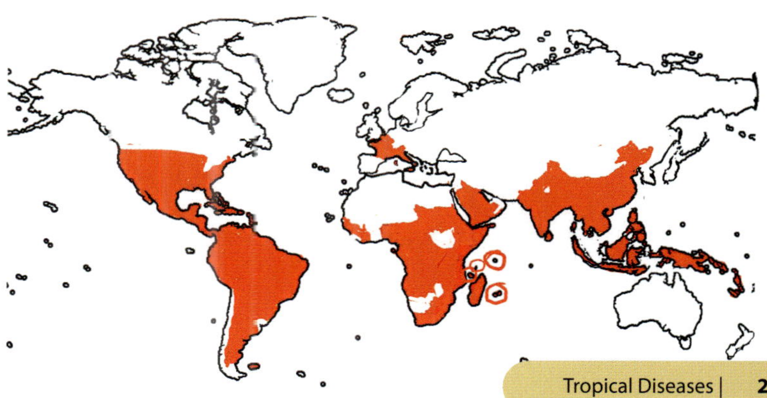

Areas with Aedes mosquitoes spreading dengue.

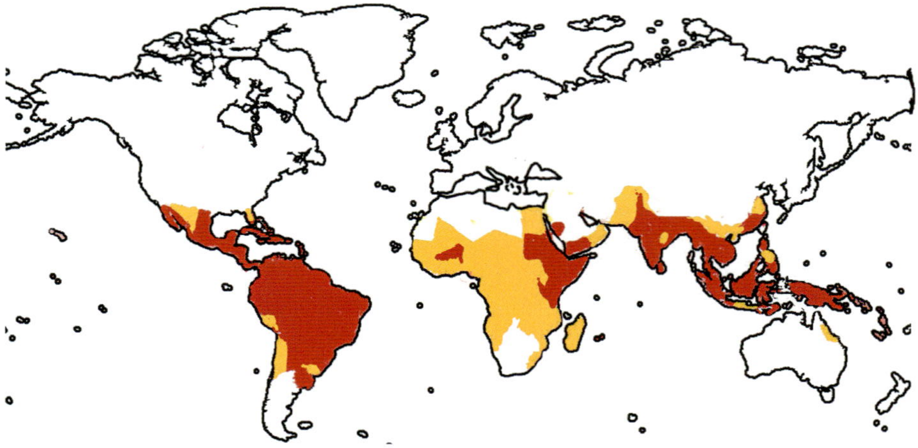

DENGUE FEVER

Dengue fever is caused by a virus transmitted by Aedes mosquitoes. Globally, around 100 million people are infected annually. The disease is common in India, Southeast Asia, Brazil and Cuba but also occurs in the Caribbean. Most cases originate in Thailand, with some in India.

The dengue virus exists in four variants, meaning reinfection is possible after recovery. Besides humans, some primates can also carry the virus. However, dengue fever does not spread directly from person to person.

Signs and symptoms

- Resembles ordinary influenza
- Acute high fever
- Headache and back pain
- Muscle and joint pain
- Sometimes red, inflamed eyes and a rash

After a few days, a measles-like rash often develops, usually located in the armpits and on the tops of the feet. Later in the illness, small bruises or well-defined skin bleeding may occur. The disease is usually benign, with recovery occurring after two to seven days of fever.

Treatment

Treatment includes analgesics and antipyretics such as paracetamol, along with plenty of fluids to prevent dehydration.

A more severe form, dengue haemorrhagic fever, can occur, particularly in children or individuals who have previously had dengue. Symptoms of this severe form include gastrointestinal issues and serious bleeding from the skin and mucous membranes. Hospitalisation is required, and sometimes intensive care is needed.

In addition to the above measures, it is recommended to confirm the diagnosis through a blood test for dengue antibodies. If you have had dengue before, take extra precautions to avoid reinfection, as the risk of developing the severe form is higher.

Whenever influenza-like symptoms arise, it is advisable to test for dengue or other diseases. A definitive diagnosis is most likely during the first three to seven days of illness.

Prevention

Avoid insect bites. A vaccine has recently become available on the market.

YELLOW FEVER

Yellow fever is caused by a virus and transmitted by mosquitoes. The disease is most common in Africa and South America. Vaccination is available and mandatory for entry into some countries where yellow fever is present. Always check vaccination requirements before arrival.

Signs and symptoms

Incubation period: 3–7 days.

- Headache
- Fever
- Chills
- Muscle aches
- Vomiting
- Stomach pain
- Jaundice
- Intestinal bleeding
- Shock

Treatment

There is no specific treatment. Monitor symptoms, treat for shock, and arrange urgent evacuation.

Prevention

A vaccine is available that, according to medical authorities, provides lifelong immunity. However, many countries impose a duration limit of 10 years.

Areas where yellow fever is prevalent.

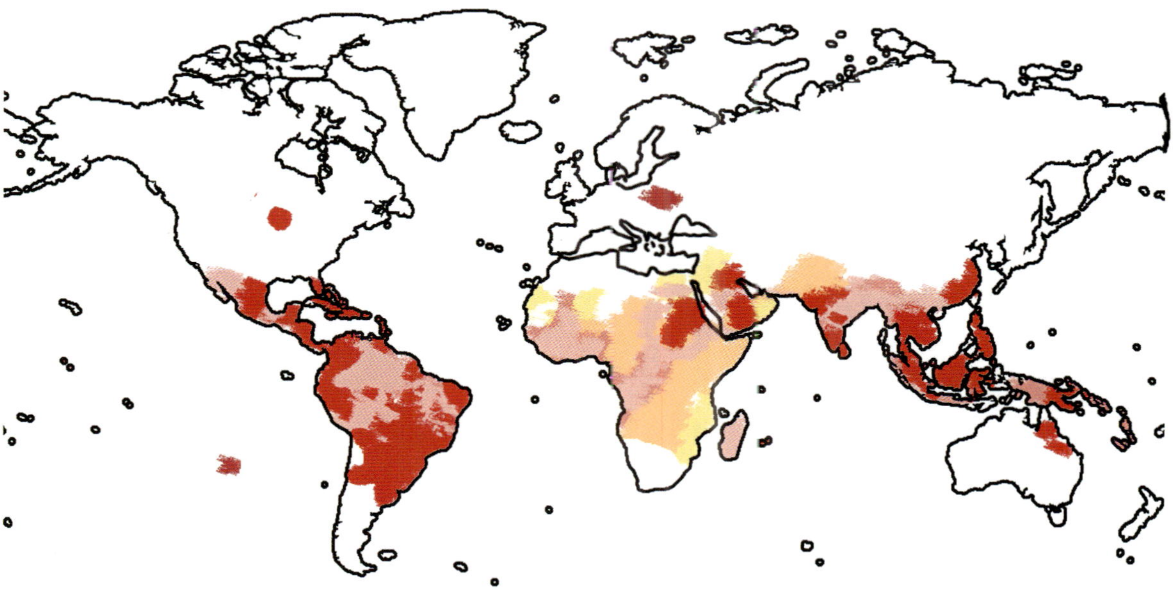

Hepatitis A is widespread and occurs in nearly every part of the world – some parts, however, more than others, as noted on the map.

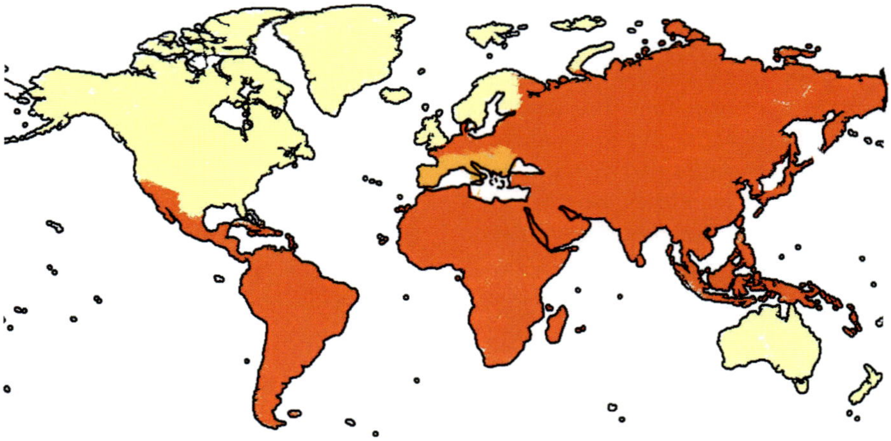

HEPATITIS A

Hepatitis A is a globally widespread viral disease, particularly common in developing countries. Most people in these regions contract the disease during early childhood, after which they develop lifelong immunity following a mild illness.

In countries with high hygiene standards, such as the USA and Europe, immunity is often lacking. This increases the risk of contracting hepatitis when travelling abroad, making vaccination an important part of the standard immunisation protocol for international travel. The virus is often present in faeces, which is why the disease is closely associated with poor hygiene.

The risk of hepatitis A infection is significant in eastern Europe, Asia, Africa, South America and parts of southern Europe. While hepatitis A typically resolves spontaneously, it is important to avoid infection during extended sailing trips or other prolonged travels.

Transmission routes:

- Poor food and hand hygiene
- Contaminated food and water
- Person-to-person contact, often within the same household
- Sexual contact

Signs and symptoms

Hepatitis A often progresses in two phases.

1. Initial flu-like phase:
   - Fever
   - Joint and muscle pain
   - Fatigue
2. Liver involvement:
   - Release of bile pigment into the bloodstream, causing yellowing of the skin and whites of the eyes (jaundice)

The disease is contagious for approximately two weeks before jaundice appears and up to two weeks after jaundice develops. Liver involvement may persist for up to three months, but most patients recover completely without specific treatment.

Treatment

There is no specific treatment for hepatitis A. Management focuses on reducing fever and providing pain relief.

Prevention

- Vaccination: Consult a specialist to ensure immunisation.
- Hygiene: Observe strict food and drink hygiene practices.

25. PREPARATIONS

Leaving the dock for a long cruise, very well prepared.

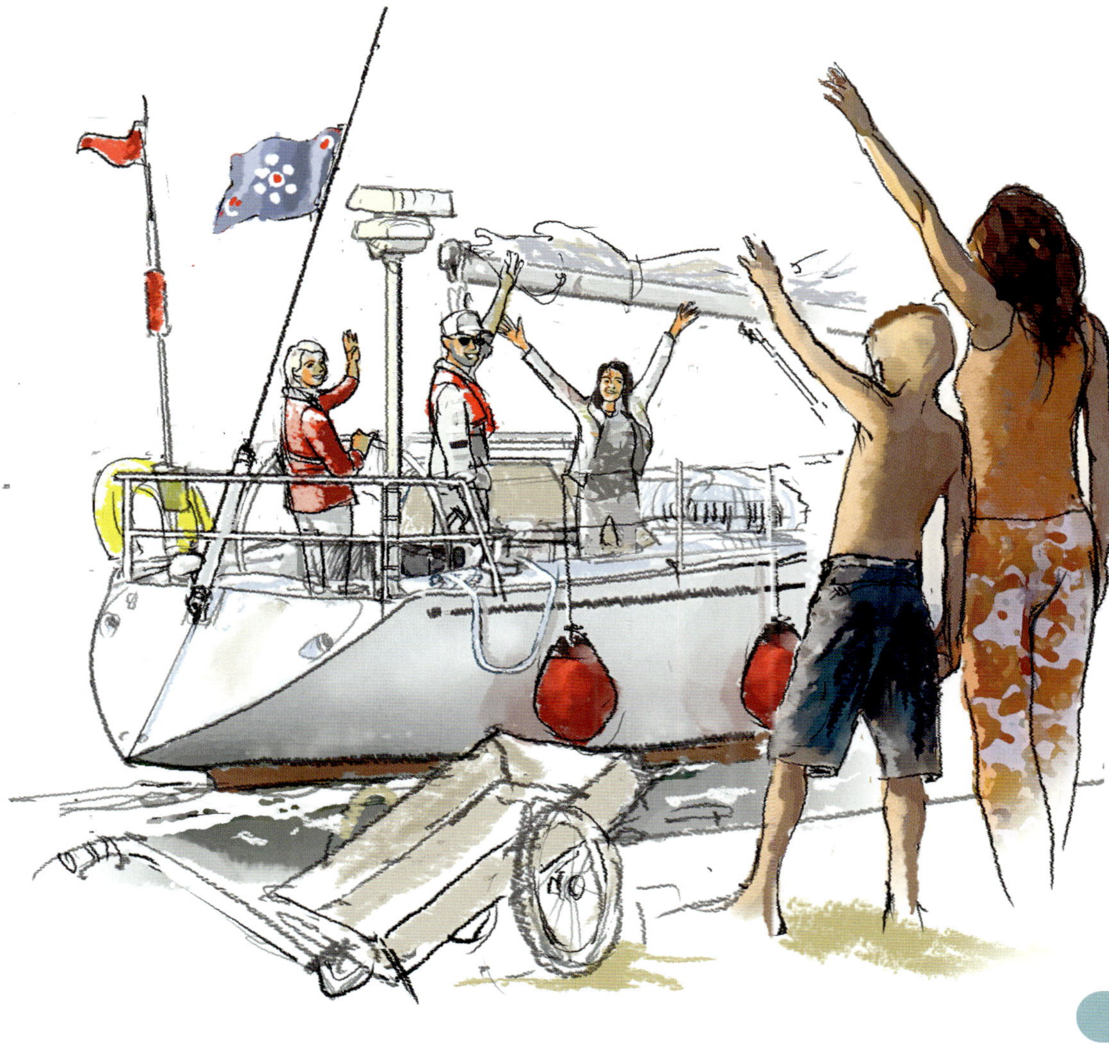

When it comes to preparations, the requirements vary significantly depending on whether you plan only day trips or longer journeys lasting months or more. Most of what is discussed here pertains to the latter category.

Long-distance sailors often carry enough supplies to almost rebuild a boat. However, we believe that proper medical training, a well-planned medical kit and a reliable ship's dispensary – essentially, spare parts for the most critical on-board element, the crew – do not always receive the priority they deserve.

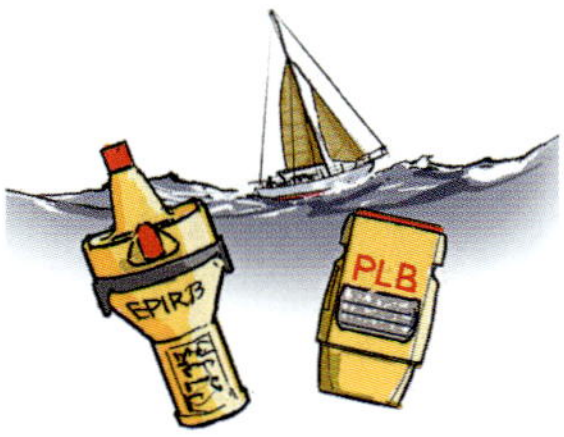

Store the EPIRB where it is easily accessible and ensure all crew members know how to use it. It is desirable that everyone working on deck has access to a PLB.

If no one on board has medical expertise and you are planning a long voyage, at least one crew member should obtain some form of medical training. This book is intended to serve as a valuable resource for such preparation, covering much of the knowledge you will need whether sailing locally or embarking on extended journeys.

EMERGENCY MEDICAL CARE ON BOARD – BOAT EQUIPMENT

Safety equipment should include approved, well-fitted lifejackets with crotch straps and safety lines. For ocean sailing, jackstays on deck are a good addition to prevent falls overboard. Avoid deck equipment that poses a tripping hazard, and practise man-overboard recovery procedures. The boat should have well-maintained, easily accessible lifebuoys. Arrange for several strategically placed hold-on handles.

The boat must also have communication equipment, medical equipment (see page 245), and a ship's dispensary (see page 247) tailored to the planned voyage.

COMMUNICATION EQUIPMENT

When sailing in local waters, the ability to quickly and reliably contact medical services and emergency centres is vital. Most coastal areas worldwide have mobile phone coverage, but ensure your phone remains dry and charged. An EPIRB is of potential great value not only when sinking but also in a medical emergency. Personal location beacons (PLBs) are important for personal safety.

For longer ocean crossings (more than three to four days), such as the North Sea, we strongly recommend a satellite phone. It allows for immediate contact for assistance anywhere, even from a liferaft. Besides emergency medical use, satellite phones are excellent for downloading weather updates.

VHF radios are another option for coastal areas and are commonly found on recreational boats, though they have limited range.

SSB radios, once used for communication with land, are now rarely monitored, so emergency calls may not be received. However, they remain effective for sending brief emails via shortwave and are valuable for social connections.

If internet access is available, contact information for all official MRCC stations can be found at https://sarcontacts.info.

Remember to have a communication plan with your relatives and friends. If official rescue stations have problems, such a plan may be the key to salvage.

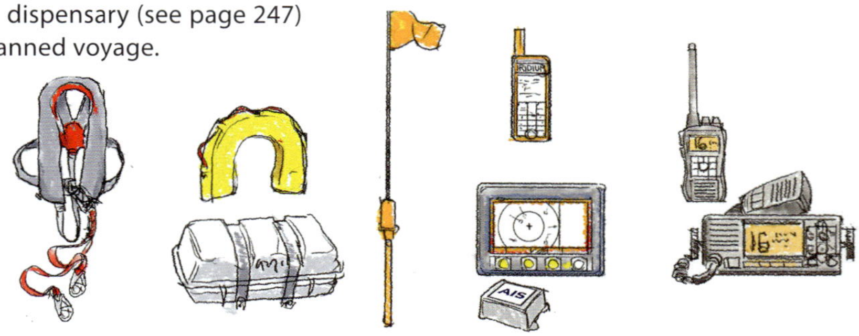

Well-functioning equipment for safety and communication is essential.

MEDICAL EQUIPMENT

The medical equipment required varies significantly depending on whether you are sailing in coastal waters or undertaking longer voyages, potentially to warmer climates or around the world.

For coastal sailing, focus on basic items such as wound-cleaning materials, appropriate dressings, burn dressings, and elastic bandages for stabilising sprains.

When it comes to long-distance sailing, medical equipment must meet a completely different set of requirements. You need to be self-sufficient and able to handle burns, wounds, sprains, fractures and so on, so that injuries and illnesses can be treated entirely on board. In severe cases, you need to manage the situation until you reach land or arrange for an evacuation at sea.

Ensure that the crew knows:

- where the medical equipment is stored and how to use it
- how to call for help and where to find contact information
- the location of a clearly posted list of emergency numbers for quick access during critical situations

MEDICAL TRAINING

It is too late to learn how to find a pulse when someone is severely injured or in circulatory shock. Practise locating both the wrist and carotid pulses on yourself and your crew. This will increase your confidence in recognising shock when the pulse you are accustomed to finding is weak or absent.

- Learn to measure respiratory rate. While simple, it can be challenging if you are doing it for the first time in a critical situation.
- If you carry an adrenaline injector, review its instructions. A crisis is not the time to read the manual.
- Review and practise with your medical equipment, ensuring everyone knows its location and use. Consider placing a clearly visible sign listing emergency contact numbers to avoid delays when time is critical.

MENTAL PREPARATIONS

The planning and preparation phase for a long voyage is both demanding and exhilarating. It is an intense part of the journey, often filled with high motivation as you anticipate long, glorious stretches of open water, palm trees, and sunsets over the sea, as well as practical and mental readiness to survive storms and even hurricanes.

However, significant technical, mechanical and mental challenges can arise during the voyage. Crew members may unexpectedly experience anxiety, fear, depression or apprehension about the task ahead.

We recommend having open discussions about these possibilities during the preparation phase to build mental readiness and a plan for addressing such challenges. The significant investments of time and money required for a long voyage mean that facing unexpected mental strain can be especially difficult.

VACCINATIONS

The need for vaccinations varies depending on your destination and prior immunisations.

Consult a vaccination clinic for advice and begin vaccinations well in advance, as some require multiple doses over months. Common vaccinations include hepatitis A and B, typhoid and cholera, as well as routine protection against tuberculosis and measles. Some countries require proof of yellow fever vaccination. Rabies vaccination is also worth considering if you plan to interact with animals. Ensure your tetanus vaccination is up to date.

If you plan to sail in malaria-prone areas, take preventive malaria medication. Although no vaccine exists, other measures can reduce your risk.

INSURANCE

Standard home insurance, including health and accident cover, is often sufficient for sailing within Europe. EU citizens can also use the blue EU card for free emergency medical care within Europe.

For longer voyages, check the validity of your insurance policy. Travel coverage typically ends 45 days after leaving home, though it can often be extended for an additional cost. This coverage is vital as it includes medically necessary transport to a hospital or even repatriation. Emergency medical evacuations without insurance can be astronomically expensive, making the premium well worth it.

CHECK YOUR OWN HEALTH

Before embarking on a longer voyage, ensure you are in good health to avoid disruptions. Even for shorter trips, address any unresolved medical or dental issues beforehand. Visit a doctor for evaluation and treatment as needed.

It is recommended to arrange exercises of the following before embarking on an adventurous cruise:

Radial and carotid pulse	Page 20
Respiratory rate	Page 13
Rescue breath with pocket mask, how to get a tight fit	Page 15
Pupil size: check normal size and reaction to light	Page 138
Bleeding control: pressure bandage, tourniquet	Page 21–2
Distal status: sensation, temperature, mobility, capillary circulation	Page 165
Move casualty away from risks (DRABC)	Page 12
Heimlich manoeuvre	Page 19
CPR: on adults and children	Page 14–15
Recovery position	Page 16
Abdomen: normal appearance and state	Page 92–3
Remove a stuck ring – the 'string trick'	Page 207

26. MEDICAL EQUIPMENT FOR SAILING

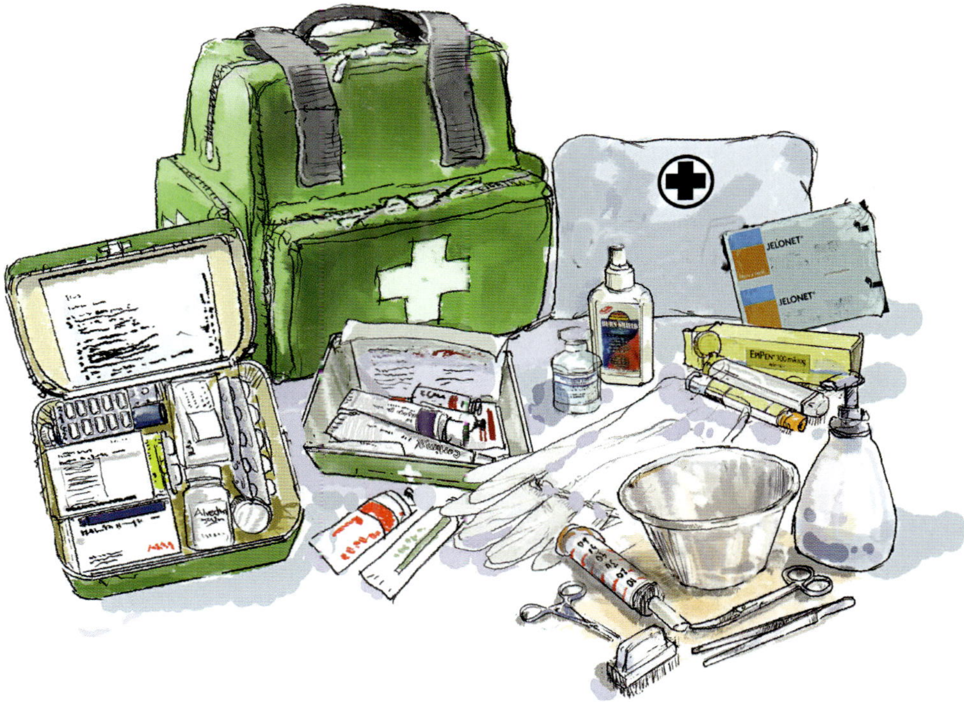

First aid kits are available in different sizes. It is worthwhile to design your own kit.

This is our guide to first aid and emergency supplies, which should be tailored to your needs.

The medical supplies should enable the skipper to handle injuries and acute illnesses that may occur during the specific voyage. These supplies might range from first aid to more comprehensive treatments for injuries requiring on-board care.

Examples of basic equipment for wound care.

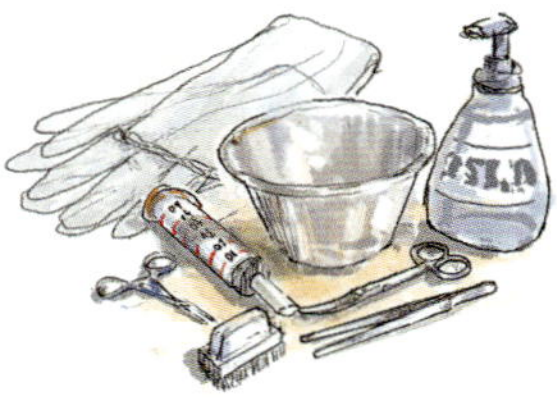

Medical equipment for coastal sailing

We recommend purchasing a pre-stocked first aid kit, available in various levels of completeness. You can supplement it with selected items from the list below for extended sailing trips.

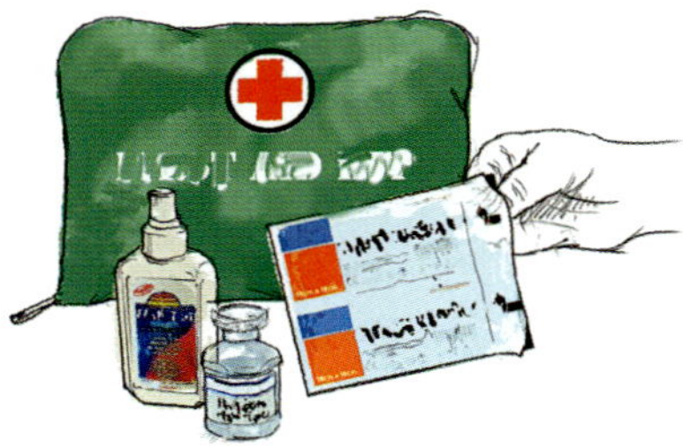

A small basic first aid kit suitable for shorter coastal cruises.

Modern water-resistant self-vulcanising synthetic foam bandages are ideal for boating.

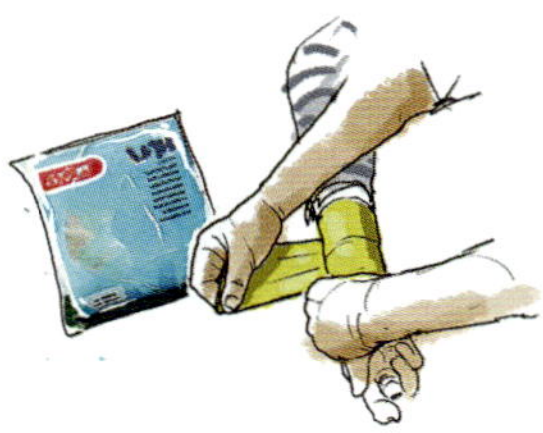

Medical equipment for long-distance sailing

For long-distance voyages, the demands are different. It is necessary to be self-sufficient and prepared to handle burns, wounds, sprains, fractures and other injuries entirely on board, or at least until you reach land or arrange evacuation.

Use warm hands for vulcanisation.

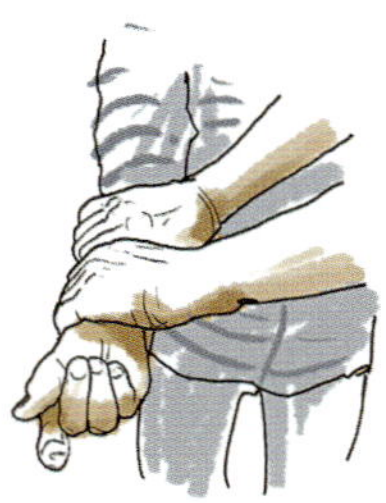

Suggested medical supplies for long-distance sailing

This comprehensive list is designed to cover injuries ranging from minor to severe.

Wound care

- Burn dressings (10×10cm): 4 packs
- Surgical tape (2.5cm): 2 rolls
- Surgical tape (5cm): 1 roll
- Suture tape (13×100mm): 30 strips (3 packs of 10)
- Suture tape (6×75mm): 25 strips (5 packs of 5)
- Non-sterile compresses (10×10cm): 150 pieces
- Physiological saline solution (20ml): 20 vials
- Physiological saline solution (500ml): 2 bottles
- Nitrile disposable gloves: 100 pieces
- Soft brush or unopened toothbrush
- Soap (unused or liquid): avoid using shared or bathroom soap
- Syringe 50ml: for wound irrigation
- Haemostats
- Tweezers
- Scalpel
- Scissors
- Self-Adherent and Vulcanizing Foam Bandage (Snögg) (6cm×5m): 1 roll
- Self-Adherent and Vulcanizing Foam Bandage (Snögg) (8cm×100cm): 4 rolls

Bandages for sprains and fractures

- Elastic bandage (10cm×4m): 6 rolls
- Elastic support bandage (8cm×4m): 2 pieces
- Stretch compression bandage (10cm× 7m): 2 rolls
- Stretch compression bandage (8cm× 7m): 1 roll
- Plaster bandages (10cm): 6 pieces
- Padding cotton (10cm): 4 rolls
- Malleable aluminium splint: 1 or 2 pieces
- Ankle orthosis: 1 piece

Supplementary / Optional

- Eye wash solution
- Long apron
- Protective gloves (silicone): 1 pair
- Insect repellent
- Sunscreen
- Sunglasses
- Sun hats
- Tick remover
- Urinary catheter (optional)
- Dental repair kit: mirror, dental cement, oral disinfectant

28. SHIP'S DISPENSARY

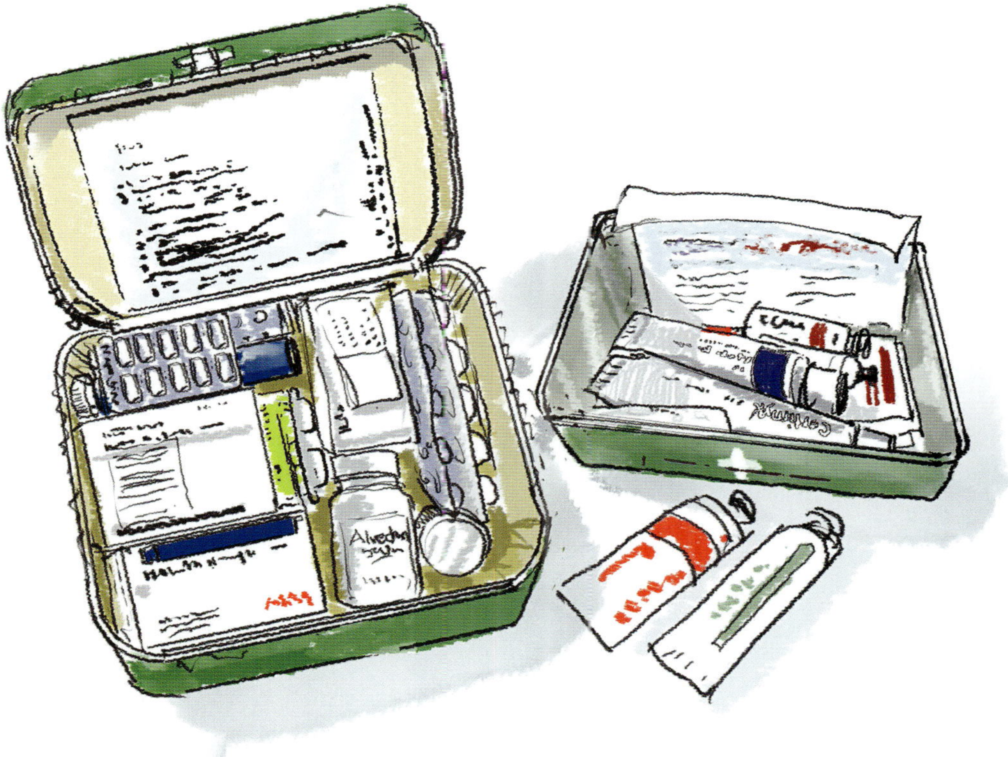

Store medications easily identified in separate boxes.

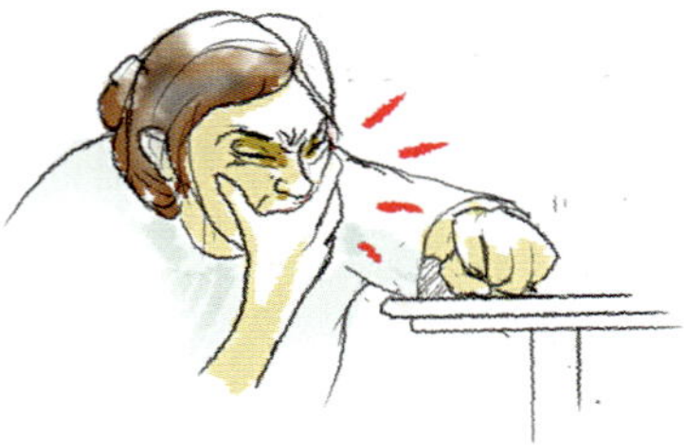

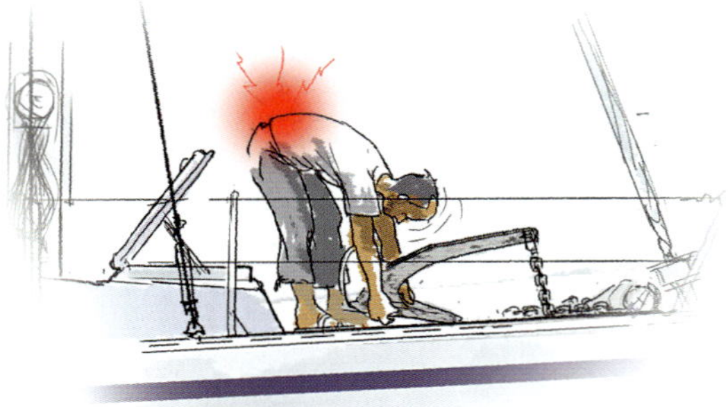

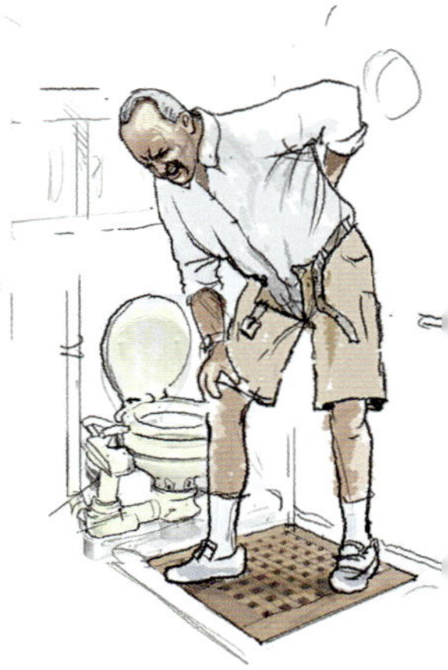

Pain is the most common symptom, all categories included.

PAIN MANAGEMENT

Pain is generally the most common reason for seeking medical attention. This section is about acute pain in trauma, severe infections or acute illness. Pain management is a matter of analysing type and intensity of pain for best choice of treatment. There are several analgesics – 'painkillers' – on the market. They have different mechanisms of action and are thus divided into specific groups: paracetamol, NSAIDs (Non-Steroidal Anti-Inflammatory Drugs) and opioids respectively. It is possible to maximise the analgesic effect by combining drugs from two or even all three groups – multimodal analgesia.

Caution

Never exceed the maximal dose for each respective analgesic. Avoid overdosage by never combining analgesics from the same group. As an example, it is possible to take paracetamol and an NSAID together with an opioid but NOT to take two different NSAIDs.

Pain ladder – a model for escalation of pain treatment.

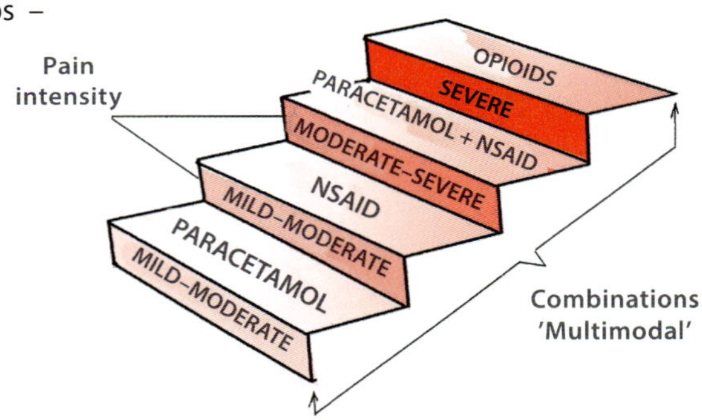

Recommended analgesics for longer cruises. Type and dose for an adult, possible to combine in multimodal analgesia for different pain intensities.

Substance	Type	Dose	Intensity of pain
Paracetamol	Paracetamol	1g every 6 hours	Mild to moderate
Ibuprofen	NSAID	400mg every 4–6 hours	Mild to moderate
Codeine	Opioid	30–60mg every 4–6 hours	Moderate to severe
Morphine	Opioid	10mg every 2–8 hours	Severe

INFECTION

Infection is the second most common reason to use the ship's dispensary. The table below summarises content and indications

Note: Choice of antibiotic and dosage may be affected by several parameters easily controlled when ashore. These general recommendations are adjusted for the specific situation out at sea and far from help.

Substance	Amount	Dose (tablets × times per day × days)	Indication
Phenoxymethylpenicillin 30 tablets	1g	1×4×10	• Erysipelas without wounds • Insect bites • Respiratory infections: tonsillitis, pneumonia • Dental infections, otitis
Flucloxacillin 30 tablets	500mg–1g	1×4×10	• Purulent wound infection • Erysipelas with wounds
Amoxicillin/clavulanic acid 30 tablets	875/125mg	1×2×10	• Open fracture • Severe wound contamination near joints • Deep soft tissue infection • Dog or cat bites • Human bites
Trimethoprim 30 tablets	200mg	1×2	• Urinary tract infection no fever
Ciprofloxacin 30 tablets	500mg	1×2	• Urinary tract infection with fever
Ciprofloxacin 20 tablets + Metronidazole 30 tablets	500mg 400mg	1×3×10 1×3×10	• Abdominal infection, e.g. diverticulitis, appendicitis • Gynaecological infection
Azitromycin 30 tablets	500mg	1x3x7	• Bacterial infections (respiratory, abdominal)

SHIP'S DISPENSARY – OUR SUGGESTED CONTENT

When sailing along our coasts at home or around Europe, we believe a minimal on-board dispensary is sufficient. It could consist of:

- Pain relief: Paracetamol + Ibuprofen
- Seasickness medication: Hyoscine hydrobromide
- Antihistamines: Chlorphenamine maleate + Desloratadine

Under these circumstances, you are rarely more than a few hours away from a port. Medical care and pharmacies are readily accessible, allowing you to obtain prescriptions and medications tailored to the current medical condition.

Long-distance sailing

A well-stocked ship's dispensary and medical supplies are essential to managing acute illness or accidents during long crossings or in remote waters. Below is the basic selection we ourselves have carried on longer voyages. Quantities are adjusted to meet the needs of one person for approximately two to three weeks.

Analgesics

Aspirin is not included due to its potential for allergies, increased bleeding risk, and risk of stomach ulcers. Avoid narcotics for individuals with a known history of substance abuse.

- Paracetamol: 500mg, 100 tablets, 2 tablets every 4–6 hours (maximum 4g in 24 hours). For pain and fever. (Note: 2 tablets is the standard adult dose; avoid in severe liver disease.)
- Ibuprofen: 400mg, 100 tablets, 1 tablet every 8 hours. For headache, joint and muscle pain, biliary colic, kidney stones.
- Diclofenac suppositories: 100mg, 10 suppositories, 1 suppository daily. For joint/muscle pain, biliary colic, kidney stones (faster effect than tablets).
- Combined Paracetamol 500mg + Codeine phosphate 30mg: 100 tablets, 1 or 2 tablets every 4 to 6 hours. Narcotic due to codeine content. If additional paracetamol is needed concurrently the total dose per 24 hours may not exceed 8 tablets (4g).
- Morphine: 10mg, 25 tablets, 1 tablet maximum every 4 hours. For severe pain. Narcotic. No risk of addiction during a short period of acute pain treatment. Can affect breathing but not at the prescribed dose.

Antibiotics

Antibiotic allergies are common. Avoid these medications for individuals with known penicillin allergies; specific prescriptions are required for such cases.

- Phenoxymethylpenicillin: 1g, 30 tablets, 1 tablet every 6 hours for 10 days. For respiratory infections, wound infections. Streptococcus.
- Flucloxacillin: 1g, 30 tablets, 1 tablet every 6 hours for 10 days. For wound infections, heavily contaminated wounds. Staphylococci.
- Amoxicillin/clavulanic acid 500/125mg, 30 tablets, 1 tablet every 8 hours for 10 days. For deep soft tissue infections, dog/cat and human bites.
- Trimethoprim: 200mg, 20 tablets, 1 tablet every 12 hours for 7 days. For bladder infections, urinary tract infections without fever.
- Ciprofloxacin: 500mg, 50 tablets, 1 tablet every 12 hours for 7 (women) to 14 (men) days. Broad-spectrum antibiotic for severe urinary or abdominal infections.
- Metronidazole: 400mg, 30 tablets, 1 tablet every 8 hours for 10 days. To be used in combination with ciprofloxacin for suspected abdominal and gynaecological infection.

- Azithromycin: 500mg, 30 tablets, 1 tablet every 8 hours. Bacterial urinary tract, respiratory and soft tissue infections.

Seasickness

Except for dimenhydrinate chewing gum, these preventive medications should be taken a few hours before departure.

- Meclizine: 25mg, 100 tablets, 1 tablet every 12 to 8 hours. For seasickness. Side effects: vision problems, dry mouth, drowsiness, and, in older men, risk of urinary retention.
- Hyoscine hydrobromide patch: 1mg, 10 patches or chewable tablets. See above.
- Dimenhydrinate chewing gum: 20 pieces.
- Promethazine: 25mg, 100 tablets.

Allergies

- Loratadine: 10mg, 30 tablets, 1 tablet every 24 hours. Antihistamine for allergic reactions.
- Betamethasone: 0.5mg, 30 tablets, 10 tablets dissolved in water. Steroid for allergic reactions.
- Salbutamol inhaler: 100mcg, 1–2 puffs when required. Bronchodilator.
- Adrenaline auto-injector: 300μg, 2 injectors, inject into the outer thigh for anaphylaxis.

Gastrointestinal

- Loperamide: 2mg, 100 tablets, 1 tablet every 12 to 8 hours. For diarrhoea.
- Bisacodyl: 30 tablets, 1–2 at bedtime. Laxative.
- Activated charcoal: 5 sachets. For acute food poisoning.
- Ezomeprazole: 20mg once a day.
- Aluminium hydroxide, magnesium hydroxide/carbonate: 30 tablets, 1 tablet every 12 to 8 hours as needed. For gastritis, heartburn.

Sedatives

Both are classed as narcotics.

- Diazepam: 2mg, 50 tablets,1 tablet every 12 to 8 hours. For anxiety, tension.
- Zopiclone: 5mg, 30 tablets, 1 at bedtime. Sleeping aid.

Eyes, ears, nose, throat

- Soothing hyaluronic acid eye drops: 5g, 1 tube. For eye irritation.
- Chloramphenical 1% eye ointment: 3.5g, 1 tube. For infected eye irritation.
- Earwax solvent. For ear canal inflammation.
- Xylometazoline nasal spray: 1mg/ml, 10ml, 1 unit. For nasal congestion.

Skin and topical use

- Hydrocortisone cream: 1%, 50g, 1 tube. For mild eczema, insect bites.
- Betamethasone cream: 0.1%, 15g, 1 tube. For severe eczema.
- Fusidic acid ointment: 2%, 15g, 1 tube. For infected skin rashes.
- Lidocaine + prilocaine gel: 5g, 3 vials. For topical anaesthesia during wound care.
- Lidocaine injectable solution: 10 mg/ml, 20 ml, 5 vials. For topical anaesthesia during wound care.

LEGAL AND PRACTICAL CONSIDERATIONS

Many of these medications are prescription-only and must be prescribed by a doctor. Questions often arise about carrying narcotic drugs like morphine on board, as well as the potential legal risks.

- Addiction: There is no risk of addiction with short-term treatment of acute pain.
- Documentation: Maintain a detailed inventory of medications on board and log their usage along with reasons for their consumption. At a control point, you can show how many were present at departure, the circumstances of use, and the remaining quantity.

To address legal concerns, we also carry a 'Customs Declaration' with the ship's name, owner, registration number, and the individual responsible for the medications. During check-ins, we declare 'no narcotics on board' but explain that these are legal, internationally approved medications necessary for on-board emergencies.

CAUTION

All medicines have side effects and should be avoided in certain situations. The list below summarises common side effects, warnings and contraindications associated with medications in the suggested ship's dispensary.

Medication for chronic disease is primarily the responsibility of the individual crew. Note that the skipper carries the final responsibility for all equipment including medication for the entire crew and for the intended route.

We recommend keeping specific instructions with medications. Check that a crew member does not have an allergy to medication before administering.

It is extremely important that all medicines are stored safely out of reach for children.

All drug doses are from the British National Formulary but may be different elsewhere in Europe.

Analgesics

Medication	Side effects	Contraindications	Warnings
Paracetamol	Very few	Renal and liver failure	Do not exceed max adult dose
Non-steroidal anti-inflammatories (NSAID) e.g. Diclofenac, Ibuprofen	Nausea, gastric ulcer, blurred vision	Gastro-intestinal bleeding, heart failure, asthma	Avoid taking together with other blood-thinners
Codeine	Nausea, biliary spasm, constipation	Biliary spasm Head injury	Avoid in respiratory failure
Morphine	Respiratory depression, nausea, sedation	Respiratory failure, traumatic brain injury – may obscure changes in consciousness	Respiratory depression. Monitor breathing. Drowsiness. Avoid driving
Loratadine	Blurred vision Drowsiness Urinary retention	Liver failure	

Sedatives

Medication	Side effects	Contraindications	Warnings
Diazepam	Sedation, respiratory depression	Sleep apnoea	Do not exceed max adult dose
Zopiclone	Sedation, respiratory depression	Sleep apnoea, Myasthenia gravis Liver failure	Respiratory depression, drowsiness. Avoid driving

Antihistamines/allergy

Medication	Side effects	Contraindications	Warnings
Adrenaline (Epi-pen)	Palpitations, tachycardia	Ongoing acute cardiac process	
Chlorphenamine	Sedation, vertigo		Avoid driving
Betamethasone	Gastritis, ulcer		Immunosuppressive. Avoid in serious infections
Salbutamol	Tremor, headache, tachycardia	Severe coronary artery disease	
Cetirizine	Drowsiness, vertigo, headache		Increased risk urinary retention in prostate enlargement. Avoid driving

Antibiotics

Medication	Side effects	Contraindications	Warnings
Phenoxyethylpenicillin Flucloxacillin Azithromycin Amoxycillin Trimethoprim Ciprofloxacin Metronidazole	Allergy Nausea, vomiting Diarrhoea	Allergy to this substance	Beware of antibiotics containing penicillin in those with a specific penicillin allergy

Sea sick/Motion sickness

Medication	Side effects	Contraindications	Warnings
Cinnarazine	Drowsiness Blurred vision		Avoid driving
Cyclizine	Drowsiness		Avoid driving
Meclizine	Drowsiness Dry mouth	Liver failure Glaucoma Epilepsy	Urinary retention in prostate enlargement (men). Avoid driving
Dimenhydrate	Drowsiness Vertigo Blurred vision Dry mouth	Asthma Glaucoma Epilepsy	Urinary retention in prostate enlargement (men). Avoid driving
Diphenhydramine	Drowsiness Vertigo Blurred vision Dry mouth	Asthma Glaucoma	Urinary retention in prostate enlargement (men). Avoid driving
Promethazine	Drowsiness		Urinary retention in prostate enlargement (men)
Hyoscine	Drowsiness Vertigo Blurred vision Dry mouth	Glaucoma	Urinary retention in prostate enlargement (men)

INDEX